The THERAPEUTICS OF FEVERS

The THERAPEUTICS OF FEVERS

Continued, Bilious, Intermittent, Malarial, Remittent, Pernicious, Typhoid, Typhus, Septic, Yellow, Zymotic, etc.

By

H.C. ALLEN. M.D.

Author of
Keynotes and Characteristics of the Materia Medica and Materia Medica of the Nosodes

B. Jain Publishers Pvt. Ltd.
New Delhi (India)

NOTE FROM THE PUBLISHERS

Any information given in this book is not intended to be taken as a replacement for medical advice. Any person with a condition requiring medical attention should consult a qualified practitioner or therapist.

Price: Rs. 90/-

Reprint Edition: 2001

Published by
KULDEEP JAIN
for

B. Jain Publishers (P) Ltd.

1921, Chuna Mandi, St. 10th, Paharganj,
New Delhi-110 055
Ph: 3670430, 3670572, 3683200, 3683300
Fax: 011-3610471 & 3683400
Website: www.bjainindia.com, Email: bjain@vsnl.com

Printed in India by

Unisons Techno Financial Consultants (P) Ltd.
522, FIE, Patpar Ganj, Delhi-110 092

ISBN : 81-7021-081-X
BOOK CODE : B-2005

PREFACE

THE author is deeply grateful to his professional colleagues, especially in India where fevers of every type are endemial, for their commendations of the monograph on Intermittent Fever. Since the publication of the first edition in 1879 an extended experience in the treatment of chronic intermittents has conclusively verified the teachings of Hahnemann, that the most obstinate and intractable cases occur chiefly in psoric or tubercular patients, and the more deep the dyscrasia the more protracted the fever. Another clinical fact which has been verified by many observing homeopathic physicians that the suppressive treatment by massive doses of quinine as practiced by the dominant school, is not only positively injurious but often fatal. Massive doses of Peruvian Bark or any of its alkaloids can only suppress the symptoms and thereby increase the sufferings of the patient.

Hahnemann's lesson in the *Chronic Diseases* on the treatment of acute syphilis must be applied to fevers of all types and acute diseases of every name and every kind, irrespective of habitat. If, as he affirms in the Organon, acute diseases "are generally only a transitory outbreak, an explosion of a latent psoric affection," the symptomatic expression of this or any other dyscrasia must be included in the anamnesis, and the remedy selected from the totality thus obtained.

This volume includes the therapeutics of typhoid, typhus, and fevers of every grade and name, from acute sporadic and epidemic intermittent to the malignant type of the malarial fevers of the tropics. But the same law of cure, the same rule of practice applies to each patient. It is the *patient* not the *fever* that is chiefly and especially to be considered. It is the individual with his or her peculiar idiosyncrasies and constitutional inheritances with which we have to deal. The symptoms of the latent psoric affection must be analyzed as fully and completely as the symptoms of the "transitory outburst," the fever paroxysm. As a rule, the family history is much more suggestive of the curative remedy than the rapid pulse and high temperature, and should be carefully studied. When discovered, the constitutional miasm—psora, sycosis, syphilis, tuberculosis—should be especially noted, for here will often be found the key with which to unlock the secret of the severity of the attack or the relapsing tendency of the fever. It is the experience of the author that if the remedy be selected from the totality of the objective, subjective, and miasmatic symptoms, the patient may be cured in any stage of the fever. It is not necessary for a typhoid or any other fever to "run its course."

The author desires to express his obligations to Drs. Geo. H. Clark, C. B. Gilbert, Wm. Jefferson Guernsey, St. Clair Smith, E. V. Ross, and P. C. Majumdar for valuable suggestions; and to Drs. C. E. Fisher and C. B. Hall for suggestions and aid in proof-reading. He is also duly grateful that he is blessed with a publisher and printer who take pride in the character and quality of their work irrespective of the dollars concerned.

THERAPEUTICS OF FEVERS

"After he has found all the existing and appreciable symptoms of the disease, the physician has found the disease itself—he has a complete idea of it, and knows all he need know to cure it."—
Hahnemann's Medicine of Experience.

THE CAUSE.

A PHYSICIAN is rarely to be met with who cannot at once, and with apparent certainty, formulate *a theory* for the *cause* of intermittent or other fevers. This universal knowledge is only equaled by the variety of theories entertained, and the failures inseparable from the attempt to treat *the theory of the cause,* and the *name of the disease,* instead of the totality of the symptoms—subjective and objective presented by the patient. The natural result of this attempt to follow the teachings and practice of Allopathy, is the charge, so often made by our medical brethren of the opposite school, that "Homeopaths are not honest in their practice;" and this charge has been more frequently based upon what they have seen of our treatment of fevers than of all other diseases combined. Allopathy affirms that Intermittent Fever cannot be cured without Quinine, because Quinine is the antidote of "Marsh Miasm," which is the *cause* of intermittent fever; and many homeopatl —departing from the law of cure, and neglecting their Materia Medica—honestly cherish a similar delusion.

The object of this work is to deal with therapeutic facts, not with speculative theories. The author has no theory to advance; and none to disprove except such as interfere with the successful homeopathic treatment of this *bete noir* of our profession. We are unable to offer an intelligent explanation of the *cause* of sporadic or epidemic intermittent fever that will bear the test of scientific investigation, and Hahnemann's *one therapeutic fact* is worth more at the bedside than all the theories that have ever been advanced.

"Intermittent fever is a neurosis. Its phenomena, as chill and heat, are distinct; their origin must also be distinct. The heat is due to the action on the sympathetic system; the chill to the spinal system."—*Lord, on Int. Fever.*

"We believe intermittent fever is a neurosis, whose seat is especially in the ganglionic system, and therefore only nerve remedies, and particularly such as act on the vaso-motor part, can cure."—*Wurmb and Caspar on Int. Fever.*

"Acute cases must always be treated by cerebro-spinal remedies; chronic cases by organic remedies."—*Burt's Characteristics.*

"Ague remedies may be divided into two classes, viz.: Quinine, Gelsemium, Eucalyptus, Nux vomica, Arsenic and Cedron, which have the power of destroying protozoa, infusoria, and cryptogamic fungi; and Eupatorium, Cornus, Salicine, Arnica, Natrum mur., and Hydrastis which have not that power, yet correspond to the periodicity of the paroxysm."—*Hale's Therapeutics,* p. 609.

Bartlett, Salisberry, and others who maintain the cryptogamic theory have many followers in our school; and here Carbolic acid, Salicylic acid, Sulphite of Soda, etc., must be used to destroy the germs.

Grauvogl's theory of splenic congestion and constitutional divisions, has many advocates. But it requires a Grauvogl to detect the constitution and splenic congestion; or a Lord, or Wurmb and Caspar, to select the cerebro-spinal or sympathetic remedy; or a Burt, Hughes, Hale, or Kafka to classify the remedies.

THE MALARIAL THEORY,

(MARSH MIASM),

Is, however, most generally accepted. The evidence advanced in its support is the prevailing occurrence of epidemics, where this poison presumably exists. It is supposed to be the result of decaying vegetable and other organic matter, and is found along rivers with low, swampy, alluvial shores, subject to frequent overflow; near bodies of stagnant water; in the neighborhood of recently dug canals, cellars, or freshly plowed virgin soil; near marshes, particularly on leeward side of prevailing winds. It is confined near the earth, seems to spread in a horizontal direction; and its progress may be cut off by walls, hedges, high banks, and dense forests. Unlike the poison of Diphtheria, Rubeola, Scarlatina, Variola, and Typhus, it is neither contagious nor infectious; but also unlike them, each attack only renders the system more liable to a subsequent one.

But, on the other hand, it has long been known that the fever may exist on a dry, or even on a sandy soil, and in rocky, mountainous regions where it is often more extensive and severe than in the adjoining low country. Ziemssen says: "On the Tuscan Appenines fevers are found at the height of 1,100 feet; on the slopes of mountains of Ceylon at 6,500 feet; on the Pyrenees at 5,000 feet; and on the Andes, in Peru, at 10,000 and 11,000 feet; while at the same time the neighboring plains are entirely free, or are only visited in a very mild form." There are large tracts of lands where all the conditions of malaria exist, and yet no intermittent fever; and other districts where no conditions of miasma are to be found, and yet ague is endemic every season. The fever occurs in a sporadic form where miasma never prevails, and the patients had never been in a malarial region. Moreover, the inhabitants of a valley where the disease prevails removing to a mountainous region where it is unknown, are often attacked with intermittent fever. The microscopist, with his most powerful lens, has never yet been able to detect the miasm; and chemical and spectral analyses are alike powerless to solve the problem. The internal cause of all fevers is in our own bodies and is *unknown,* and because unknown we cannot expect to find its opposite, for we must know the poison before we give an antidote.

On such evidence—quite as strong against as in favor of the malarial theory—we may be pardoned if we doubt the existence of such an agent in the production of intermittent fever. And when we are asked to abandon the *certainties* of our *law of cure,* and accept a treatment based upon the antidoting of an unknown poison, as homeopaths we should respectfully decline. We know quite as much of the nature of those poisons which produce scarlatina, diphtheria and typhus as we do of that which produces intermittent fever; yet the success of the so-called antidotal treatment is not such as would warrant any homeopath in abandoning the teaching of his Materia Medica for it. This search after a hypothetical cause, and the adoption of a treatment based upon its supposed discovery, has been the fatal Scylla upon which has stranded many a homeopathic success. The element of accuracy once removed, our practice degenerates into empiricism.

THE PSORIC DIATHESIS.

Another cause for intermittents, and especially for *the most obstinate types*—a cause almost universally neglected or overlooked by the majority of homeopathic physicians—is found in the inherited dyscrasia of the patient, the psoric or tubercular diathesis. Hahnemann says (Chronic Diseases, page 75):

> Intermittent fever, even when there are no cases about, either sporadic, epidemic or endemic, the form, duration and type of the fever are very various; quotidian, tertian, quartan, quintan or every seven days.

Every evening, chills with blue nails.

Every evening, single chills.

Every evening, heat with a rush of blood to the head, with red cheeks, also at times an intervening chill.

Intermittent fever of several weeks' duration, followed by a moist itching eruption lasting several weeks, but which is healed again during a like period of intermittent fever, and alternating thus for years.

Epidemic intermittent fevers probably never seize a man who is free from psora, so that wherever there is susceptibility to them, it is to be accounted a symptom of psora.

This is true, not only of intermittents but of typhoid, typhus and all types of continued fevers. All fevers that tend to a protracted, low or malignant type, occur in the psoric or tubercular patient, and the more deeply psoric the more malignant the attack.

SIMILIA IS A NEVER-FAILING GUIDE.

It would, no doubt, be a great satisfaction to be able to explain *the cause* of intermittent fever; and it would be equally gratifying to be able to tell **why all persons, subjected to the same exposure, are not attacked**; just as it would be a satisfaction to be able to explain the cause of many phenomena in physical science existing all about us. Such knowledge might aid us in a sanitary way in preventing the disease or modifying its severity; but it could never be of the slightest benefit in its homeopathic treatment. When once we depart from Hahnemann's method of individualizing each case, we enter upon the sea of doubt and uncertainty upon which our allopathic brethren, without a compass, have ever sailed.

"If our school ever gives up the strict inductive method of Hahnemann, we are lost, and deserve only to be mentioned as a caricature in the history of medicine."—Constantine Hering.

Hale—in condemning the indiscriminate use of Quinine—says: "Unless the physician is absolutely certain that the attack is due to miasmatic poisoning, he should wait until the disease shows its true character." How is it possible for the physician to be "absolutely *certain*" that he is dealing with miasmatic poisoning? And how can that knowledge change the symptoms presented by the patient, or enable us with more ease, or greater certainty, to select the remedy? There is a very nice distinction between *certain* and *sure.* I am *certain* the sun will rise; I am *sure* it has risen. The successful treatment of intermittent fever requires that the physician should not only be *certain,* but *sure.* I am *sure* I have a sick man to treat who presents certain symptoms; but I am not *certain* that he has been poisoned with miasma or has been within a hundred miles of it; and I am quite *uncertain* whether the "cerebro-spinal" or "sympathetic" is affected; or *whether* to select, or *how* to select, a cerebro-spinal or organic remedy. There are many remedies which affect both nervous systems; my patient requires but *one. But of this I am sure, that the objective and subjective symptoms of which he complains are in every respect similar to those produced on the healthy subject by Cinchona.* For me and my patient this simple fact is all sufficient. It approximates a mathematical demonstration. There are no doubts or uncertainties about it. My patient does not have to wait until I can demonstrate the truth or falsity of some favorite theory, which, whether right or wrong, could never change the characteristics of his case, so far as the selection of the remedy is concerned.

EXAMINATION OF THE PATIENT.

The first step in individualization—the keystone of the homeopathic arch—begins with an examination of the patient. It is impossible to examine a patient *in general* and prescribe for him *in particular.* Before we can select a remedy for a given case we must first ascertain the particular symptoms of which the patient complains, which form the picture of the disease; and this is often a most difficult task.

Hahnemann says: "The totality of the symptoms which characterize a given case, being once committed to writing, the most difficult part is accomplished."

Dunham says: "Do you say that this is an easy matter? Gentlemen, it is the most difficult part of your duty. To select the remedy after a masterly examination and record of the case is comparatively easy. But to *take* the case requires great knowledge of human nature, of the history of disease, and, as we shall see, of the *Materia Medica.*"

"Make haste slowly" never had a better illustration in medical science than in this advice; as no disease demands a closer observance of instructions, or a more strict adherence to principle for its successful treatment, than intermittent and other fevers.

The symptoms occurring before and during the *chill, heat, sweat* and *apyrexia;* the *time* of occurrence of paroxysm; the *parts* of the body in which the chill first makes its appearance; the *regularity* of its stages; the *degree* or *absence* of *thirst,* and *time* of its appearance; as well as the *constitutional ailments aroused by the fever,* are all to be carefully noted.

"Till the present time, pathology has only been acquainted with one single *intermittent fever,* which has been called *ague.* It admits of no other difference than the interval which exists between the paroxysms; and upon this are founded the particular denominations, quotidian, tertian, quârtan, etc. But besides the variety which they present in regard to the periods of their return, the intermittent fevers exhibit yet other changes that are much more important. Among these fevers there are many which cannot be denominated agues, because their attacks consist solely of heat; others are characterized by cold only, succeeded or not by perspirations; while yet others freeze the body of the patient, and inspire him notwithstanding with a sensation of heat, or even create in him a feeling of cold, although he seems very warm to the touch; in many, one of the paroxysms is confined to shivering or cold, which is immediately succeeded by a comfortable sensation, and that which comes after it consists of heat followed by perspiration or not. In one case, it is heat which manifests itself first, and cold succeeds; in another, both the cold and heat give place to apyrexia; while the next paroxysm, which sometimes does not occur before an interval of several hours, consist merely of perspiration; in certain cases no trace of perspiration is perceptible, while in others the attack is composed solely of perspiration, without either heat or cold, or of perspiration that flows during the heat alone. There exist, likewise, innumerable differences relative to the accessory symptoms, the particular kind of headache, the bad taste in the mouth, the stomach sickness, the vomiting, the diarrhea, the absence or degree of thirst, the kind of pains felt in the body and limbs, sleep, delirium, spasms, changes of temper, etc., which manifest themselves before, during or after the cold, hot, or sweating stages, without taking into account a multitude of other deviations. These are usually intermittent fevers that are very different from one another, each of which demands naturally that mode of homeopathic treatment most appropriate to it individually. It must be confessed that they may almost all be suppressed (a case that so frequently occurs) by large and enormous doses of Cinchona or Quinine—that is to say, Cinchona prevents their periodical return and destroys the type. But where this remedy is employed in intermittent fevers, where it is inappropriate (as in the case with all epidemic intermittents, which pass over whole countries, and even mountains), the patient is not at all cured, because the character of the disease is destroyed; he is still indisposed, and often much more so than he was before; he suffers from a peculiar chronic bark complaint, often incurable, and yet this is what physicians term a cure."—Note to § 233, Organon.

The type of fever—intermittent (tertian, quartan, etc.), remittent, bilious, malarial, typhoid, etc., etc.—at most is but a single symptom, and of little, if any value, as a symptom in the selection of the remedy. We must take all the evidences of disturbed health, both local and general, on which to make a selection.

The physician of the "rational" (?) school searches only for general conditions. To be able to diagnose *ague* and its quotidian, tertian, or quartan form, or bilious, or remittent fever, is enough for him; it satisfies the supposed demands of science, and enables him to prescribe Quinine or some preparation of Cinchona (see Organon, p. 195). Either the ready facility of the generalizing practice with the entire absence of consistency in its application, or a praiseworthy, yet unsuccessful attempt to utilize the pathological theories of Allopathy, have induced many very excellent men of our school to abandon, if they ever possessed, a knowledge of Hahnemann inductive method, for this "short cut" to success. This can be better illustrated by the following comparison of

GENERALIZING.

Arsenicum.

If the paroxysm varies widely from the typical form; if there is no chill or no sweat; if there are unusual gastric, hepatic, intestinal or cerebral disturbances; well-marked capillary congestion, and the patient is half sick during the apyrexia; we may be sure that the malarial poison has made a profound impression on the sympathetic ganglia. Arsenic, not Quinine, the typical remedy for this state.—W. H. Holcombe, *U. S. M. & S. J.*, Jan., 1872.

INDIVIDUALIZING.

Cinchona.

The paroxysm is preceded by headache, nausea, hunger, anguish, and palpitation of the heart. Thirst before the chill and during the sweating stage. Chills alternating with heat, skin cold and blue, headache, nausea and absence of thirst. During hot stage, dryness of the mouth and lips, red face and headache. After the heat, *thirst* and *profuse sweat*. Ringing in the ears, with dizziness and a feeling as if the head was enlarged.—*Johnson's Key*.

There are many remedies that would fulfill the requirements of Dr. Holcombe's Arsenic case. Each one of Dr. Burt's organic remedies is apparently well indicated. On the other hand, there is but a single remedy that will meet the requirements of Dr. Johnson's. It does not aid us in finding the remedy to know that the paroxysm is not of the typical form, or that gastric or cerebral disturbance be present, or that malarial poison has profoundly impressed the sympathetic ganglia, or even to know that he feels as he did in his former attack. We want a statement of the case in graphic, figurative language, not in the abstract terms of science. We want a clear statement of the objective and subjective phenomena which precede, accompany or follow the various stages of the paroxysm.

Quinine.

A simple, fresh, uncomplicated case of intermittent fever, with distinct cold, hot, and sweating stages, and perfect apyrexia, is promptly cured by moderated doses of Quinine. —B. F. JOSLIN, *Hom. News. S. J.*, Jan., 1872.

Arsenicum.

Tertian intermittent fever; first chill, then heat, then perspiration. Thirst during the whole paroxysm, *drinks often; but little at a time;* during cold stage, pain in the small of the back and lower limbs; tongue blue; great prostration and debility after the paroxysm. Arsenic cured. —B. F. JOSLIN, *Hom. News.*

"A simple, fresh, uncomplicated case of intermittent fever," etc., may be promptly cured by twenty-five or thirty other remedies as well as Quinine; but Arsenic, alone, will cure that of Dr. Joslin's. To know that Quinine, or any other remedy, has cured intermittent fever *is of no value to the homeopath;* unless he be given the particulars in which *this fever,* cured by Quinine, *differed from other similar fevers;* and generalization can never give him this knowledge.

"There are diversities in the form in which intermittent fever appears in different persons and in different epidemics; that these forms require different remedies, and that thus there is a form which is capable of being cured by Arsenic, and by nothing else; a form capable of being cured by Quinine and by nothing else; and so of other drugs. In this view, when a case of intermittent fever presents itself, the question can never be: Is Arsenic a better remedy for this disease than Quinine is? Does it offer greater chances of a cure? There can be no better or worse. The question is between right and wrong; suitable and not suitable. The question should be always: Which remedy corresponds to this particular case, and is, therefore, indicated in it?" *Dunham,* Vol. II, p. 201.

THE GENUS EPIDEMICUS.

As the prevailing cough which occurs during epidemic whooping-cough is relieved by the genus of the epidemic; or the acute angina occurring when diphtheria is prevalent is also most readily controlled by the remedy which controls the epidemic; so also may our attention be directed to the curative remedy in intermittent fever by carefully observing the character of the prevailing disease. This is especially the case in sea-side intermittents which so often find their simillimum in Arsenicum, Gelsemium, or Natrum muriaticum. Where the epidemic breaks out after an overflow of a river, Baptisia, Bryonia, Capsicum or Rhus may frequently be called for; or during epidemic dysentery occurring at autumn Colchicum may relieve every case. Cinchona, Eucalyptus, Eupatorium, Ipecacuanha, Malaria officinalis and other drugs are often thought of in this connection, when a careful study will lead to the remedy required.

Hahnemann calls attention to this feature of disease in the following:

"Epidemics of intermittents occurring in places where such fevers are not epidemic, partake of the nature of chronic diseases, and are composed of a series of acute attacks. Each epidemic possesses a peculiar uniform character, common to all individuals attacked by the epidemic disease. By observing the complex of symptoms peculiar to all patients, this common character will be found to point out the homeopathic (specific) remedy for all cases in general. This remedy will also usually relieve patients who, previous to this epidemic, had enjoyed good health, and who were free from developed psora."

WHEN TO ADMINISTER THE REMEDY.

Although this has never been a question of much controversy, yet the prevailing practice has been to administer Aconite, Gelsemium, Veratrum viride, or some other favorite during the paroxysm, for the double purpose of "doing something" and "controlling the fever." Every observing physician who has had much experience in the treatment of intermittent or other fevers will testify that this plan rarely has any perceptible effect upon the paroxysm, unless it be to render it more obscure. This "doing something" can be successfully accomplished with Sac lac., if it be absolutely necessary to do anything. The easiest, safest, most satisfactory and scientific method is that of Hahnemann, and no cause for regret will ever follow its adoption.

Hahnemann says, Organon, § 236: "In these cases, the medicine is generally most efficacious when it is administered a short time after the termination of the paroxysm, when the patient has partially recovered from it. During the intermission the medicine will have time to develop its curative effect in the organism, without violent action or disturbance; while the effect of a medicine, though specifically adapted to the case, given just before the next paroxysm, would coincide with the renewal of the disease, thereby creating such counteraction and distress in the organism, as to deprive the patient of much strength, and even to endanger life.* But if the medicine is given just after the termination of the attack, when the fever has entirely subsided, and before the premonitory symptoms of the next paroxysm have time to appear, the vital force of the organism is in the most favorable condition to be gently modified by the medicine, and restored to healthy action."

§ 237: "If the feverless interval is very brief, as in some severe fevers, or if it is disturbed by the after-effects of the preceding paroxysm, the dose of homeopathic medicine should be administered when the perspiration diminishes, or when the subsequent stages of the paroxysm decline."

§ 238: "One dose of the appropriate remedy may prevent several attacks, and may actually have restored health; nevertheless, we may perceive threatening indications of a new attack, and in this case only, the same medicine should be repeated, provided the complex of symptoms continues to be the same."

If, after the exhibition of the proper remedy, the next paroxysm be *earlier* and *more severe*, or *later* and *milder* than preceding one, the action of the remedy should not be interfered with; wait for succeeding paroxysm, which may be lighter still or not return at all.

§ 245: "Perceptible and continued progress of improvement in an acute or chronic disease, is a condition which, as long as it lasts, invariably counter-indicates the repetition of any medicine whatever, because the beneficial effects which the medicine continues to exert is rapidly approaching its perfection. Under these circumstances every new dose of any medicine, even of the last one that proved beneficial, would disturb the process of recovery."

---

* There are proofs of this, unfortunately, in the too frequent cases where a moderate allopathic dose of Opium, administered to the patient during the cold stage of the fever, has quickly deprived him of life.—Note to Organon, p. 195.

To many, as it was to Hahnemann for years, this is one of the most perplexing problems in practice. Those who have given it a trial are convinced not only of the soundness of Hahnemann's conclusions, but of its superior success in practice. Those who have never tried it can never know its scientific value.

THE SIMILLIMUM.

The selection of the remedy is the question of questions—the one of vital import to the physician as well as his patient. Once unmistakably found, a cure will as certain result. The potency question, in comparison, sinks into insignificance. The more perfect the simillimum, the quicker and surer the cure. On the other hand, if the remedy be not the proper one, no matter how high or how low the potency, how crude the drug, or how massive the dose, we will utterly fail; or, at most, only partially cure by suppressing the attack. We are slow to learn the great lesson inculcated by Hahnemann from the first to the last page of the Organon: **that it is quality, not quantity, that cures**; that *the proper selection of the remedy* is of much greater moment than the quantity to be given; that *disease is not an entity, and cannot be expelled from the system by* **quantity**; *nor can quantity ever take the place of, or atone for, an improper or imperfect selection of the remedy;* neither Arsenicum, Cinchona, Quinine in any form—crude, low or potentized—can ever cure a Nux vomica fever.

Dunham says: "The selection of the remedy for a case of sickness, is a process of comparison. We compare the symptoms of the case with the symptoms which drugs have produced in the healthy; and we select the drug of which the symptoms are most similar to those of the patient. We seek a parallelism between drug symptoms and those of the patient. The symptoms of a case of sickness, like the physiological phenomena of healthy persons, are not always and during all time the same; they vary from day to day, from hour to hour or from minute to minute. Indeed, it might properly be said that life is, in so far as every physiological process is concerned, a series of oscillations within physiological limits; now action is vehement, now mild; waste is now in excess, now in deficit.

"Just so it is with morbid phenomena or symptoms, whether they be of natural, or of artificial or drug disease. We are then instituting comparison between, so to speak, oscillating and continually shifting series of phenomena.

"Now, the point of importance here is that oscillation and shifting require time, and that, therefore our summary of the symptoms must cover not merely the moment of time at which we observe the patient, but also some previous time during which the symptoms may have been different from those of the present time. This remark applies both to the drug and the case. It is necessary not simply for the purpose of getting a full picture of the case, but also to make certain that there is a complete parallelism between the case and the drug we think of giving the patient.

"Two lines, each an inch long, may appear to be parallel. If we would be certain whether or not they are so, let us project each line until it is a foot long. We shall then more easily see the divergence or convergence if there be any. Just so, at some particular moment, the symptoms of a case and of a drug may appear to be very similar; but if we compare the succession and order of the symptoms, for the space of a day or two, with the succession and order of the drug symptoms, we may notice a marked difference.

"This is illustrated by comparing the symptoms produced by two drugs in the healthy prover. There is a period in the action of each, when, to my mind, the symptoms of Aconite and Carbo vegetabilis are very similar, and yet, taking a broader view of these drugs, we can scarcely find any more unlike.

"Shall I shock any of my hearers by stating this necessity for taking into consideration the course and succession of symptoms in selecting a remedy, and shall I be told that strict Homeopathy requires that a prescription shall be made for the symptoms that are present, the remedy to change when the symptoms change? I believe that some conscientious physicians too closely follow this method—too closely for the best success. Let us take a practical instance; a case of intermittent fever. The patient has certain symptoms which precede and usher in the chill. Then, for two hours or more, he has the symptoms which constitute the chill; then, after an interval, those which constitute the hot stage; then those of the sweating stage; after which comes a period of from ten to forty hours, constituting the apyrexia, during which the patient probably may have some symptoms which serve to characterize his case, and individualize it. We may see the patient during one or all of these periods. His symptoms at the different times are certainly very different. Is it our custom, is it good practice, to give the patient a different remedy, corresponding to each of these stages; or, would the nicest faculty of selection lead us to select for each stage the same remedy, to which a survey of the whose case would bring us? The former is not our custom.. It would not be good practice. We could not so select. On the contrary, we extend our lines of symptoms—unless they correspond with the complete paroxysm and apyrexia—and then we can judge of their parallelism. We seek a remedy which produces just such cold, hot and sweating stages, in just such order and with just such concomitant symptoms, and that likewise produces such symptoms in the apyrexia. Do you point me to cases in which no such parallelism is found, and yet a successful prescription is made? I reply that, as I said at first, we are like the Israelites, and must make bricks whether we have straw or not. We must prescribe from our Materia Medica as it is. Where we can do no better, we must prescribe on a few symptoms, or an inference or an analogy, rather than refuse to prescribe at all. Yet nobody will deny the greater certainty of the prescription where such a parallelism can be established. In such a case then we follow the patient along a series of violent oscillations, between cold, heat, sweat, and the normal state again, and this we do, to a greater or less extent, in very many illnesses in which the oscillations are not so violent. I believe that a broad enough consideration of this subject would lead physicians to abstain from alternation of remedies even in the few instances in which Hahnemann sanctioned it, and would deter them from the error, as I deem it, of leaving a patient several remedies to be taken, variously, as different phases of sensation or objective phenomena succeed each other. But to be able to prescribe in this large-viewed way for your patient, you must have studied the Materia Medica in the same comprehensive way; you must have studied the connection and succession of the symptoms. A mere repertory study for the case in hand will not suffice. * * * * * Seeking the means to cure the patient then, we look among drug provings for a similar series of phenomena. Let us suppose that we find one, which corresponds pretty well. Not exactly, however, for here are certain symptoms characteristic of that drug of which the patient has not complained. We examine the patient as regards those symptoms. No! his symptoms in that line are quite different. We try another similar drug, comparing its symptoms with the patient's, and questioning the patient still further; and thus comparing and trying proceed until we find a fit. This is a mental process, so expeditious sometimes that we are hardly aware how we engage in it. But it shows how difficult it is to take a case unless we have some knowledge of the Materia Medica, and how much an extensive knowledge of the Materia Medica aids us in taking the case; and this explains why the masters in our art have given us such model cases.

"To cure an intermittent fever we must:

1. Study the patient during the apyrexia, to form an exact idea of the functional action, regular or otherwise, of all the organs.

2. Observe all the symptoms of the pyrexia in its three stages of cold, heat and sweat.

3. Particularly note if a stage is absent, and which among them is the most marked.

4. Expressly depend upon the bizarre, singular, exceptional phenomena, because they, above all, are characteristic, and figure in the first rank of the symptoms to which the drug must correspond in order to cure."—A. CHARGE, M. D.

The more time and care devoted to a careful and thoughtful examination of the patient, the less guessing and alternating and changing of remedies afterwards; a case well taken is already half cured. The following:

ANALYSIS OF A CASE

Is an example of the comparative or cancellation method of selecting the remedy:

Symptom	Remedies
Time.—Paroxysm every other day, in the afternoon.	Common to many remedies.
Prodrome.—Violent yawning and stretching.	Ant. t., Arn., **Ign.**, Ipec., Quinine, Rhus.
Chill—Especially along the back and arms, for an hour, *with thirst,* followed by	Arn., Caps., Carbo v., **Ign.**
Heat.—(Without thirst) over whole body, with cold feet; accompanied with internal shuddering, not disappearing until the	Caps., Cinch., **Ign.**, Led.
Sweat has broken out, the sweat lasting several hours (without thirst).	**Ign.**, Ipec., Puls.
Dull, aching pain in the pit of the stomach; heaviness in the limbs, with pain in the joints.	Bry., **Ign.**, Rhus.

During apyrexia, great weariness and bending of the knees.	**Ign.**
Sleep sound, with snoring breathing.	**Ign.**, Nux m., Op.
Tongue coated white; lips chapped and dry. Taciturn, indifferent, starting.	Ars., **Ign.**, Nat. m.
Countenance pale.	Fer., **Ign.**, Sec.

THE POTENCY.

The greatest calamity that in practice can befall a homeopathic physician, is to acquire a routine habit of thinking that a remedy can cure only certain conditions or diseases, and no others. This usually is the first step in a routine habit of prescribing, and keeps time and pace with that other habit of thinking that, "the potency I use is the only successful one." The objections that "there is no power in potentized drugs, hence I have never used them;" or, "I do not believe they can possibly cure, or I would use them," or, "I cannot understand how they are made," are daily offered as objections by the allopath to our low potencies and even drop doses of the tincture. Truth is truth, whether we believe it or not. The potency, whether high or low, will never be affected in the slightest degree by such objections. Faith can have no place in science, where a fact can be demonstrated by experiment. The question of potency can only be settled by the experimental test; and every practitioner must make the experiment for himself. Those who never use but one potency can never have any experimental knowledge of any other. Hahnemann asked to have his great discovery, under the rules he laid down, subjected to the test of practice, and the failures published to the world. Submit the potency question to the same test, write out the case, *in extenso,* with the remedy and potency, and publish the failures; the profession can then decide whether it was in the selection of the remedy used, or in the potency. Columbus had no difficulty in making the egg stand. The calling of hard names can neither decide the question, nor reconcile the conflicting views. In the interests of science, published facts, which bear on their face the stamp of reliability, should, both in justice to ourselves and our patients, be accepted as such, irrespective of potency, instead of being met with the weapons used by the contemporaries of Hahnemann and Jenner. **Hahnemann decreased the dose as he increased his knowledge of Materia Medica. Can we adopt a better rule?**

"Boastful homeopathic physicians often claim that they can cure *any* case of ague with the high potencies. But those who have practiced many years in malarious districts know that such assertions are false. I need only refer you to the writings and experience of such men as Holcombe, Ellis, Douglas, Marcy, Pulte, and hundreds of others in this country; also Hughes, Baehr, Roth, Kafka, and others, in England and on the continent."—*Hale's Therap.*, p. 610.

"Every case of intermittent fever, *can, has and must be cured,* with the potentized remedies, under the law of the similars *homeopathically.*"—*Lippe.*

This statement is endorsed by the writings and experience of such men as Hering, Raue, Guernsey, Wells, Dunham, Bayard, Joslin, Bell, Gallupe, H. V. Miller, Baer, Wilson, and many others in this country; also Hahnemann, Gross, Bönninghausen, Müller, and others, in England and on the continent.

Dunham says: "Nothing will gain the confidence of a patient so surely as *success*. His confidence, once gained by *success,* cannot be shaken by the form of your dose! Yes; it may, though! If he sees that while your doctrines require you to give small doses, you yet dissemble and juggle, and, by using large pills and lozenges and mixtures, try to make it appear that you are giving as large doses as your Old-School neighbor, he will suspect that your faith in the system you profess is not really strong, and he will have doubts of both you and your system. The sick man who feels that you are *curing* him, cares not a straw for the logical improbabilities of your doctrines, nor for the scientific difficulties attending the explanation of the action of your little dose. Large or small—much or nothing—if under your auspices his health return, he will have faith equally in yourself and in your methods.

"Patients are like soldiers; they believe in a man who believes in himself. We say this with all humility, for, in a matter of science, belief in one's self is faith in the laws one has undertaken to carry out in practice. And if the physician shows confidence in his methods, his patients will yield themselves implicitly to his guidance. The prejudice in favor of large and many doses is a relic of the past ages, when the practitioner was paid, not for his skill and personal services, but for the medicines he furnished."

A homeopathic cure is as beneficial to our patients as an allopathic one; and if it be quicker, surer, safer, and more pleasant, why not cure him homeopathically.

CHARACTERISTIC.

I am convinced that in the treatment of fevers, as well as of many other affections, we pay too much attention to the local manifestations of disease—to the local symptoms of the drug—and too little to the *general symptoms of the patient* and the constitutional action of the remedy. For this reason we fail to get a true picture of the disease—the totality of the symptoms, objective and subjective—and are apt to fall into the routine practice of treating the disease instead of the patient. This is especially true in that large class of chronic intermittents, in which the *psora* of Hahnemann—the constitutional dyscrasiæ of the German pathologists—becomes such an important factor.

In "masked intermittents," also, where the character of the disease is not marked by the usual chill, heat, and sweat, our only guide is the constitutional symptoms of the patient. In this way we may relieve a multitude of ailments, as well as intermittents, for whose local symptoms and tissue lesions we have as yet been unable to find an analogy in our drug provings. For this reason, and to make the book a more complete work of reference, I have added some of the leading peculiarities of each remedy under the term

CHARACTERISTIC:

Which is defined in Organon, § 153:

In the search for a homeopathic specific remedy, that is to say, in the comparison of the collective symptoms of the natural disease with the list of symptoms of known medicines, in order to find among these an artificial morbific agent corresponding by similarity to the disease to be cured, the *more striking, singular, uncommon, and peculiar* signs and symptoms of the case of disease are chiefly and almost solely to be kept in view; for it is *more particularly these that very similar ones in the list of symptoms of the selected medicine must correspond to,* in order to constitute it the most suitable for effecting the cure. The more general and undefined symptoms: Loss of appetite, headache, debility, restless sleep, etc., demand but little attention, when of that vague and indefinite character, if they cannot be more accurately described, as symptoms of such a general nature are observed in almost every disease and from almost every drug.

Dunham says: "The fact cannot be too often called to mind, nor too strongly insisted upon, that our most characteristic indications for the use of a drug, which presents well-defined general symptoms, as Arsenic does, and indeed as every well proved drug does, are derived not from its local action upon any organ or system, not from a knowledge of the particular tissues it may affect, and how it affects them, but upon the general constitutional symptoms and their conditions and concomitants. If this were not so, in the presence of how many maladies, of the intimate nature of which we are wholly ignorant and which nevertheless we cure, should we be utterly powerless for good.

"A case will serve to illustrate not merely this point but also another, viz.: the detection and treatment of what is sometimes called 'masked intermittents,' by which is meant a disease clearly resulting from marsh-malaria, but which nevertheless does not manifest itself by the customary paroxysm of chill, heat and perspiration, which constitute intermittent fever.

"A precocious child in Dutchess Co., twelve years old, had complained for more than eighteen months of a severe pain in left ear. She was brought to my office for treatment, with the statement that for this affection she had been treated, both locally and constitutionally, for an inflammation of the middle ear, by some of the most distinguished surgeons of the city of New York but with no good result. I could discover no distinct signs of local lesion, but nevertheless supposed it to be a case of otalgia, and from a very close correspondence of the case, as described to me, with the symptoms of Chamomilla, gave that drug. She got no better. I then learned, that she had been under the care of a good homeopathic physician, who, if it had been simple otalgia, would surely have cured her. This fact induced me to scrutinize the case very carefully before I prescribed again. Visiting the patient repeatedly at her residence, at different times in the day, I found that the attacks of pain were regularly and distinctly paroxysmal; that they were attended by the peculiar thirst so characteristic of Arsenic, by the restlessness and anguish, and followed by the prostration, equally characteristic. Furthermore, concomitant symptoms of an Arsenic gastralgia and diarrhea were also present. It then occurred to me that this was probably a case of masked intermittent. The situation of the house and the topography of the neighborhood favored the idea. On the strength of the symptoms recited, I gave Arsenic 200. Within five days the pains had ceased to appear, but in their stead came a regular paroxysm of chill, fever and sweat, indicating the existence of quotidian intermittent fever. These paroxysms recurred for four days, gradually diminishing in intensity. They then ceased, leaving the patient well.

"Whatever, then, may be the local name of the disease, whatever pathological name it may bear, if the general symptoms correspond to those of Arsenic, in the way that I have pointed out, do not hesitate a moment to give that drug."

THE CLINICAL CASES

Of former editions have been replaced very largely by remedies. They were intended to illustrate the sphere of action, as well as the selection of the remedy, and at the same time dispel the delusion honestly entertained by many, "That patients will not *wait* for the homeopathic remedy to act, hence, must resort to Quinine." Patients *wait* for the prompt action of the homeopathic remedy in croup, cholera, diphtheria, dysentery, pneumonia and yellow fever! The *remedy* is not at fault; it acts just as promptly in fever as in any other disease.

TYPHOID, TYPHUS, CONTINUED FEVERS.

There is perhaps no disease the homeopathic physician is called to face, that has received more patient investigation, more caretaking scientific research, than typhoid fever and its allied affections. From the time of Louis, Andral, Skoda, Rokitansky and Virchow in Europe, to the more recent work of Wood, Flint, Osler, Raue and others in America, the entire field has been apparently well covered. In history, etiology, symptomatology, differential diagnosis and prognosis, all that could be revealed by the scalpel and the microscope has been found, all that thousands of autopsies could disclose has been seen. Yet the brilliant results of these investigations—in which all rejoice, for they are the common heritage of the profession—augment pathology to the front rank, establish effects in place of causes, regard the products of morbid action as the disease itself and on this "fatal error" and its resultant teaching is reared the fabric of therapeutics.

But why should the condition of the glandular structure of the ileum and its post-mortem revelations be considered *the disease,* any more than the dry, cracked tongue, the sordes on the teeth and lips, the petechia, sudamina, decubitus or other objective symptoms, quite as much the result of deranged vitality as the ulceration of Peyer's patches or the bacillus of Eberth? Future investigations will increase our knowledge and broaden our views of the pathology of typhoid, but the quick sands of an imperfect ever-changing pathology can never be the basis for a safe practice or a stable therapeutics. This is corroborated by the fact that notwithstanding the discovery of the pathological lesion the mortality under the practice of the dominant school remains unchanged. With this fact staring us in the face, why should the professed homeopath abandon his law of cure—the therapeutics of the Master—for the uncertainties of the schools? We can expect no better results from such treatment—the cold bath or ice pack to reduce the temperature, animal extracts and stimulants to maintain strength, etc.—than are obtained by other schools. The same methods must yield the same mortality.

The law of similars points to a better way, a natural method of cure, and an unequaled success is vouchsafed to those who follow it; not to those who simply *believe* in it, but to those who *obey its every mandate.* The prescribing of homeopathic remedies for the pathological lesions of typhoid is very far from being homeopathic treatment. The nearer we approach allopathic methods, the more certainly we obtain their results; while the highest success and the lowest mortality are only to be attained by the accurate selection of the similar remedy and strict compliance with the requirements of law.

THE ANAMNESIS.

In the Organon, §§ 83-104 inclusive, is to be found the most complete instruction for "the taking of the case" recorded in medical literature. It is the personal experience of the most astute and accurate observer the history of medicine has produced, and should be mastered and applied by the physician ere he undertakes the duties and assumes the responsibilities of a case of typhoid fever; for *life often depends upon the first prescription.* It is not often that the disease can be crushed by the first blow, for its cause may have been slumbering for months; but if the first remedy be the simillimum the entire future course is comparatively clear. Hence the first step, the **complete and thorough examination of the patient,** is the key to success, and is all-important to both patient and physician. It was in this that the early giants, the pioneers of Homeopathy—Hahnemann, Gross, Bönninghausen, Hering, Lippe, Wesselhœft, Wells, Guernsey, Bayard and others—made their wonderful records and won their unparalleled success in the treatment of fevers. *Here is where the real cure-work is to be done.* Too much weight cannot be laid upon this part of the first prescription nor too much time given it; it is the first element of success, its neglect the most frequent cause of failure in typhoid.

Yet from an extended personal experience we are warranted in the assertion that not ten per cent. of the homeopathic profession have ever read, much less applied in practice, this most essential instruction of Hahnemann, rules so vital to success that neglect of their strict observance is little less than criminal. A strict individualization is the keystone of the homeopathic arch, and without it the selection of the similar remedy must be largely empirical. It is an axiom that neither Arsenic, Bryonia nor Rhus either singly, in combination, or alternation can ever check the course of a Baptisia typhoid; and this is equally true of every remedy in the Materia Medica. Natural law abhors substitution.

It is also axiomatic that *the similar remedy* will cure, or cut short a typhoid or other fever in any stage; but it must be the similar. Hence how essential that the taking of the case the *first step* in its selection be thoroughly done and "the symptoms committed to writing." Then the physician may *know,* not *think,* he has the simillimum. Unless the record be written the selection is difficult if not impossible; yet how few comply with this all-important first duty.

If the first remedy be the simillimum and it only palliates—relieves for a time but does not cure—the constitutional miasm has been overlooked or neglected and must be included in the totality of the symptoms in the next anamnesis. Study the family history. It has been truly said that Aconite, Belladonna or Mercury should not be given in typhoid, as it would mar the symptom picture and delay the cure; for these remedies rarely correspond with this type of fever. The same may be said of any remedy in the Materia Medica. It is the want of similarity, not the remedy that is at fault.

At the close of Hahnemann's masterly instruction: "How to examine the sick," he says: *"After the totality of symptoms has been committed to writing, the most difficult part is done."* This has been so well expressed by Dr. P. P. Wells in his valuable work on Typhoid Fever, and endorsed by Dr. Carroll Dunham, that we reprint, even at the expense of repetition, for it is a page from the personal experience of an able clinician:

The first duty of the physician in the treatment is a *thorough examination* of all the elements of his case. This cannot be too strongly insisted on, or too carefully performed. In no other disease is this so important, though it is indifferent in none. Having honestly discharged this duty, and ascertained not only that he has the fever to combat, but all the elements it now reveals, let him consider them well and carefully before he decides on his first prescription, and be ***positively sure*** that it is ***right*** before he ventures on the first dose, for no subsequent effort in the case is of equal importance. If the first prescription be wrong, no subsequent pains may be sufficient to remedy the consequences of the blunder. A confusion of the case from this source has often been realized which no skill could remove. If the *first* prescription be right all the subsequent course is comparatively easy. If wrong there is only vexation, difficulty and anxiety before the physician; and to the patient and his friends, it is too likely there is only a certain fearful looking for of pain, danger and death. Let it never be forgotten that *time* here is of no account, if the question be of time or a wrong prescription. Let whatever of time the case may require for accuracy be given to it, no matter to what extent, for it is infinitely better for the patient that we do nothing than that we do wrong.

The exactly similar remedy once found should not be changed until the change of symptoms forms a new picture of the disease, to be again met by its simillimum. The temptation sometimes is strong to change, or interpolate, or alternate another remedy to meet a new symptom or an apparently new condition, and every honest physician intent on doing the best for his patient will have to meet it. Here is where Hahnemann's insistence on a written record becomes invaluable, for a single symptom is no more the entire disease than a single organ is the entire patient. If the first remedy was selected because it covered the totality of symptoms it must have been right, and should be allowed time to act, as a premature or hasty change generally would be made without due study of the entire case for a remedy less similar, hence less appropriate, and the result would be a serious if not a fatal injury to the patient with bitter regret for the physician when it was too late to correct the error. Hahnemann and every true follower learned this rule of practice after years of experience; let us begin where they left off and profit by their errors. This rule applies to the treatment of all diseases, acute and chronic, but more especially to typhoid than any other acute disease.

Typhoid like all other ailments is prone to develop from exposure to any depressing or exhausting morbid influence, either mental or physical, when the vital force is least able to resist the onset. Hence at puberty, when vitality is weakened by or expended in a rapid growth, susceptibility is greater and resistance less, an attack of continued fever is to be dreaded and extra vigilance on the part of the physician is demanded. The same is true at the climacteric, and from the severe mental strain of business and financial reverses.

THE NAME: ITS USE AND ABUSE.

Typhoid (low, stupor) fever is designated by groups of symptoms which appear sporadically, epidemically, sometimes annually, and assume the type to which this name is given.

Typhus, a more severe form—ship-fever, camp-fever, war-typhus, etc.—more contagious and malignant, due to bad sanitation where persons already exhausted by exposure, ill-treatment, etc., are crowded together in ill-ventilated rooms or prisons, tenement houses, holds of vessels, or when some chronic organic disease assumes a febrile type.

The groups of symptoms by which we name the fever are termed *diagnostic;* those by which we select the remedy *therapeutic*. The more valuable the symptoms for the purpose of diagnosis the more worthless they become for therapeutics; for the diagnostic are based on the name—the pathology—which we do not treat, the therapeutic on the characteristics of each individual patient.

Hahnemann says, Organon, note § 73: The homeopathic physician does not acknowledge the names gaol fever, bilious fever, typhus fever, putrid fever, nervous fever or mucous fever, but cures all these diseases individually according to the symptoms they present, their several peculiarities.

While we have no "specifics" for typhoid, typhus or any other fever, any remedy in the Materia Medica may be called for by the individuality of the patient. In some epidemics the same remedy may for a time fit many cases—be the genus epidemicus—but under the law of similars we cannot have a remedy for the pathological name of any fever. The name of so-called bilious, typhoid or typhus is utterly worthless for the selection of the remedy. That our friends of other schools prescribe for the fever, the name, is the best possible reason why we as homeopaths should follow the opposite course, should be guided by our principles, for we wish to obtain different results. Still we can never neglect pathology. We need it just as we need anatomy, physiology, sanitary science; we need it for prognosis, sanitation, dietetics, quarantine, but not as a factor in the selection of the curative agent. Symptomatic pathology must be made more comprehensive so as to include the constitutional miasms of Hahnemann, for appendicitis, diabetes and Bright's diseases in man are perhaps as often due to sycosis as pelvic cellulitis and salpingitis in woman.

THE TRUE CAUSE OF TYPHOID.

Since the first edition of "Intermittent Fever," more than twenty years ago, the author has devoted much time to the investigation of the true cause of typhoid. The labor has been expended in the therapeutic verification of the truth of Hahnemann's theory of chronic diseases in the line of symptomatic pathology, until the suspicions of former years have ripened into the conviction that when he promulgated his psoric theory he "builded better than he knew." He did not fully realize that he had made a discovery in therapeutics co-equal with the law of cure and the dynamic remedy. Neither did he even dream that as valuable and indispensable in the cure of chronic diseases as his psoric theory has become, it is of even more value in the management of acute diseases.

The author has verified its truth in hundreds of cases, all forms and types of acute and chronic disease, especially in all types of fevers, and in the last twenty years has not seen a case of continued fever of any type—from mild ague to malignant hemorrhagic typhoid and typhus—that has not occurred in a patient with a psoric or tubercular history. And the more pronounced the psoric miasm (diathesis, dyscrasia), the more severe and fatal the disease. The more the vital force (vitality) is weakened by the psoric and tubercular diathesis, the more susceptible the patient becomes to all external dynamic morbid influences, and consequently the less the vital resistance to the onset of typhoid or other fevers; and this may be equally true of sycosis and syphilis.

Still, ever since its publication in 1830, Hahnemann's work on chronic diseases, like the law of cure and the dynamic remedy, has met with ridicule and vituperation from the dominant school, and we regret to say the majority of professed homeopaths have neither examined the truth, demonstrated its falsity, nor accepted its teaching. And strange as it may seem in both schools of practice, those who have studied it least, and know little or nothing of its practical value in the cure of the sick, have been its most bitter opponents. Will this attempt to introduce and apply it in acute diseases meet a similar reception?

Hahnemann defines these acute diseases in:

Organon, § 73: As to acute diseases, they may be classed under two distinct heads. They first attack single individuals, and arise from some pernicious exciting cause to which they have been exposed. Errors in diet, either excess in eating or drinking, or a want of proper food, severe physical impressions, extremes of cold or heat; fatigue, dissipation, strains, etc.; psychical irritations, severe mental emotions, are the most frequent causes. *But in reality they are generally only a transitory outburst, an explosion of a latent psoric affection,* which returns to its former dormant state when the acute affection is not too violent, or when it has been promptly cured.

In the Organon and Chronic Diseases Hahnemann mentions only three constitutional miasms or diatheses—sycosis, syphilis, and psora—including under the latter what we know at present as the tubercular diathesis, which, while an aggravated form of psora, the later investigations in pathology and the discovery of the tubercular bacillus entitle it to the rank of another and a distinct miasm, dyscrasia or diathesis with which we have to deal in acute affections. Sporadic influenza, so-called La Grippe, is generally an "outburst" of a latent tubercular diathesis.

This psora is the only real, true and fundamental cause that produces all the other countless forms of disease, which under the names of nervous debility, hysteria, hemicrania, hypochondriasis, mania, melancholia, madness, imbecility, epilepsy, and convulsions of all kinds, rickets, caries, softening of the bones, cancer, fungus hematodes, malignant organic growths, gravel, calculus, gout, hemorrhoids, jaundice, dropsy, cyanosis, amenorrhea, dysmenorrhea, hemorrhage from the nose, lungs, stomach, kidneys, bladder, bowels, uterus, of asthma and ulceration of the lungs, of impotence and sterility, megrim, deafness, amaurosis, cataract, paralysis, defects or loss of the senses, pains of every kind, etc., appear in our works on pathology as peculiar, distinct, and independent diseases.—*Organon,* § 80.

An outburst of latent psora may, according to the exciting cause, produce any acute disease, any form of fever. Hence the value of a well taken anamnesis; for a patient in whose personal or family history any of these diseases may be traced, or who has a record of asthma, hay fever, croup, bronchitis, pneumonia, appendicitis, peritonitis, eczema, or other skin disease, either active or suppressed; erysipelas, glandular swellings, tonsilitis, quinsy, especially at change of seasons; acne, catarrh, otorrhea, typhoid or other fevers, or a marked susceptibility to every epidemic influence, has this constitutional dyscrasia. A person whose vital force is handicapped by a psoric inheritance is peculiarly susceptible to psychic impressions. Here a severe mental shock, anger, chagrin, fear, mortification, grief, financial reverses, loss of honor or reputation, all dynamic in character, may convert a mild into a severe or even fatal typhoid. And thus far science has no instrument sufficiently delicate to measure a dynamis which would have little or no effect on a healthy individual.

THE TENDENCY TO RELAPSE.

The tendency to relapse is found in all acute diseases, and in most fevers this "outburst of latent psora" assumes a periodicity—occurring every 3, 5, 7, 14, 21, 28 days—and pertains to the *patient,* not the *fever.* In the mild forms it is this periodic return of the paroxysm to which the name quotidian, quartan, tertian, etc., has been given; in typhoid, typhus and some malarial fevers the relapse assumes a weekly or monthly aggravation.

The first prescription selected for the totality of the symptoms of any febrile attack may be Aconite, Arnica, Baptisia, Belladonna, Gelsemium, Rhus, etc., and may not only remove the group for which it was given, but apparently restore the health of the patient when the original cause which still remains uncared for produces a return of fever.

As the falling apple arrested the attention of Newton, this relapsing tendency of acute diseases set Hahnemann thinking, and he says:

> I spent twelve years in investigating the source of this incredibly large number of chronic affections, in ascertaining and collecting certain proofs of this great truth, which had remained unknown to all former or contemporary observers; to establish the basis of its demonstration and find out at the same time the principal anti-psoric remedies.—*Organon, foot note,* § 80.

After the first relapse, when the symptoms are taken for the second prescription, the lines of comparison must be extended so as to include the miasm—the inherited tendency—and the family history should be carefully examined, for here will be found the key with which to unlock this tendency. It may be appendicitis, typhlitis, quinsy, croup, pneumonia, ague or typhoid fever; the name is not important, the patient is everything. It may be and often is Sulphur in which "complaints that are continually relapsing" is a marked characteristic.

When Sulphur or the best selected remedy fails to relieve or permanently improve, Psorinum or Tuberculinum, selected upon the symptoms and peculiarities of the family history and inherited diathesis, will cut short the acute attack and prevent a future relapse. This has been verified in scores of patients and all forms and types of fever and is entirely reliable. It is one of the most precious gifts bequeathed us by the genius of Hahnemann; but, like his theory of chronic diseases, it may never be applied in typhoid or other fevers, and for the same reason, viz., we do not believe it, hence we will not investigate it; and we will not investigate it because we do not believe it.

The author's attention was first called to the use of the anti-psoric remedy in typhoid by a case in the *American Homeopathic Review,* by Dr. P. P. Wells, in 1863. But it was not until 1876 that the hint was put into practice. The following is the case:

A girl, aged 10, light complexion, slender, mixed nervous and lymphatic temperament, whose mother had frequent attacks of facial erysipelas, and the father was psoric or scrofulous. There was in the early stage no notable characteristic, except the rapidity with which the case reached the state usually met in the last stage of the severe forms of the fever. On the sixth day, through an uninterrupted downward course, the patient had come to insensibility; profound coma with staring eyes; involuntary unnoticed evacuations of feces and urine; subsultus; when the eyes were open reaching after objects and picking at the bed clothes; entire loss of hearing and apparently of sight; diarrhea, liquid, brownish and very offensive; pulse 130, small, weak, quick. In consultation with Dr. A. F. Haynel, on whose advice the patient got four globules of Psorinum 30. In twelve hours, having had no other dose, and no other medicine, she answered questions loudly put, the diarrhea was less frequent, the pulse 120. The dose was permitted to act, and the improvement progressed for forty-eight hours, when she again became insensible with involuntary evacuations and an increase of the remaining symptoms, though slighter than before Psorinum was taken. She now got Sulphur 3d cent. a half grain. The improvement was prompt, the convalescence rapid and complete. No other dose of medicine was required or given.

SANITATION—THE SICK ROOM.

The sanitary surroundings of the fever patient cannot be too scrupulously guarded. The temperature, as far as possible, should be adapted to the comfort of the sick, the room freely ventilated in the day time, especially when the sun shines, and at all times an abundance of fresh, pure air maintained. Other things being equal, a room with a southern exposure is preferable. If a cool, or even a cold, room should be preferred by the patient, the attendants and nurses should protect themselves with sufficient clothing; for if there be a rule as to temperature it is that which is most grateful to the patient.

To disinfect the room flood it with fresh air, protecting the patient from drafts and undue exposure. The so-called disinfectants in general use—Chloride of Lime, Carbolic Acid, Platt's Chlorides, etc.—are a chemical abomination, worse than useless, often positively injurious. It is a bungling attempt to destroy a theoretical germ by chemical agents, and should never be permitted in the sick room. If other disinfectants than pure air be required, the similar dynamic remedy meets every requirement of science.

Bathing is essential in every stage of typhoid, especially during the fever exacerbation. The warm or tepid bath is most beneficial and generally most grateful. The bath cloth or wet towel, not a sponge, should be used; and if very sensitive or perspiring, under the clothes. Never use the cold or ice bath to reduce the temperature; it is always harmful, often fatal.

The bedding should be well aired and frequently changed, as quietly and gently as possible.

Never waken a sleeping patient; but never forget that the stupor of delirium is not sleep.

Hering says: Tubs or pans of water under the bed will, in most cases, prevent decubitus. Try it.

The wet compress—cold or warm, as the patient prefers—on the abdomen, when painful or sensitive to touch, will be both grateful and beneficial. I generally apply a towel wet with cold water and wrung dry over the abdomen or around the body in this region, covered with dry woolen cloth to protect the clothing and retain the heat, and allow it to remain until it dries before renewing or changing. In a few minutes it becomes warm and grateful, often bringing refreshing sleep to a nervous patient.

THE DIET OF THE TYPHOID.

"All roads lead to Chicago." Every physician, irrespective of the school of practice or the condition of the patient, has a favorite diet on which he relies in typhoid. The conditions and indications are essentially the same in all cases, viz., the diseased mucous membrane of the digestive tract and the ancient academic demands of the schools to "sustain the strength of the patient" until the fever expends its force or runs its course. Apparently the diet of fever patients, one of the most essential factors in the treatment, is without rule, reason or science; although nature's indications are as clear and her demands as imperative as the law of similars in therapeutics, or of gravitation in astronomy.

Absolute rest of the digestive organs is just as necessary for safe and speedy recovery in continued fevers as it is in iritis, in a surgical wound or in a broken bone. If food can neither be digested nor assimilated enforced feeding is very unwise, to use no stronger term. No fever patient will starve for want of food that cannot be appropriated.

Nature endeavors to make this plain. She points to the heavily-coated or dry, parched tongue, the complete revulsion at the sight or even the smell of food, the rapid pulse and rise in temperature after eating, with entire loss of appetite, as a protest against the custom which is worse than useless; in fact, it may be the straw that overpowers the vital force and hastens what we are trying to prevent, a fatal issue. We do not compel the inflamed eye to perform its duties, when light, its normal pabulum, only irritates the organ; we order a dark room and absolute rest. Then why force the sensitive and inflamed glandular structure of the digestive tract to work when it is incapable of performing its functions, or when even a partial attempt may produce severe irritation, a troublesome relapse or a fatal hemorrhage?

Pure water, ad libitum, is the best and safest *diet* for the fever patient, *until the tongue is clean, the appetite—nature's call for food—returns, and the pulse and temperature are nearly normal.* The best results are generally obtained by *hot* water if it can be taken; if luke-warm, it often nauseates. Cracked ice or melted ice is injurious, and if cold water is given the patient it should be cooled by ice around the outside of the vessel. Ice water should not be used internally or externally in typhoid, typhus or yellow fever.

This diet may, and sometimes does, become monotonous, when it may be varied to suit the taste of the patient by adding the juice of orange, grape, raspberry, strawberry, watermelon, currant, etc., but not lemon or vinegar. As the tongue cleans and appetite returns rice water, unseasoned dried apple water, or toast water may be allowed. Stale bread well toasted should be put into boiling water while hot and allowed to cool in an earthen vessel. Barley, cracked wheat, or oatmeal gruel well cooked may be allowed later. The late Dr. Woodruff, of Detroit, fed his fever patients on codfish water. The so-called Extract or Essence of Beef is an abomination, contains no nourishment for the typhoid patient, is always injurious and harmful, and in typhus and yellow fever often fatal. Alcoholic stimulants are rarely advisable, although Hering recommends pure American or Hungarian wine *during convalescence,* but prohibits port. It is a better and safer practice, however, to correct abnormal hunger or a total want of appetite by the indicated medicine rather than by diet or stimulants. The abnormal cravings of the fever patient may be at times the guiding characteristic of the case, and like the cravings of pregnancy, the drug habitue or the alcoholic should be corrected by the similar remedy rather than by indulgence, which is not always safe.

THERAPEUTICS OF FEVERS

ACONITUM NAPELLUS.

Characteristic.—Aconite is most frequently indicated in recent cases occurring in young persons, especially *girls of a full plethoric habit, who lead a sedentary life;* persons easily affected by atmospheric changes; dark hair and eyes, rigid muscles.

Complaints from exposure to *dry, cold air;* dry north or west winds (land winds); drafts of air while in a perspiration; bad effects of checked perspiration.

On rising from a recumbent posture, the red face becomes deathly pale, or he becomes faint or giddy and falls over; he fears to rise again; often accompanied by vanishing of sight and unconsciousness.

GREAT FEAR AND ANXIETY OF MIND, with great nervous excitability; afraid to go out, to go into a crowd where there is any excitement or many people, to cross a street.

His countenance is expressive of fear; his life is rendered miserable by it; is sure his disease will prove fatal; predicts the day he will die; fear of death during pregnancy.

This mental anxiety, worry, fear accompanies the most trivial ailment.

Music is unbearable, makes her sad (**Sab.**—during menses. **Nat. c.**)

Restless, anxious, does everything in great haste; must change position often; everything startles him.

Hahnemann says: "Whenever **Aconite** is chosen homeopathically, you must, above all, observe the moral symptoms, and be careful that it closely resembles them; the anguish of mind and body; the restlessness; the disquiet not to be allayed."

Aggravation.—In the evening and night the pains are insupportable; in a warm room; when rising in bed; lying on affected side (**Hep., Nux m.**).

Amelioration.—During the day; in the open air (**Alum., Mag. c., Puls., Sab.**); while at rest (except at night in bed); after perspiration; from wine.

Relation.—Aconite is the acute of **Sulphur**, and both precedes and follows it in acute inflammatory conditions.

Abuse of **Aconite** requires **Sulphur.**

Type.—Quotidian; quartan. No regularity; periodicity not marked. Apt to become synochal, or inflammatory symptoms with congestion of local organs, as head and chest, may form a complication.

Time.—Usually in the evening.

Cause.—Dry, cold north or west winds; hot days and cool nights; getting wet (**Dulc., Rhus**); suppressed perspiration by uncovering or sitting in a draft; *by fright;* rheumatic exposure.

Chill.—*Ascends from feet to chest;* with internal heat and sensation of hot water in the head; chilly *when uncovered or even touched;* chilliness on *the slightest movement, even by lifting of bed clothes* (**Nux**); cold sensation in blood vessels (**Ars., Rhus**).

Coldness, with **redness and heat of one, coldness and paleness of the other cheek (Cham., Ipec.).** Chill with *one hot cheek;* contracted pupils; anxiety; or *body chilly,* with *red face. hot cheeks, hot forehead* and *ear lobules;* face hot, hands and feet cold. *Chill in extremities to head and face; heat, vice versa.*

Heat.—With thirst. *Towards evening, dry heat in the face,* *with anxiety; high fever;* DRY, BURNING HEAT, which extends from head and face; burning heat, with chilly shiverings running up the back. *Great fear; nervous excitability;* RESTLESSNESS and ANXIOUS TOSSING ABOUT; excessive anguish and oppression. *Cough during heat,* with palpitation and pleuritic stitches in the chest (cough during chill and heat, **Bry.**—cough before and during the chill, **Rhus**). *Red face while lying,* and *pale face and fainting when rising up. Great thirst for large quantities of water; everything else tastes bitter* (thirst for large quantities in every stage, **Bry., Nat. m.**—only during heat, **Ipec.**). Can not bear to be covered, yet fears to be uncovered (**Camph., Sec.**). *Long lasting dry heat.*

Sweat.—*Must be covered as soon as sweat begins; covered* or *affected parts sweat most profusely* (**Ant. t.**) or *perspiration only on side on which he lies* (**Cinch., Nit. ac.**); sweat on single parts only (**Bry.**). Profuse warm perspiration over whole body, by which nervous excitability, restlessness and anxiety are relieved (sweat brings relief of all suffering, **Nat. m.**). General warm steaming sweat. Most on parts covered. Profuse during sleep. Worse while sweating.

Tongue.—Coated white; papillæ red and elevated. "Strawberry tongue."

Pulse.—During chill, intermittent, thread-like; during heat, quick, full, hard, bounding. *Cold sensation in the blood vessels.*

Apyrexia.—*Never clear.* Loss of appetite; sleep restless and disturbed by dreams; *very anxious* about recovery; weak and exhausted by slightest exertion; either mental or physical.

Is rarely indicated, *per se,* as the remedy to cure. Cause, often the characteristic indication; then it acts promptly and cures permanently.

Unless indicated by the exciting cause, is nearly always injurious in the early stages of typhoid.

"Aconite is never given first to subdue the fever, and then some other remedy to meet the case; never to be alternated with other drugs for the purpose of controlling the fever. If the fever be such as to require Aconite, no other drug is needed. If other drugs seem to be indicated, one should be sought which meets the fever as well; for many drugs besides Aconite produce fever, each after his kind."—*Dunham,* I, p. 87.

Analysis.—CAUSE; nearly always guiding; exposure to dry, cold winds, drafts of air, effects of checked perspiration, getting wet when heated.

Chill.—From extremities to chest and head; one cheek red and hot, the other cold and pale (**Cham., Nux**); < slightest movement or lifting of bed clothes (**Nux**).

Heat.—**Skin dry and hot**; face red, or pale and red alternately; *burning thirst for large quantities of cold water;* **intense nervous restlessness, tossing about in agony**; becomes intolerable towards evening and on going to sleep; *long lasting.*

Sweat.—Must be covered soon as it begins.

"Aconite will sometimes be found serviceable in relieving oppression of the heart and respiration, when this is great during the paroxysm *It is the one exception to the rule which requires the remedy for this fever to be given in the intermission.* Where this oppression is great, and the other symptoms do not contradict it, a few pellets of the appropriate potency may be dissolved in water and a teaspoonful given every fifteen, twenty or thirty minutes, according to the symptoms, till relief is obtained. This, if the remedy be in place, will not impede the action of the specific remedy for the case.

This remedy will be the more appropriate if the oppression be accompanied by the characteristic loud complaining, and the equally characteristic fear of death."—*Dr. Geo. H. Clark.*

ACTEA RACEMOSA.

Characteristic.—Anxious, indifferent, melancholic, taciturn.

Sensation as if *a heavy black cloud had settled all over her* and enveloped her head so that all is darkness and confusion.

Delirium: with nausea, retching, dilated pupils; incessant talking, changing from one subject to another; saw wires encaging him; visions of rats and animals; dreams of negroes. devils, etc., waking from sleep frightened; fear of death.

Head and neck retracted.

Nervous, intense restlessness.

Menses: irregular; exhausting (**Alum., Coc.**); delayed or suppressed by mental emotion, from cold, from fever; with chorea, hysteria or mania; increase of mental symptoms during; severe left-sided infra-mammary pains (**Ust.**).

Spasms: hysterical or epileptic; reflex from uterine disease; worse during menses; chorea < left side.

Violent pains in muscles of neck and back; feel stiff, lame, contracted; spine sensitive, from using arms in sewing, typewriting, piano playing (**Agar., Ran. b.**).

Rheumatism affecting the bellies of the muscles; pains stitching, cramping. Excessive muscular soreness.

Rheumatic dysmenorrhea.

Sharp, lancinating, electric-like pains in various parts, sympathetic with ovarian or uterine irritation; in uterine region, dart from side to side.

Aggravation.--During menstruation: the more profuse the flow the greater the suffering.

Type.—Yellow fever; cerebro-spinal fever.

Chill.—Down the back from 11-12 M. Chill, then heat, then sweat, alternating with dryness of skin, 5 P. M. Chill, cold tremors from the back; hot flushes, then sweat on the abdomen.

ÆSCULUS HIPPOCASTANUM.

Characteristic.—Most suitable to persons with hemorrhoidal tendencies, who suffer from gastric, bilious or catarrhal troubles.

Despondent, gloomy; very irritable; loses temper easily and gains control slowly; *miserably cross* (**Cham.**).

Constant backache—*severe, dull, aching pain*—affecting the sacrum and hips, *sacro-iliac articulations,* worse when walking or stooping forward.

Back gives out at that point when walking, must sit or lie down.

Venous congestion (portal and hemorrhoidal); *fulness in various parts,* as from an undue amount of blood; heart, lungs, stomach, brain, pelvis, skin.

Mucous membranes of mouth, throat, rectum are swollen, burn, feel dry and raw.

Coryza; thin, watery, burning; rawness, and sensitive to inhaled cold air.

Follicular pharyngitis, especially in hemorrhoidal subjects; violent burning, raw sensation in throat; dryness and roughness of throat.

Frequent inclination to swallow, with burning, pricking, stinging and dry constricted fauces (**Apis, Bell.**).

Rectum: *dryness and heat of;* feels as if *full of small sticks;* knife-like pains shoot up the rectum (**Ign., Nit. ac., Sulph.**); hemorrhoids blind, painful, burning, purplish; rarely bleeding; sore, with fulness, burning and itching.

Constipation: hard, dry stool, difficult to pass; with dryness and heat of rectum; *severe lumbo-sacral backache.*

Aggravation.—Backache and soreness from walking and stooping; motion; inhaling cold air; swallowing liquids.

Type.—Quotidian; tertian; double tertian. Periodicity marked. Autumnal fevers. Remittent. Malarial.

Time.—4 P. M. (Lyc., Puls.) Evening. Fever without chill from 7 to 12 P. M.

Prodrome.—Yawning, stretching and bursting headache. Without thirst.

Chill.—At 4 P. M., with goose-flesh, relieved by heat of fire (**Ign.**); along the spine; runs up the back, or creeping up and down the back (**Gels.**), with heat and burning in the rectum and anus. Severe chilliness, with rigor; cannot get warm.

Heat.—Flushes of heat over the face, occiput, neck and shoulders, or over the whole body. In evening fever from 7 to 12 P. M., no thirst, skin hot and dry, palms and soles burn, disposed to yawn and stretch; head aches as if it would burst. Photophobia. Lungs feel engorged; heart beats violently.

Burning in the mouth and profuse salivation. Burning dryness and constriction of the throat, constant inclination to swallow, profuse saliva and frequent spitting of mucus from the mouth.

During paroxysm burning of throat and pharynx as from a live coal; great thirst with inability to swallow from painful dryness of throat.

Sweat.—Profuse, hot, and comes on with the heat, not after it: on head and face. The congestions of head, face and chest decline and abdominal symptoms disappear during sweating stage.

Pulse.—Soft, slow and feeble. Functional disturbances of heart from hemorrhoidal complications; hearbeat full and rapid; can feel pulsations over whole body (**Nat. m.**).

Tongue.—Coated white or yellow; tip sore as if ulcerated; feels scalded. Taste sweet with ropy mucus; metallic, coppery, with salivation.

Apyrexia.—Constipation and hemorrhoids, with the characteristic backache, dryness and burning of the rectum. Painful dryness and burning of throat and pharynx with difficult swallowing.

In France, during the continental wars of the Empire, the blockade of the European ports by the English navy was so rigid that Peruvian bark—the recognized specific for intermittent fever—was effectually excluded.

It was during this time that a vigorous search by the faculty for a substitute for bark, brought into experimental use many remedies, and among others Arsenic and Æsculus.

The *Bulletin des Science Médicales,* in 1808, Vol. II, p. 560, published a large number of cures obtained by the bark of the horse-chestnut. Dr. Ranque reports 43 cases; Dr. Cazin 2 cases of tertian and one of double tertian; and Dr. Lacroix in an epidemic of intermittent fever in the department of Loire et Cher, successfully treated over 200 cases with Æsculus alone.

Analysis.—The hemorrhoidal diathesis with lumbo-sacral backache, and the dry, burning throat, pharynx and rectum are most marked.

Chill.—*At 4 P. M.* (**Anac., Lyc., Puls.**); coldness without shivering; thirsty but unable to drink from pain in throat.

Heat.—With hot sweat of entire body.

ÆTHUSA.

Characteristic.—Especially for children during dentition in hot summer weather; **children who cannot bear milk.**

Great weakness: children cannot stand; unable to hold up the head (**Abrot., Cal. p., Sil.**); prostration with sleepiness.

Idiocy in children: incapacity to think; confused.

Features expressive of great anxiety and pain, with a drawn condition and well-marked linea nasalia.

Herpetic eruption on end of nose.

Complete absence of thirst (**Apis, Puls.**, rev. of **Ars.**).

Intolerance of milk: *cannot bear milk in any form;* it is vomited in large curds as soon as taken; then weakness causes drowsiness (compare **Mag. c.**).

Indigestion of teething children; *violent, sudden vomiting* of a frothy, milk-white substance; or yellow fluid, *followed by curdled milk and cheesy matter.*

Regurgitation of food an hour or so after eating; copious greenish vomiting.

Epileptic spasms with *clenched thumbs,* red face, eyes **turned downwards,** pupils fixed and dilated; foam at the mouth, jaws locked; pulse small, hard, quick.

Weakness and prostration with sleepiness; after vomiting, after stool, after spasm.

Aggravation.—After eating or drinking; after vomiting; after stool; after spasm.

Chill.—Violent, without thirst, through whole body with general and external coldness.

Coldness of abdomen, objective and subjective (**Tab.**); with red face; with horripilation; with rigors and stiffness of limbs; with delirium; chin and corners of mouth feel cold.

Heat.—General; skin hot and dry; with complete absence of thirst.

Sweat.—From least exertion; profuse, cold; on going to sleep (**China**); cannot bear to be uncovered during (**Acon., Nux**); relieves malaise and delirium.

Analysis.—The fever usually occurs in nursing children, during dentition, in the morning; with marked lassitude, prostration and delirium. The complete absence of thirst, the intolerance of milk and other gastric phenomena make its selection easy.

AGARICUS.

Characteristic.—Persons with light hair; skin and muscles lax.

Old people, with weak, indolent circulation.

Drunkards, especially for their headaches; *bad effects after a debauch* (**Lob., Nux, Ran.**).

Delirium: with constant raving; tries to get out of bed (**Bell., Hyos.**); in typhoid or typhus.

Headaches: of those who readily become delirious in fever or with pain (**Bell.**); of persons subject to chorea, twitchings or grimaces; from spinal affections.

Chilblains that itch and burn intolerably; frostbite and all consequences of exposure to cold, especially in face.

Involuntary movements *while awake,* cease during sleep; chorea, from simple motions and jerks of single muscles to dancing of whole body; trembling of whole body (twitching of muscles of face, **Myg.**).

Sensation: as if ice touched or ice-cold needles were piercing the skin; as from hot needles.

Burning, itching, redness of various parts; ears, nose, face, hands and feet; parts red, swollen, hot.

Uncertainty in walking, stumbles over everything in the way; heels pain as if beaten when standing.

Spine sensitive to touch (**Chin. s., Ther.**); worse mornings.

Pain: sore, aching, in lumbar and sacral regions; during exertion in the day time; *while sitting* (**Zinc.**).

Spinal irritation due to sexual excesses.

Nervous prostration after sexual debauches.

Epilepsy from suppressed eruptions (**Psor., Sulph.**).

Every motion, every turn of body, causes pain in spine. Single vertebræ sensitive to touch.

Prolapsus, post-climacteric; bearing-down pain almost intolerable (compare **Lilium, Murex, Sepia**).

Extremely sensitive to cold air (**Cal., Kali c., Psor.**).

Complaints appear diagonally; upper left and lower right side (**Ant. t., Stram.**), upper right, lower left (**Ambr., Brom., Med., Phos., Sul. ac.**).

Relations.—Similar: to **Act., Cal., Can. Ind., Hyos., Kali p., Lach., Nux, Op., Stram.**, in delirium of alcoholism; **Myg., Tar., Zinc.**, in chorea.

Aggravation.—After eating; after coitus; cold air; mental application; before a thunderstorm (**Phos., Psor.**).

Time.—From 10-11 A. M.; from 12-1 P. M.

Chill.—Shiverings, from above downwards (**Ver.**); general, over the body; in the open air; on the slightest movement; from raising the bed clothes; shaking chill with gaping.

Chill in back as if cold water was running down, if he leans back in the chair.

Chilly feeling: with yawning; limbs cold and blue; weakness; ill-humor; no appetite.

Heat.—Almost wanting; chiefly on upper parts of body; in face and upper part of body.

Burning heat, has to uncover lower limbs; blood seems to run glowing through the vessels; turning in bed or lifting the covers produces chilliness.

Sweat.—*Profuse;* oily, but not offensive (**Cinch.**); all night; during sleep; from slight exertion or bodily effort; on front of body, especially about the legs. The face, neck and chest were wet with cold perspiration. The sweat, though profuse, is not debilitating. Viscid, and great prostration.

ALUMINA.

Characteristic.—Adapted to spare, dry, thin subjects of scrofulous habit, who suffer from chronic diseases; dark complexion; anxious, mild, tearful disposition; constitutions with lack of vital heat; old people; hypochondriacs.

Dry, tettery, itching eruption, worse in winter (**Petr.**); intolerable itching of whole body when getting warm in bed (**Psor., Sul.**); scratches until it bleeds, which then becomes painful.

Time passes too slowly; an hour seems half a day (**Can. I.**).

Inability to walk, except with the eyes open, and in the daytime; tottering and falling when closing eyes (**Arg. n., Gels.**).

Abnormal appetite; craving for starch, chalk, charcoal, cloves, coffee or tea-grounds, acids, and indigestible things (**Cic., Psor.**); *potatoes disagree;* cause colic.

Chronic eructations for years; worse in evening.

All irritating things—salt, wine, vinegar, pepper—immediately produce cough.

Constipation: *no desire for, and no ability to pass stool until there is a large accumulation* (**Melil.**); **with great straining, must grasp the seat of closet tightly; stools hard, knotty, covered with mucus; or soft, clayey, adhering to parts (Plat.)**; of nursing infants, from artificial food; **inactive rectum,** *even soft stool requires great straining* (**Anac., Plat., San., Sil., Ver.**); of old people (**Lyc., Op.**); of pregnancy (**Sep.**).

Urine voided while straining at stool, or cannot pass it without such straining.

After menses; *exhausted mentally and physically* (**Carb. an., Coc.**).

Leucorrhea; **acrid, profuse, running down to heels in large quantities** (**Lyc., Lys., Onos., Syph.**); > by cold bathing; < during the day.

Aggravation.—Generally in cold air; out-doors; on alternate days; while sitting; *eating potatoes, soups; at new and full moon.*

Amelioration.—Generally in warmth; in mild weather; walking; while eating (**Psor.**); in wet weather (**Caust., Nux, Lach., Sulph.**).

Alumina is the chronic of Bryonia.

Relation.—Complementary to Bryonia. Follows Bry. well.

Type.—Tertian. Chronic; relapsing. No regularity.

Time.—Chilliness at 4 P. M., lasting till evening. Evening paroxysm from 5 to 8 P. M.

Chill.—*With great thirst; with nausea* (**Arn., Caps., Ign.**). Internally cold and chilly, with desire for warmth of stove without relief from heat (**Lach.**—relieved by heat of stove, **Ign.**), and stretching and bending of the limbs; *worse after warm drinks,* and *after eating warm soup* (after cold drinks, **Ars., Caps., Eup. perf.**). Chilliness of whole body, feet cold as ice the whole day, with heat of head, *external chilliness* and *external heat,* especially *dark redness of the cheeks.* Frequent repetition of *chills in the evening,* every other day. Chills near the warm stove. Violent chilliness in evening, especially feet and back, that could not get warm near stove. Chilly during the day, heat all night (chill lasting 12 hours, **Canth.**). Chill increased by slightest motion (**Acon., Bry.**—increased by uncovering, **Amm., Nux, Sep.**).

Heat.—*Without thirst; heat, with anxiety at night, and sweat.* Heat in evening beginning in and spreading from face and head, frequently *only of right side of body.* Heat < by motion (**Bry.**—> by motion, **Caps.**).

Sweat.—*At night, in bed, toward morning;* most profuse in face, *often only on right side of face* (**Nux, Puls.**). Sweat upon every motion (**Bry., Sep.**), followed by cold shivers as if taking cold. Sometimes entire inability to sweat (**Hep.**).

Tongue.—Clean. Appetite good. Longing for fruit and vegetables. Longing for indigestible things. Aversion to meat (**Arn.**).

Apyrexia.—*Continual empty eructations which afford relief. Great lassitude of the whole body;* great exhaustion and inclination to lie down; unconquerable disposition to lie down.

If patient has had frequent attacks of painter's colic. Rarely indicated, but when acquired, chronic constitutional ailments will almost always be present. Often completes a cure begun by Bryonia, and should always be thought of as the next remedy if symptoms correspond.

Analysis.—The constitutional symptoms of this anti-psoric remedy are guiding. In fever accompanying myelitis or other diseases of the cord.

Chill.—With thirst and nausea, < by least motion, warm drinks, warm soup.

Heat.—Without thirst; often only right-sided; < by motion; with sweat.

Sweat.—< by motion; of right side of face.

AMBRA GRISEA.

Characteristic.—For children, especially young girls who are excitable, nervous and weak; nervous affections of old people, nerves "worn out."

Lean, thin, emaciated persons who take cold easily.

Great sadness, sits for days weeping.

After business embarrassments, unable to sleep, must get up (**Act., Sep.**).

Ranula with fetid breath (**Thuja**).

Sensation of coldness in abdomen (**Æth., Cal.**).

The presence of others, even the nurse, is unbearable during stool (while urinating, **Nat. m.**); frequent, ineffectual desire, which makes her anxious.

Discharge of blood between periods, at every little accident —a long walk, after every hard stool, etc.

Leucorrhea; *thick, bluish-white mucus,* especially, or only, at night (**Caust., Merc., Nit. ac.**).

Violent cough in spasmodic paroxysms, with eructations and hoarseness; worse talking or reading aloud (**Dros., Phos.**);

evening without, morning with expectoration (**Hyos.**); whooping-cough, but without crowing inspiration.

Aggravation.—Warm drinks; warm room; lying down; at night; too little sleep; the presence of others during stool.

Amelioration.—After eating; cold air; cold room and drinks.

Type.—No periodicity.

Time.—In the forenoon. Fever, without chill, 7 to 8 P. M.

Chill.—Of *single parts of body,* with heat of face. Chill, with lassitude and sleepiness, > *by eating* (sweat > by eating, **Anac.**); chills before dinner. Skin of whole body, except face, neck and genitals, cold (ice cold genitals, **Sul.**). Coldness of left hand, with headache.

Heat.—In face and over the whole body every quarter of an hour, most violent from 7 to 8 o'clock in the evening.

Sweat.—Profuse night-sweat, < after midnight, the body being warm. Sweat every morning, **worse on affected side** (**Ant. t.**). Profuse sweat of abdomen and thighs (during exercise).

Analysis.—Chill: *of single parts,* > by eating.

Sweat.—Profuse, *of affected parts;* < *on affected side.*

Should not be given in the evening, apt to produce nightly aggravation.

AMMONIUM MURIATICUM.

Characteristic.—Suitable to those who are fat and sluggish; **or body large and fat but legs thin** (see **Lyc.**).

Watery, acrid coryza, excoriating the lip (**Cepa**); mouth and lips sore and excoriated (**Nat. m.**).

Stools: like scrapings of meat or copious, consisting of coagulated blood; green, slimy, yellow, watery or undigested.

The various affections of the bowels have much flatus (**Aloe, Carbo v., Lyc., Pod.**).

Obstinate constipation accompanied by much flatus.

Hard, crumbling stools require great effort in expulsion; crumble from the verge of anus (**Mag. m.**); vary in color, no two stools alike (**Puls.**).

Hemorrhoids: sore and smarting; with burning and stinging in the rectum for hours after stool (**Æsc., Sul.**); especially after suppressed leucorrhea.

During menses: *diarrhea and vomiting; bloody discharge from the bowels* (**Phos.**); neuralgic pains in the feet; flow more profuse at night (**Bov.**—on lying down, **Kreos.**).

Leucorrhea; like white of egg, preceded by griping pain about the navel; brown, slimy, painless, *after every urination.*

Sensation of coldness in the back, between scapulæ (**Lachn.**).

Hamstrings feel painfully short when walking; tension in joints as from shortening of the muscles (**Caust., Cimex**).

Offensive sweat of the feet (**Alum., Graph., Psor., Sil.**).

Blood seems in constant ebullition. Chills alternating with heat every half hour.

Aggravation.—From uncovering during fever paroxysm (**Acon., Nux**).

Type.—No periodicity.

Time.—3 till 4 A. M.—5, 6 and 7 P. M.

Septimani.—Chill and fever followed by profuse sweat every seventh day (**Cinch., Sul.**).

Prodrome.—Thirst; sleeplessness.

Chill.—Without thirst. Chilliness evenings after lying down, and *as often as she awakes,* lasting entire night. Violent shivering, without subsequent heat (without subsequent heat or sweat, **Bov.**). Chill running up the back; warm covering does not relieve the coldness. Chill with external coldness day, evenings and nights; *worse from uncovering, dares not uncover on account of chilliness* (**Nux**). *Chill alternating* **every half hour,** *with heat and bloated red face* (yellowish, mahogany-red, **Eup. perf.**). Severe pain in lumbo-sacral region.

Heat.—With thirst; over the whole body, with redness of face and a kind of stinging heat in skin, especially over whole chest (**Apis, Nit. ac.**—itching over whole body, **Led., Petr.**).

Flushes of heat frequently coming on, always ending in sweat, which is most profuse in face, palms of hands and soles of feet.

Sweat.—Without thirst; day and night; following heat. Increased transpiration; every movement makes him sweat (**Bry., Sul., Ver.**—when sitting quietly, **Staph.**). Sweat on the lower part of the body. Night-sweat, most copious after midnight and towards morning, in bed. Fever paroxysms begin with chilliness, then heat, and end with sweat.

Analysis.—Chill < by uncovering (**Nux**); alternating *every half hour* with heat and bloated red face. The intestinal flatus, meat scrapings and stools of coagulated blood indicate it in enteric or continued fever.

ANACARDIUM ORIENTALE.

Characteristic.—Adapted to ill-natured, nervous, hysterical persons, in whose diseases mental symptoms predominate.

Sudden loss of memory; everything appears as in a dream; patient much troubled about his forgetfulness. Hypochondriasis.

Disposed to be malicious, seems bent on wickedness; *irresistible desire to curse and swear* (**Lac c., Lil., Nit. ac.**—wants to pray, **Stram.**).

Suspects every one and everything around him; when walking he felt anxious as if some one were pursuing him; lack of confidence in himself and others; weakness of all the senses.

Strange temper, laughs at serious matters, and is serious over laughable things; thinks herself a demon; swears.

Sensation as of a hoop or band about the part (**Cac., Carb. ac., Sul.**).

Headache; relieved entirely when eating (**Psor.**), when lying down in bed at night, and when about falling asleep; worse during motion and work (**Arg. n., Bry.**).

Swallows food and drink hastily; symptoms disappear while eating (**Kali p., Psor.**).

Stomach: sensation of fasting "all gone," comes on only when stomach is empty, and is > by eating (**Chel., Iod.**); > during process of digestion (rev. of **Bry., Nux**).

Great desire for stool, but with the effort the desire passes away without evacuation; rectum seems powerless, paralyzed, with sensation as if plugged up (irregular, peristaltic or overaction, **Nux**).

Amelioration.—By eating (**Psor.**).

Type.—Quotidian; tertian; quartan.

Time.—4 A. M. Afternoon. *Every P. M., at four o'clock, fever without chill* (**Lyc.**).

Chill.—Especially in the open air, relieved in the sunshine (**Con., Sec.**). Shivering over the back and whole body, as from cold water being thrown upon the person, with heat of face (**Rhus, Ant. t., Arn.**). Repeated icy cold creeping; feeling of chilliness of limbs, hands and feet, which causes trembling; internal chill even in a warm room; worse in open air. Shaking chill, with ill-humor and restlessness. Forehead cold and cheeks red. External heat with internal chill. Internal heat with cold sweat. Heat of left side only.

Heat.—From 4 P. M. till evening, daily > *by eating;* heat of upper part of the body; with hot breath, cold feet with internal shiverings; external heat, especially of face and palms; abdomen and knees weak; heat over whole body, but complains of being cold. If any thirst, between heat and sweat (**Cinch.**—between cold and hot stage, **Sabad.**).

Sweat.—Night-sweats; frequently waking up from sleep with general sweat. At nights he sweats on the *chest* and *abdomen.* Clammy sw t in the palms, especially the left. *Sweat > by eating.* Sweats when sitting. Dyspnea and distressing shortness of breath (during chill, **Apis**).

Tongue.—Is white and rough; taste, like herring brine; *bitter taste after smoking.* Flat, offensive taste in the mouth. Apt to choke when eating or drinking. Eats and drinks hastily.

In fevers of nursing children, which return every afternoon at four o'clock, Anacardium vies with Lycopodium; but the fever is not so severe in character, all stages being of a milder grade. *Child is very irritable, a slight offence or contradiction makes him excessively angry* (**Bry. Cham.**).

Analysis.—The mental symptoms predominate. The patient is irritable, nervous, hysterical, malicious, profane. The paroxysm occurs at 4 P. M.; and all stages are *relieved by eating.*

ANGUSTURA.

Characteristic.—Very much fatigued, feels it most in the thighs.

Caries and very painful ulcers, which affect the bones and pierce them to the marrow, particularly if the patient has longing for coffee and a very touchy, sensitive mind; *very susceptible,* will not bear the slightest joke (**Ign.**).

Timid; dyspeptic.

Traumatic tetanus (**Hyper.**).

Aggravation.—From touching the affected part; 3 P. M., in afternoon.

Type.—Periodicity not marked.

Time.—3 P. M.—(Apis, Ars., Chin. s.)

Cause.—Fevers occurring in tropical countries; after traveling through swamps in a hot climate (**Ced.**).

Chill.—Violent chill every afternoon at 3 P. M. (**Apis**) *Shivering with goose-flesh, without thirst,* for several days in succession. Severe cold sensation over back; cold hands, fingers and feet; drawing pain in elbows, knees and toes (pains in ankles and wrists, **Pod.**). Chill lasts half an hour. Creepings up the back, with restlessness extending to inner parts, causing trembling with warm lips without thirst. Coldness, followed by heat the same day; recurring now in the evening, then at noon, then in the morning, with thirst in the beginning of the fever, and vomiting of bile.

Heat.—Warmth of the whole body, except head, towards evening, so that she is unable to sleep again after 3 A. M. (worse at 3 A. M. and 3 P. M., **Thuja**). Cold cheeks. The heat ascends (**Sep.**). Flushes of heat with anxiety.

Sweat.—Perspiration at night in bed. Sweat only in the morning; on the forehead.

Analysis.—This remedy, like Cedron, is adapted to fevers of tropical climates. The paroxysm in each occurs at 3 P. M. (**Apis**), and is severe and prostrating.

ANTIMONIUM CRUDUM.

Characteristic.—Gastric complaints from *over-eating;* stomach weak, digestion easily disturbed; **thick, milky-white coating on the tongue.**

Young people *disposed to obesity* (**Calc.**). Old people with morning diarrhea suddenly get costive; alternate diarrhea and constipation (**Nux**).

Sensitive to cold; < after taking cold.

Child is fretful, peevish, **cannot bear to be touched or looked at**; sulky, does not wish to speak (**Ant. t., Iod., Sil.**); angry at every attention.

Great sadness, with weeping.

Loathing life; abject despair, suicide by drowning.

Anxious, lachrymose mood, the slightest thing affects her (**Puls.**). Irresistible desire to talk in rhymes or repeat verses.

Headache: after river bathing; from taking cold; alcoholic drinks; deranged digestion, acids, fat, fruit; suppressed eruption.

Longing for acids and pickles.

Gastric and intestinal affections: from bread and pastry; acids, especially vinegar; sour or bad wine; *after cold bathing;* over-heating; hot weather.

Constant discharge of flatus, up and down, for years; belching (**Alum.**), tasting of ingesta.

Mucus: in large quantities from posterior nares by hawking; from anus, *ichorous, oozing,* staining yellow; *mucous piles.*

Disposition to abnormal growths of skin; finger nails do not grow as rapidly; crushed nails grow in splits, like warts, and with horny spots.

Large horny places (corns) on soles, which are very sensitive when walking, especially on stone pavements.

When symptoms re-appear, they change locality, or go from one side of body to the other.

Aversion to cold bathing; child cries when washed or bathed with cold water; causes headache; suppressed menses; colds or fevers from swimming or getting wet (**Rhus**).

Cannot bear *heat of sun;* < from exertion in sun; *exhausted in warm weather.*

Aggravation.—After eating; *cold bathing;* sour wine or acids; *heat of sun or fire;* extremes of heat or cold.

Amelioration.—During rest; in the open air; a warm bath.

Type.—Quotidian; double quotidian; tertian. Remittent of children. Continued: typhoid.

Time.—12 M. or afternoon. *Sweat at same hour every other day.*

Prodrome.—Ushered in by gastric disturbances; with **great melancholy, sadness, and a woeful mood.**

Chill.—*Without thirst* (**Apis, Puls., Cinch.**). Violent shaking at noon; or chill in the afternoon with shivering in the back; chill with sweat at same time; chill and shivering over the back, feet cold as ice, with sweat on rest of body; **chilliness predominates (Meny.)**; even in a warm room, cold and chilly during the day (chill worse in warm room or near a stove, **Apis**—chill < external heat, motion, **Ipec.**). Painful coldness of nose during inspiration, as if inhaling cold air. **Great** desire to sleep (wants to sleep during hot stage, **Apis**). Drawing pain in sacrum.

Heat.—When sweat sets in with the heat; great heat for an hour, then sweat ceases suddenly, followed by dry heat for two hours, or even all night. *Heat with sweat.* Heat with thirst followed by sweat. Great heat from the least exercise, especially in the sun. Heat at night, before midnight, with cold feet. During heat, pain in chest. Vomiting during the heat (**Nat. m.**).

Sweat.—Sets in simultaneously with or immediately after the chill (**Pod.**). Sweat in the morning when awaking which causes shrivelling of tips of fingers (**Canch., Ver.**). Sweat which returns at precisely the same hour every other morning. Sweat alternating with chilliness, or vice versa. Sweat soon disappears, dry heat remaining. After sweat is over heat and thirst return.

Tongue.—**Thickly coated: milky white is characteristic.** Taste bitter. *Great desire for pickles.* Saliva saltish. Hunger, which eating does not relieve.

Pulse.—Irregular; rapid, then slow; changing every few beats.

Apyrexia.—*Predominance of gastric symptoms* (**Ipec., Puls., Nux**). Want of appetite, nausea, vomiting and bitter taste in mouth (**Ipec.**); tension and pressure in region of the stomach; belching with taste of ingesta, pain in bowels with diarrhea, or constipation: *aversion to food; longing for acids, particularly pickles* (longing for salt, **Nat. m.**); *disgust for drink and food; increasing sweat.*

Antimonium crud.	**Pulsatilla.**
Prodrome.—Great sadness, and a *woeful mood.*	**Prodrome.**—Thirst and *diarrhea at night.*
Chill.—Predominant, followed by *sweat,* then *heat;* or chill and sweat simultaneous; or chill and sweat, or sweat and heat, alternating.	**Chill.**—*Heat* and *sweat* in usual order, but apt to run into each other. One-sided coldness. No two chills alike.
Tongue.—*Thickly coated; milky-white.* Diarrhea or constipation. No thirst in any stage.	**Tongue.**—Coated with yellow mucus; feels sore, as if scalded. Diarrhea.. Thirst before chill.

Antimonium crudum will often relieve, where Pulsatilla or Ipecacuanha seem indicated and fail. One of the few remedies where sweat follows chill and is followed by heat. Gastric symptoms usually present; acts promptly and cures completely.

Relapses often occur from derangement of stomach. Quotidian or tertian fever with *loathing, nausea, vomiting, cutting in bowels and diarrhea* or constipation (**Puls.,** but no constipation).

Analysis.—The sad, woeful, suicidal mood. The gastric derangements from over eating. Tongue thickly coated; milky-white.

Aversion to food and drink.

Craving for acids, especially pickles.

Paroxysm mixed: chill predominates; followed by sweat, then heat; or chill and sweat, or sweat and heat; no thirst in any stage.

Frequent relapse from gastric derangement, in all types of fever, especially from over eating during typhoid convalescence.

ANTIMONIUM TARTARICUM.

Characteristic.—Adapted to torpid, phlegmatic constitutions: the hydrogenoid (of Grauvogl).

Intermittents or other fevers from exposure in damp cellars or basements (**Aran., Ars., Tereb.**).

Child: clings to those around; wants to be carried; cries and whines if any one touches it; will not let you feel the pulse.

When patient coughs there appears to be a large collection of mucus in the bronchi, and it seems as if much would be expectorated but nothing comes up.

Face cold, blue, pale, covered with cold sweat (**Tab.**).

Nausea, vomiting, want of appetite and constipation in intermittents (**Ant. c.**).

Vomiting: in any position except lying on right side; until he faints; followed by *drowsiness and prostration;* of cholera morbus with diarrhea and cold sweat, a dose after each attack (**Ver.**).

Asphyxia: mechanical, as apparent death from drowning; from mucus in bronchi; from impending paralysis of lungs; from foreign bodies in larynx or trachea; with *drowsiness and coma.*

Child at birth pale, breathless, gasping; asphyxia neonatorum. Relieves the "death rattle" (**Taran.**).

Great sleepiness, *or irresistible inclination to sleep,* with nearly all complaints (**Nux m., Op.**).

Aggravation.—In damp, cold weather; in evening; lying down at night; motion; warmth of room; change of weather in spring. (**Kali s.**).

Amelioration.—Cold open air; sitting upright; eructations; expectoration; lying on right side (**Tab.**).

Type.—Quotidian; tertian; quartan. Apt to become remittent or typhoid. Epidemics of winter or early spring. *In tertian fever attacks anticipate several hours.* Yellow fever.

Time.—9 A. M., severe rigor without shaking. **3 P. M.**, or evening at 6 P. M. *All periods;* no regularity.

Cause.—Rheumatic exposure, living or working in cellars or basements, underground habitation or employment.

Prodrome.—Yawning and stretching (Cinch., Eup.). When gaping, mouth remains open for a while, could not shut it.

Chill and **Heat,** *without thirst,* alternating during the day (**Ars.**—chill and sweat, or sweat and heat alternating, **Ant. c.**). Chill as if cold water were dashed over one (**Rhus**), with goose-flesh, gaping, want of thirst; drowsiness following heat with dullness in head. Chill with trembling and shaking over whole body. Backache with the chill. He looks pale and is so chilly on going into the open air that he trembles (chilly when going from open air into a room, **Ars.**—see **Rhus**). *Cold skin. Trembling and chilliness always from within outward. Short chill and long lasting heat, with somnolency and profuse sweat on forehead.* Chill with external coldness, coming on at all times of the day, with somnolency; mostly with trembling and shaking. Chill lasting 45 minutes followed by vomiting, headache, heat and thirst; after drinking, retching.

Heat.—*Violent short heat succeeding a long chill, aggravated by every motion* (feels chilly if he moves, **Nux, Apis**). Thirst not constant during the hot stage, but marked between heat and sweat. Heat long and severe with much sweat, intense thirst and delirium, sometimes occurs in tertian type.

Sweat.—*Profuse all over;* may last all night; follows long after, in the afternoon during the sleep, or profuse sweat the following night, with increased secretion of urine. **Affected**

parts sweat profusely (Amb.). Sweat often, *cold, clammy, sticky;* < by sweating, but rather better after (**Ipec.**).

Tongue.—Characteristic, *red edges,* or *red* and white in alternate streaks; papillæ red and *raised as in scarlatina;* tongue bright red and dry in the centre, covered with a thick, white, pasty fur. Food tasteless; tobacco has no taste. *Craving desire for apples;* acids (desire for juicy fruits, **Ver.**).

Pulse.—Much accelerated by slightest motion; strong and full during chill; feeble, slow and very weak as the heat passes off.

Apyrexia.—The *gastric, rheumatic, soporous* character of the intermittents of Antimonium tart. will not fail to call our attention to this polychrest. In spring and autumn, especially with children, fevers are prone to take on a remitting type, attended with nausea, vomiting and drowsiness. Gastric symptoms are very pronounced, as in Antimonium crud. Nausea and vomiting may be present; if so, it is very prostrating. Weakness and exhaustion, with great depression of spirits. Weariness and lassitude with no appetite.

Analysis.—Working or living in basements or damp underground rooms (Ars., Aran.).

During paroxysm, cannot keep his eyes open; irresistible sleepiness and deep, stupefied sleep; when awake, hopelessness and despair.

Violent but not long lasting heat succeeding a long chill, aggravated by every motion.

Long-lasting heat, after a short chill, with somnolency and sweat on the forehead.

Affected parts sweat profusely.

In some epidemics occurring in winter and early spring it often amounts to the *genus epidemicus;* especially when gastric and typhoid fevers predominate, or when every fever is inclined to become remittent or typhoid.

ANTHRACINUM.

In the septic fever of carbuncle, malignant ulcer and complaints with *ulceration, sloughing and intolerable burning.*

When Arsenicum or the best selected remedy fails to relieve the *burning pain* of carbuncle or malignant ulceration.

Hemorrhages: blood oozes from mouth, nose, anus or sexual organs; black, thick, tar-like, rapidly decomposing (**Crot.**).

Gangrenous ulcers; felon, carbuncle, erysipelas of a malignant type.

Felon; the worst cases, with sloughing and terrible burning pain (**Ars., Carb. ac., Lach.**).

Malignant pustule; *black or blisters:* often fatal in twenty-four or forty-eight hours (**Lach., Pyr.**).

Carbuncle; *with horrible burning pains;* discharge of ichorous offensive pus.

Dissecting wounds, especially if tendency is to become gangrenous; septic fever, marked prostration (**Ars., Pyr.**).

Suspicious insect stings. If the swelling changes color and red streaks from the wound map out the course of lymphatics (**Lach., Pyr.**).

Septic inflammation from absorption of pus or other deleterious substances, with burning pain and great prostration (**Ars., Pyr.**).

Bad effects from inhaling foul odors of putrid fever or dissecting room; poisoning by foul breath (**Pyr.**).

Type.—Continued fevers; septic, typhoid or typhus, with rapidly sinking pulse, loss of strength, fainting and delirium.

Prodrome.—Restless sleep, great debility and depression for many days.

Chill.—With debility; headache followed by loss of appetite and general malaise.

Cause.—*Septic infection;* sewer gas, odors of the post mortem or dissecting room, absorption of pus or decayed animal tissue.

Chilliness, with great prostration, pain in back and limbs, increased fever and weakness; anxiety, restlessness, vertigo, dull headache and delirium; skin dry, later covered with cold sweat.

Pronounced chill, followed by colic, nausea, vomiting, and in two or three days with collapse, cyanosis and death.

Generally subnormal temperature.

Fever.—With thirst; with diarrhea; with sweat.

Sweat.—General, debilitating, sticky. In severe cases copious, cold sweats.

Tongue.—Dry; thickly coated with a brown fur; taste sweetish, or lost.

Pulse.—Frequent, small, soft, almost imperceptible; red or discolored lines over the veins or lymphatics.

Analysis.—The septic cause first. The tendency to produce malignancy.

The marked prostration with subnormal temperature.

The intense burning pain which the best selected remedy fails to relieve.

APIS MELLIFICA.

Adapted to the strumous constitution; glands enlarged, indurated; scirrhous or open cancer.

Women, especially widows; children and girls who, though generally careful, become awkward, and let things fall while handling them (**Bov.**).

Bad effects of acute exanthems imperfectly developed or suppressed (**Zinc.**); measles, scarlatina, urticaria.

Ailments from jealousy, fright, rage, vexation, bad news.

Irritable; nervous; fidgety; hard to please.

Weeping disposition; cannot help crying; discouraged, despondent (**Ant. c., Puls.**).

Sudden, shrill, piercing screams from children while waking or sleeping (**Hellebore, Tuberculinum.**).

Edema: bag-like, puffy swelling *under the eyes* (over the eyes, **Kali c.**); of the hands and feet; dropsy, without thirst (**Acet. ac., Apoc.**).

Extreme sensitiveness to touch (**Bell., Lach.**).

Pain: **burning, stinging, sore**; suddenly migrating from one part to another (**Kali bi., Lac c., Puls.**).

Incontinence of urine, with great irritation of the parts; can scarcely retain the urine a moment, and when passed scalds severely; frequent, painful, scanty, bloody.

Constipation: sensation in abdomen as if something tight would break if much effort were used.

Diarrhea: of drunkards; in eruptive diseases, especially if eruption be suppressed; involuntary from every motion, as though *anus were wide open* (**Phos.**).

Relations.—Complementary: Nat. mur.

Disagrees, when used either before or after Rhus.

Ars. and Puls. follow Apis well.

In dyspnea Natrum follows where Apis only partially cures.

Aggravation.—After sleeping (**Lach.**); closed, especially warm or heated rooms are intolerable. Worse from getting wet (**Ant. t., Cal., Rhus**), but better from washing or moistening the part in cold water.

Amelioration.—Open air; cold water or cold bathing; uncovering.

Type.—Quotidian or double quotidian. Tertian most common. Congestive, continued, remittent, typhoid, typhus, yellow.

Time.—3 P. M. and **3 to 4 P. M.** (4 P. M., **Lyc.**); 4 P. M., fever, *without chill;* 5 P. M., rarely, ***then night and morning paroxysms.***

Prodrome.—Sudden vomiting.

Chill—With thirst, *always* (**Alum., Arn., Ign., Carbo v., Caps.**). Chill sudden, begins *in front of chest, abdomen, knees,* and runs down the back (reverse of **Eup. purp.**); chill **worse in a warm room;** from **external heat (Ipec.).**

Cannot bear heat of stove (> by heat of stove, **Ign.**—> by external heat, **Ars.**); chilliness *renewed from the slightest motion* (chill increased by motion, **Caps.**—*cannot bear to move or be uncovered in any stage,* **Nux**). Chill, with *cold feet* and *fingers, heat of face* and *hands,* and *oppressed breathing* (during sweat, **Anac.**). **Oppression of chest as though patient would smother.** Falls into a *deep sleep* as the severity of the chill passes off, and breaks out with urticaria (urticaria before and during chill, **Hep.**—during heat and sweat, **Rhus**—during heat only, **Ign.**). Sensation of cold without external coldness of the skin; cold limbs and feet, with burning toes and burning cheeks.

Heat.—*Rarely with thirst;* heat with inclination to uncover (**Acon., Sec.**); more or less violent headache and generally a continuous deep sleep (**Op.**); chilliness on moving or uncovering *during heat* (**Arn., Nux**). *Burning, hot, dry skin all over,* particularly felt in *abdomen, epigastrium* and *chest* and *hands,* with *muttering* and *unconsciousness; alternate dry and hot skin,* or cool in some places and *hot in others, with occasional spells of sweating.* **Great oppression and burning in the chest, with smothering.** Itching, burning nettle-rash, in this stage (**Ign., Hep.**). *The heat of the room is intolerable.* Sensation of heat through whole body, especially on chest and region of stomach, without heat of skin.

Sweat.—*No thirst in sweating stage. Sweat after trembling and fainting, then nettle-rash. Perspiration may alternate with dryness of the skin.* Sweating stage often absent, or of a light grade. Weak and trembling. Sleep, or sleepy.

"This stage is usually wanting, and is characteristic of Apis fever in old protracted cases."—CARROLL DUNHAM.

Tongue.—Clean in old cases. In acute attacks, dry, red, with a raw, sore, painful tenderness; does not care to talk or protrude it. *Swelling and burning of lips during entire paroxysm.* No appetite, nor desire for food; craves milk, which relieves.

Apyrexia.—Soreness and pain under ribs of left side, in region of spleen; great soreness of all the limbs and joints; feet swollen; urine scanty; restless; sleepless; urticaria and great debility. In old cases, badly treated by domestic and patent medicines. Natrum mur. often indicated if Apis fails to permanently cure. In either acute or chronic cases occurring as sequelæ of eruptive diseases.

"Chills and fever in seasons when the flies sting with unusual vigor."—HERING.

Apis.	Bryonia.
Time.—3 P. M.; 3 to 4 P. M.	**Time.**—All periods.
Prodrome.—Free from pain. Sudden vomiting.	**Prodrome.**—Stretching and drawing in the limbs; headache, vertigo, and *great thirst.*
Chill.—*With thirst* always in chill, absent in heat and sweat. Begins in *front of chest, abdomen, knees.* Oppression of chest as though he would smother. *Sleep* and *urticaria* as chill passes off.	**Chill.**—With *great thirst* in all stages. Begins in *tips of fingers, toes* and *on the lips.* Violent, dry, racking cough, with pleuritic stitches. Stitching pain in hypochondrium.
Heat.—Oppression of chest with burning, smothering. Heat worse in the chest, abdomen, epigastrium. Urticaria. Sleep.	**Heat.**—Cough, with pleuritic stitches. Heat as if blood in the veins was burning; headache and vertigo.
Sweat.—This stage is usually wanting. Sleepy. Urticaria.	**Sweat.**—Profuse, sour, easily excited by exercise. Thirsty. Irritable.
Apyrexia.—Soreness in spleen—in all limbs and joints; feet swollen; urine scanty; urticaria.	**Apyrexia.**—Constipation of dry, hard, lumpy stools. *Exceedingly irritable;* everything makes him angry.

Analysis.—The time 3 P. M. is guiding.

Chill with thirst < in warm room, and from external heat. Chilliness with heat of hands and feet, the opposite of Belladonna, which has cold hands and feet and heat of head and face.

No thirst with heat or sweat.

Burning, oppression, smothering sensation in chest with chill and heat.

Sweat with urticaria.

ARANEA DIADEMA.

Characteristic.—Headache and confusion of the head, < *by smoking,* and ceases entirely in the open air (Tab.).

Sudden violent pains in the teeth of the whole upper and lower jaws, at night, immediately after lying down.

Toothache every day at same hour.

Aggravation.—In cold rainy weather; damp dwellings; cold bathing; sleeping in damp wet rooms; lying down.

Amelioration.—From tobacco smoke; in the open air.

Type.—Quotidian, tertian. Remarkable periodicity in every type. Paludal origin; pernicious; dengue.

Time.—At precisely same hour, *every day, or every other day* (**Ced., Sabad.**). **Great regularity of paroxysm.**

Cause.—Rheumatic exposure: getting wet; working in the rain, working while standing in water (**Ant. t., Cal., Led., Rhus**); from living or working in basements; working in cellars or underground places (**Ars.**).

Chill.—*Long-lasting,* often 24 hours; chill predominates. Constant chilly feeling, *worse on rainy, cold days; from bathing with cold water; from damp dwellings.* Chill as soon as he touches the cold sheets of the bed, followed by heat but no sweat. Chill violent, shaking; severe internal coldness as if frozen (Helod.). Chilly all the time, day and night, in midsummer. Bone pains for four weeks; fever attacks, consisting almost wholly of coldness. Chill without *heat, sweat* or *thirst.*

Headache, which ceases entirely in the open air. Great exhaustion; lassitude. Painful feeling of coldness in lower incisors every day at same hour.

Heat.—Slight, preceded by chill. Evening heat, with fullness and heaviness in epigastrium as from a stone; qualmishness in pit of stomach, and heaviness of the thighs so that she is scarcely able to drag her limbs along. Forearms and hands so heavy that he imagines he cannot lift them. *This stage often wanting.*

Sweat.—Wanting.

Tongue.—Slightly coated; taste, nauseous, bitter, > by smoking.

Apyrexia.—Clear. Spleen enlarged. Menses eight days too early, too strong and too copious.

The paroxysm of Aranea is often unattended by either heat or sweat consisting only of coldness, which is persistent and severe, and *not > by anything.* It is usually without thirst in any stage; if any thirst, usually during the heat.

A CASE.—A teamster 43 years old, 6 feet 2 inches in height, and well developed, never been sick before, slept on some straw on the bar-room floor in Frankfurt, on a winter night. In the morning *felt stiff in his limbs, tired and sick. Chill began at 7 p. m., and lasted till precisely 8 in the morning, every day at same hour, without heat or sweat,* with cough, loss of appetite, sleeplessness, and great exhaustion, which distressed him most because it interfered with his occupation. Being yet unskilled in Homeopathy, and not having the least confidence in it in fever and ague, I gave him two-grain doses of Quinine every two hours at first, then every hour during the day, until he had taken forty powders without the least improvement; on the contrary, his general weakness had increased. I now consulted the original provings, and found that according to the law of similarity *Aranea diadema* must be the remedy. He received five drops of second dec. attenuation every hour. Next day the patient exclaimed: "Now you have hit the right medicine; after the second hour I felt warmth again in my whole body, and the first time for three weeks I slept some hours at night again, without any chill." The cure was complete in six days, and for seventeen years he had no relapse.—GRAUVOGL, p. 204.

Like many of our colleagues of the present day, Grauvogl's

lack of confidence in homeopathic treatment of fever and ague (in his early investigations) was only equaled by his imperfect knowledge (at that time) of the true curative sphere of Quinine in the same disease. Here was a fever with *chill prolonged* and *predominant; heat and sweat absent.* It could never be cured by Quinine, which has all three stages, but *particularly heat and sweat,* prominently developed. Possibly, owing to its rheumatic character, Quinine would not seem even to suppress it, and there certainly was enough given (80 grs.) to fairly test its suppressing power.

CASE No. II.—A tall, robust, heavily bearded man who, from the nature of his business, was exposed to all sorts of weather. For weeks past, though feeling tolerably well throughout the day, attending regularly to his daily round of duties, every night, as soon as he stepped into bed, he was seized with a severe chill which lasted perhaps for two hours, followed by heat but no sweat. Thinking the cold sheets upon which he lay had something to do with it he substituted blankets, but without improvement. *Aranea* with its remarkable symptoms, "toothache every day at same hour" loomed up before me, and here was a similar one, *"Chill as soon as he touches the bed,"* and Aranea 30, a dose night and morning for four days. Chills ceased after the fourth dose, and no relapse.—C. C. SMITH, M. D., *Hom. Phys.*, vol. 5, p. 236.

Analysis.—Rheumatic exposure.

Regularity of paroxysm.

Severe, long-lasting, bone searching chill; internal coldness as if frozen (Heloderma).

Heat and sweat slight or wanting.

ARNICA MONTANA.

Characteristic.—Hydrogenoid constitution. Dark hair; rigid muscles. Plethoric; red face. Especially adapted to those who remain long impressed by even slight mechanical injuries.

Nervous, cannot stand pain; whole body over-sensitive (Cham., Coff., Ign.); **sore bruised feeling all through the body, as if beaten.**

Everything on which he lies, seems too hard; complains constantly of it, and keeps moving from place to place, in search of a soft spot (must move continually to obtain relief from the pain, Rhus—See Bapt., Pyr.).

Heat of upper part of body; coldness of lower.

The face, or head and face alone is hot, while the body is cool.

Diseases of traumatic origin, muscles chiefly involved; with stupor from concussion; from blunt instrument (Symp.).

Unconscious; when spoken to answers correctly but unconsciousness and delirium at once return (falls asleep in the midst of a sentence, Bapt.).

Fears being touched or struck by persons coming near him.

Belching; eructations; foul, putrid, like rotten eggs.

Constipation: *rectum loaded,* feces will not come away; ribbon-like stools from enlarged prostate or retroverted uterus.

Cannot walk erect on account of a bruised sore feeling in pelvic region (Bellis).

Soreness of parts after labor; prevents post-partum hemorrhage and puerperal complications.

Retention or incontinence of urine after labor (Op.).

Tendency to small painful boils, one after the other; extremely sore (small boils in crops, Sulph.).

Relation.—Complementary: to Acon., Hyper., Rhus.

Similar: to *for soreness as if bruised;* Bap., China, Nat. m., Phyt., Pyr., Rhus, Ruta, Staph.

Arnica follows well: after, Acon., Apis, Ars., Ham., Ipec., Ver.; is followed by, Sul. ac. and Psor.

Antidotes abuse of quinine and other suppressive measures.

Aggravation.—At rest, when lying down; from wine.

Amelioration.—From contact, motion (Rhus, Ruta).

Type.—Tertian; quartan. CONGESTIVE. Malaria intermittens. Cerebral typhoid; typhus.

Time.—Not characteristic; usually 4 A. M., 8-10.30 A. M.; *afternoon or evening,* 5-8 P. M.

Prodrome.—Thirst for large quantities of cold water, sometimes with vomiting (**Eup. perf.**). Much yawning and stretching; drawing pain as if in the periosteum; aching in wrists; skin blue; drinking refreshes (**Nat. m.**).

Chill.—With thirst, and, if he drinks a great deal, vomits afterwards (**Ars.**). Chill, as if cold water were poured over him (**Rhus**—as if cold water were dashed over him, **Ant. t.**). Chill with **pain in muscles of back and extremities as if bruised; aching in bones** (**Nat., Rhus**); *soreness of the whole body* (whole body feels soré, **Bapt.**). Chill *felt most severely in* PIT, OF STOMACH. *Chill after every sleep; with heat and redness of one cheek;* with burning of *head alone,* or *face alone, rest of body being cold.* Internal chill with external heat (**Ars., Thuja**). Chilliness on one (right) side; on side on which he lies. **Chilly, with heat and redness of one cheek. Shivering over the whole body and the head, at same time heat in the head and redness and heat in the face,** *accompanied by a coolness of the hands, and a feeling as if the hips, the back and anterior surface of the arms* were **being bruised.** *Morning chill while in bed;* begins before she rises and lasts four hours. Chilly from the slightest movement of the bed-clothes (**Acon., Rhus**—constant desire to be covered up, **Nux**). Skin of arms and hands mottled blue (Nux).

Heat.—*Thirst* continued, but less than during chill, except early in the morning, when it is violent. Dry, general heat, with *indifference, stupor* and such *weakness,* that when he attempts to sit up he faints (**Acon.**). **During heat,** *slightest lifting of bed-clothes, or even moving in bed, makes him chilly* (**Apis, Nux, Rhus,** same in all stages of paroxysm). *Great internal heat, with coldness of hands and feet.* **The heat becomes intolerable to him (Apis, Puls.),** *and he tries to un-*

cover himself, but upon uncovering he feels chilly. Dry heat over the whole body after waking early in the morning. Burning heat in one spot, which is cold to the touch; alternate heat or coldness here and there over the entire body.

Upper part of body warm, lower part cold.

Sweat.—*Sour, fetid, offensive,* like *mouldy earth;* in old cases, sometimes cold and clammy. The exhalations smell sour; the night-sweat is sour. Worse when sweating (**Ant. c., Ipec.**). Partial sweat on front of body; on plantar surface of hands and forearms. General sweat about midnight followed by faintness. Headache (which begins in hot stage) and soreness continue, but pain and drawing in the periosteum, which occurs before the chill, disappear gradually (*all pains disappear with sweat,* **Nat.**).

Tongue.—*Never clean.* Dry yellow, or dirty white coating, and often, in acute cases, with a brown streak down the middle. **Breath sour, fetid.** Taste *bitter,* **putrid, of rotten eggs.** Longing for alcoholic drinks; for acids. Repugnance to food.

Pulse.—Variable; full, hard, or weak and slow; in evening strong pulsations through whole body.

Apyrexia.—Headache, *soreness and bruised feeling of muscles* continue; **eructations tasting like rotten eggs.** *Yellow face; bitter taste; aversion to meat;* and, especially in chronic cases, debility and aversion to exercise. The apyrexia is not marked in recent attacks, but is always a characteristic in chronic cases where large quantities of Quinine have been taken, then the soreness and bruised feeling are always indicative.

All three stages, chill, heat, and sweat are well marked; and in each stage the same characteristic of the remedy is usually found.

Arnica.	**Eup. perf.**
Prodrome.—Drawing pains as if in the periosteum.	**Prodrome.**—Pain in back and bones of extremities, as if broken.
Thirst.—For large quantities of cold water, which refreshes him.	**Thirst.**—He cannot drink enough, but drinking hastens chill, and produces nausea.
Chill.—*With thirst,* pain in muscles of back and extremities, as if *bruised;* great soreness of whole body.	**Chill.**—*With thirst,* but drinking causes nausea. Headache, with intense pain in back and bones, *as if broken.*
Heat.—*Less thirst,* but increased soreness of flesh; must lie down, yet bed feels too hard; he cannot find a soft place and keeps constantly changing position in search of one.	**Heat.**—*Less thirst,* but increased cephalalgia and bone pains. *Vomiting of bitter bile before heat begins* (Lyc., sour vomiting).
Sweat.—Generally absent in recent attacks. In old cases, sour, and offensive.	**Sweat.**—Generally absent, scanty if any. Headache continues for several hours after fever is gone; sweat relieves all pains except cephalalgia (all pains, Nat. m.).
Apyrexia.—Bruised feeling and soreness continue through every stage, and persist during apyrexia.	**Apyrexia.**—Bone pains begin before the chill, but disappear with disappearance of sweat. None in apyrexia. Loose cough; night-sweats.

In the Materia Medica Pura, Hahnemann recommends Arnica as a remedy that in its pathogenesis corresponds with the Quinia cachexia; and clinical experience for many years has confirmed his observation. Arnica is probably more frequently indicated in cases maltreated with Quinine than any other remedy; and here lies its chief value in the treatment of fevers. It is also a fact, that in acute cases, where Arnica is indicated, relapses are more frequent perhaps than with any other indicated remedy. It apparently antidotes the previous maltreatment, but some other remedy is required to complete the cure. The patient does not feel well, but can scarcely tell why, and in four or five days has another paroxysm. This paroxysm, however, will differ materially from the preceding ones, Arnica having apparently paved the way for Apis, Arsenicum, Ipecac, or Natrum muriaticum (which follow Arnica well) to complete the cure. Arnica is often the best remedy with which to begin the treatment of a case maltreated by Quinine or patent "ague cures." Psorinum or Sulphur may prevent tendency to relapse.

The "key note" of Arnica is the same in fevers as in all other diseases (Quinine drugging always an additional indication), viz.: **Bruised, sore, weary; great weakness, and must lie down in consequence, yet bed feels too hard; hence frequent change of position in search of a soft place, which may cause pain.** In old cases, where Arnica is indicated, the symptoms of apyrexia should be carefully studied.

Analysis.—Frequent suppression of urine.

Prodrome; thirst and drawing pains in bones and periosteum.

Chill; with thirst; bruised, sore, weak; bed feels hard, frequent change of position in consequence.

Heat; motion or slightest uncovering makes him chilly; *heat intolerable.*

Sweat; sour, offensive, like mouldy earth.

ARSENICUM ALBUM.

Characteristic—Great prostration, *with rapid sinking of the vital forces.* Fainting.

The disposition is:

a. Depressed, melancholic, despairing, indifferent.

b. Fearful, restless, anxious, full of anguish.

c. Irritable, sensitive, peevish, easily vexed.—Dunham.

Mentally restless, *but physically too weak to move;* cannot rest in any place; changing places continually; wants to be moved from one bed to another, and lies now here, now there.

Anxious fear of death; thinks it useless to take medicine, *is incurable,* is surely going to die; *dread of death,* when alone, or, going to bed.

Burning pains > by heat, is very characteristic.

Burning pains, the affected parts burn like fire.

Excessive anxiety; great anguish; extreme restlessness; fear of death.

Burning thirst, without special desire to drink; the stomach does not seem to tolerate, because it cannot assimilate, cold water; it is wanted but he cannot drink it.

Great thirst for cold water; *drinks often but little at a time,* simply to moisten the dry mouth and lips; eats seldom but much.

Teething children are pale, weak, fretful, and want to be carried rapidly.

Cannot bear the smell or sight of food (Colch., Sep.).

Desires: acids, beer, brandy, wine, coffee, warm food, milk, fruits and vegetables.

Aversions: sweets, meats, fatty things, farinaceous food; loathes even the thought of food.

Gastric derangements: after cold fruits; ice cream; ice water; sour beer; bad sausage; alcoholic drinks; strong cheese.

Bad effects from decayed food or animal matter, whether by inoculation, olfaction or ingestion.

Diarrhea *after eating or drinking;* stool scanty, dark color, offensive odor, **followed by great prostration.**

Rapid emaciation: with cold sweat and great debility (Ver.—of affected parts, Tub.).

Excessive exhaustion from least exertion.

Exhaustion is not felt by the patient while lying still; when he moves he is surprised to find himself so weak.

Skin: dry and scaly; cold, blue and wrinkled; with cold, clammy perspiration; like parchment; white and pasty; black vesicles and burning pain.

Breathing: asthmatic; must sit or bend forward; springs out of bed at night, especially after twelve o'clock; *unable to lie down for fear of suffocation;* attacks like croup instead of the usual urticaria.

Relation.—Complementary: All. s., Carbo v., Phos., Pyr.

Aggravation.—After midnight (1-2 A. M.; 1-2 P. M.); from cold; cold drinks or food; when lying on the affected side or with the head low.

Amelioration.—From heat in general (rev. of Sec.) except headache, which is temporarily > by cold bathing (Spig.).

Type.—Quotidian; tertian; quartan; double tertian and quartan. Anticipating (Bry., Cinch., Nux). Every fourteen days. Yearly (Lach., Nat.). Irregular, both in type and stage (Nux). Remitting and relapsing both tend to typhoid and typhus, especially after abuse of Quinine.

Septic, typhoid, typhus or yellow fever.

Time.—All periods—*mostly afternoon paroxysms,* **1 to 2 P. M.; 12 to 2 A. M.**; 3 to 6 P. M.; 5 P. M.; 12 M. *Every fourteen days* **(Cal., Cinch., Puls.).**

Anticipates, **one hour every other day.**

Yearly return of complaints (Carbo v., Sul., Thuja).

Fever without chill—2 A. M.; 4 P. M.; 10 P. M.

Afternoon intermittents of nursing children, *without chill, must be covered,* and *very thirsty; fever lasting all night.*

Prodrome.—"Sleepiness night before paroxysm."—H. V. Miller.

Yawning and stretching; malaise; debility; weakness; headache; vertigo; *great weariness and inclination to lie down;* slight creepings over the back after drinking; cutting pain in chest and bowels like knives, and watery diarrhea; shuddering. Every morning stretching of limbs, gaping, emptiness in head, anxiety, thirst, and immediately after drinking chilliness and crawling.

Chill.—*Without thirst; irregularly developed; never clearly defined; simultaneously,* or *alternating with heat; mingling of heat and chilliness;* **all ameliorated by external warmth**

(**Ign.**—*aggravated* by external heat, **Apis, Ipec.**). Irregular chills at any time of day. *Shuddering when walking in the open air.* Generally little if any thirst during chill, then prefers hot drinks; if thirsty, *frequent drinking but little at a time,* but drinking increases the chilliness and causes shuddering, nausea and vomiting (drinking hastens and aggravates chill and causes nausea, **Eup. perf.**—causes headache, **Cimex**—every drink causes shivering and chill, **Caps.**); oppression of the chest (**Apis**); coldness of abdomen (**Men.**); blue nails and lips (**Nux**); tastelessness of food; shuddering without thirst, worse in the open air. *Internal chill, with external heat and red cheeks;* coldness of body and dryness of the skin; burning heat of skin, cold to the touch; headache.

Coldness of the whole body; pale, sunken face; very sickly appearance; lips pale, rigor, pains in limbs, back and chest; breathing impeded, restless, trembling.

Crawling in the evening, with stretching of limbs and anxious restlessness. Chill gradually increasing to shaking rigor.

Concomitants of chill: colic and nausea, diarrhea, unconsciousness, drawing, tearing in limbs, thighs feel as if beaten, cramps and contraction in chest, difficult breathing, desire to urinate and frequent urination; hunger.

With the shivering and coldness, aggravation of other complaints. Coldness and chilliness renewed after drinking and after eating.

"Chill in forenoon not relieved by anything; external coldness, with cold, clammy sweat."—HERING.

Chill or chilliness without thirst; if there be thirst during chill except for hot drinks, do not give Arsenic.—H. N. GUERNSEY.

Heat.—The hot stage of the fever is *intense, long lasting, dry, burning* and *pungent to the touch,* with *inclination to uncover* (**Apis, Sec.**) and **insatiable thirst for cold water;** *drinks little and often, with vomiting after drinking, several* *times.* Internal, burning, dry heat at night, must be uncovered. Burning heat as if *hot water were poured over one,* or as if *hot water were coursing through the blood-vessels* (**Bry., Rhus**). Oppressed breathing (**Apis**); **great restlessness,** and pressing, burning pain in region of the spleen. Burning pain in stomach and bowels. **During chill and heat, aggravation of previously existing symptoms.** Heat following the chill is *dry, burning, unbearable,* lasts three or four hours, with painful pressure and tension in both hypochondria; fulness in epigastrium; pressing pain in forehead; *restlessness, anxiety and unquenchable thirst;* sometimes a great desire for acids and acid drinks.

Sweat.—This stage is as variable as that of chill—*with* **unquenchable thirst for large quantities of cold water** (**Cinch.**), *which causes vomiting.* Sweat, with cessation of all the previous symptoms (**Nat.**—of all except headache, which is increased, **Eup.**). Sweat; sometimes *offensive and sour smelling.* Sweat during first sleep, or during entire night; **cold, clammy sweat.** *Sweat with excessive thirst.* Sweat with thirst, coming on *several hours after the heat,* or, *which is oftener the case, there is no sweat at all, the dry heat continuing all night.* **After the paroxysm**—*with or without sweat*—**great weakness and prostration** *and a desire for stimulants, wine or coffee.* There is more headache than in the hot stage, unless there be copious sweat (most intense in hot stage, **Nat.**). **Drinks large quanties in sweat; little and often in chill and heat.**

With the various stages of the fever always appear other symptoms.

Tongue.—Sides furred with red streak down the middle (**Ant. t.**) and red tip; yellowish-white; brown; bluish. Water tastes bitter; desire for acids; brandy. Aversion to food (aversion to meat, **Arn.**).

Pulse.—Weak, small, easily compressible. Very frequent

in morning, slower at night. Pulsations through whole body (**Arn., Nat.**). Burning or cold sensations in the blood-vessels (Rhus).

Apyrexia.—*Never clear of symptoms. Great debility;* lassitude; weakness of all the limbs and constant inclination to lie down (**Arn.**). Face *pale, sunken, sallow, clay-colored, bloated;* dull aching in region of liver and spleen, painful on pressure, with sensation as if swollen. Abdomen bloated (**Apis**); *fetid, watery, diarrheic stools,* which are *very debilitating;* urine scanty and turbid. Constant desire for acids or something refreshing. The patient is constantly chilly and must be in a warm room. *General anemic appearance* (**Eup., Cinch., Fer.**). Skin pale, often covered with cold perspiration. *Icterus after the fever. Fevers contracted at sea-shore watering places,* coming on in the autumn, or "wintered over" and not coming on until spring (**Gels.**).

"The paroxysm is not complete. One (especially the cold) stage is generally wanting."—CARROLL DUNHAM.

The following admirable analysis of the indications for Arsenic in intermittent (or other) fever is by Dr. Wurmb in *Homeopathische Clinische Studien,* I, p. 179:

"Arsenic is one of those few drugs whose action is distinguished not alone by its intensity, but equally by its extent; it involves the entire organism. Every system, every organ of the body, every nervous filament, is so subjected to its powerful influence that we are not able to say which of its symptoms are primary, which are secondary, and where the focus of its action chiefly lies. We see the entire nerve-life attacked in all directions, from the slightest excitement to the most violent irritation; from the mere sensation of weakness to actual paralysis, and then we see, likewise, another series of disturbances arise from its action, which advance in regular gradation from the most inconsiderable acceleration of the circulation to the most violent febrile storm; from the slightest irregularity in the vegetative sphere to a cachectic dyscrasia; yes, even to decomposition and destruction of the organic substance.

"In addition, we remark the striking similarity between the symptoms of chronic arsenical poisoning and those of the intermittent cachexy, as well as the fact that Arsenic has the property of causing the periodical recurrence of symptoms in so high a degree as to surpass in this respect all other drugs; in a word, no other drug known to us has such a power of affecting so intimately and so variously those organs that are especially affected in intermittent fever, and none corresponds so well as Arsenic does to all the requirements of a remedy for intermittent.

"Arsenic is indicated in cases which are distinguished not only by weakness in the vital power and deterioration of the organic substance, but also and at the same time by symptoms of excitation of the circulation, or of the nervous system alone, or of both together. Again, it seems to be more especially indicated the more malignant the influence from which the disease has sprung. Marsh-miasm is the chief of these influences; in this originate the most serious and most dangerous cases of fever, and in these Arsenic is often the only remedy that will rescue the patient. Again, the longer the disease has lasted the more is Arsenic generally indicated, because the more deeply have the organs and tissues been affected, the more nearly has the patient's condition approached that known as the intermittent cachexia, and which so nearly resembles the arsenical cachexia. Especially is this the case when the liver and the spleen have become swollen.

"The intermittents which find their homeopathic remedy in Arsenic present in their paroxysms the following peculiarities: The paroxysms are general, violent and of long duration; the stages are either distinctly developed and equally proportioned to each other, or else, as is most frequently the case, one of the stages is absent or is very feebly present; if the latter be the case, it is generally the cold stage which fails, and the hot is all the more violent. The more intense the heat, the longer it continues, the higher the degree of development of the accompanying excitement in the vascular system, and the more burning and insatiable the thirst, the better is Arsenic indicated. The sweating stage may be altogether wanting, or the perspiration may be very copious; it breaks out generally several hours after the hot stage and lasts a long time.

"With the paroxysms are associated many distressing accessory symptoms, which are connected, some with the disturbances in the nervous system, some with those of the vascular system, *e. g.*, spasms, pains, delirium, paralyses and the anguish and restlessness that are so characteristic of Arsenic.

"The apyrexia is not pure, but is disturbed by symptoms of the most various kinds; restlessness, sleeplessness, spasms, digestive disorders, feeling of weakness and general prostration, and it is especially characteristic for Arsenic that after every paroxysm there is a notable increase of prostration."

Arsenicum.	**Cinchona.**
Time.—Characteristic; 1 to 2 P. M.—12 to 2 A. M. Anticipates. "Sleepy, night before the paroxysm."—H. V. MILLER.	**Time.**—Not characteristic. 5 A. M.—5 P. M. Anticipates or postpones. "Restless sleep, night before the paroxysm."—HAHNEMANN.
Prodrome.—*No thirst.* Headache, with vertigo and *pale face;* pain in bowels and watery diarrhea.	**Prodrome.**—*Great thirst.* Canine hunger, headache with *flushed face* and palpitation of the heart.
Chill.—Irregular; mingling of heat and chilliness; chills alternating with heat; *ameliorated* by external heat. Thirst slight, if any, for hot drinks.	**Chill.**—Regular; violent chill over whole body, with icy cold hands and feet; external heat *increases* chill. *No thirst during chill.*
Heat.—*Dry, burning, intense, as if hot water were coursing through the blood vessels. Great restlessness; uncovering brings relief. Insatiable thirst; drinks little and often.*	**Heat.**—*With distended veins and congestive headache,* often *delirium.* Wants to uncover, *but chilly when uncovered. Rarely any thirst;* if any at close of heat. Hunger instead of thirst.

Arsenicum.	Cinchona.
Sweat.—*Rarely occurs,* light if any; *but cold and clammy. Unquenchable thirst* for *large quantities* of cold water, with vomiting after drinking.	**Sweat.**—*Debilitating, profuse. On being covered, he sweats profusely all over. Sweating during sleep. Thirst returns; for large quantities, or little and often.*
Tongue.—Sides furred, with red streak down the middle. Tongue brown; blue; desire for acids; *aversion to food.*	**Tongue.**—White; yellow. Thick, dirty coating; taste too acute; food tastes bitter; too salt; *hungry.*
Pulse.—Weak, small and easily compressible. Frequent in morning; slower at night.	**Pulse.**—Hard; full; quick. Uncommon distention of blood-vessels.
Apyrexia.—*Great weakness and prostration;* pale; sunken face; fetid, watery diarrhea; **abdomen** bloated; great desire to lie down.	**Apyrexia.**—*Sweats easily; exhausting night-sweats;* pain in both hypochondria; complete loss of appetite.

Arsenicum is often given (by some homeopaths) in alternation with Cinchona or some of its alkaloids in this disease; but with the above comparison, to those who differentiate, there ought to be little danger of confounding them. *Where one is indicated the other never is.* Fowler's solution, and massive doses of the lower triturations of Arsenicum, frequently repeated, are wholly unnecessary in the treatment of intermittent or any other fever. If the remedy be indicated, the potentized drug will effect a more prompt and radical cure.

Arsenicum is probably more often indicated than any other remedy, in the so-called "dumb ague," "masked intermittent," so often met with after abuse of Quinine. Also, in the afternoon intermittents of nursing children—who never have chills, and from whom it is impossible to obtain many indications—it frequently suffices to complete a cure. The general constitutional symptoms are guiding.

In typhoid and continued fevers no remedy perhaps is so often abused as Arsenicum, when it is too frequently repeated in the 3x or 6x for "typhoid fever" not for the symptoms of the patient. In the characteristics of Arsenicum will be found such complete indications for its use in any stage of typhoid, typhus or yellow fever that the baneful effects of a routine practice may be avoided.

Analysis.—Time, 1-2 P. M. or 12-2 A. M. is always guiding

Chill.—Light, irregular, mingling with heat, > by externa heat. Thirst, if present, for warm drinks.

Heat.—Dry, burning, intense; great restlessness; uncovering >; unquenchable thirst, drinks little but often.

Sweat.—Often wanting; if any cold and clammy; great thirst for large quantities of cold water, with vomiting after drinking.

The mental restlessness, physical weakness and profound prostration are always present in every form of fever.

Anxiety, fear of death, fears disease is incurable, < when alone or when retiring.

Incomplete stages; obscurity of either chill, heat or sweat.

ARGENTUM NITRICUM.

Acute or chronic diseases from unusual or long-continued mental exertion.

Always think of Argentum nit. on seeing withered, dried-up, old-looking patients (thin, scrawny, Sec.).

Emaciation, progressing every year; most marked in lower extremities (Am. m.); marasmus.

Apprehension when ready for church or opera; diarrhea sets in (Gels.).

Time passes slowly (Can.); impulsive, wants to do things in a hurry; must walk fast; is always hurried; anxious, irritable, nervous (Aur., Lil.).

Great longing for fresh air (Amyl, Puls., Sulph.).

Headache: congestive, with fulness and heaviness; with *sense of expansion;* habitual, gastric, of literary men; *from dancing;* hemicrania, pressive, screwing in frontal eminence or temple; ending in bilious vomiting; < from *any exhaustive mental labor;* > *by pressure or tight bandaging* (Apis, Puls.).

Flatulent dyspepsia: belching after every meal; stomach, as if it would burst with wind; belching difficult, finally air rushes out with great violence.

Belching accompanies most gastric ailments.

Diarrhea: green mucus, *like chopped spinach in flakes;* turning green *after remaining on diaper; after drinking;* after *eating candy or sugar;* masses of muco-lymph in shreddy strips or lumps (Asar.); with much noisy flatus (Aloe).

Diarrhea as soon as he drinks (Ars., Crot. t., Throm.).

Urine passes unconsciously day and night (Caust.).

Chilly when uncovered, yet feels smothered if wrapped up; craves fresh air.

Aggravation.—Cold food; cold air; eating sugar; ice cream: *unusual mental exertion.*

Amelioration.—Open air; craves the wind blowing in his face; bathing with cold water.

Type.—Continued, remittent, typhus, yellow fever, especially the second stage.

Chill.—Without thirst. Chilliness with nausea; constant, up the back and over the shoulders; < after meals (Nux); coming into the room from the open air; with cold extremities. General chill followed in a short time by general heat; chill returns on uncovering, even during heat; no thirst.

Evening chill followed by sweat.

Temperature, subnormal.

Chill from being uncovered, yet feels smothered if wrapped up.

Heat.—Without thirst, with aversion to uncover (Arn., Nux).

Always kept covered because easily chilled.

General heat following general chill with perceptible pulsations in the left temporal artery.

Sweat.—Sweat and chilliness, as soon as he gets warm in bed.

Profuse sweat, it stands out on the face in beads.

Night sweats.

Had to leave a window open day and night, for when it was shut patient became restless.

Septic fever following scarlatina.

Pulse.—Dicrotic; finally feeble, small, could not be counted.

BAPTISIA TINCTORIA.

Characteristic.—For the lymphatic temperament.

Great prostration, with disposition to decomposition of fluids (Pyr.); ulceration of mucous membranes.

All exhalations and discharges *fetid*, especially in typhoid or other acute diseases; breath, stool, urine, perspiration, ulcers (Psor., Pyr.).

Aversion to mental exertion; indisposed, or want of power, to think.

Perfect indifference; does not care to do anything; inability to fix mind on work.

Stupor; falls asleep while being spoken to or in the midst of his answer (when spoken to, answers correctly, but delirium returns at once, Arn.).

Face flushed, dusky, dark-red, with a stupid, besotted, drunken expression (Gels.).

Can swallow liquids only (Bar. c.); least solid food gags (can swallow liquids only, but has aversion to them, Sil.).

Painless sore throat; tonsils, soft palate and parotids dark red, swollen; putrid, offensive discharge (Diph.).

Dysentery of old people; diarrhea of children, especially when very offensive (Carbo v., Pod., Psor.).

Cannot go to sleep because she cannot get herself together; head or body feels scattered about the bed; tosses about to get the pieces together; thought she was three persons, could not keep them covered (Petr.).

In whatever position the patient lies, the parts rested upon feel sore and bruised (compare, Arn., Pyr.).

Decubitus in typhoid (Arn., Carb. ac., Pyr.).

Relation.—Similar: to Arn., Ars., Bry., Gels., in the early stages of fever with malaise, nervousness, flushed face, drowsiness, and muscular soreness.

When Ars. has been improperly given or too often repeated in typhoid, typhus, or yellow fever.

After Baptisia: Crot., Ham., Nit. ac., Pyr. and Tereb., act well in hemorrhage.

Type.—Quotidian; double quotidian; intermittent or remittent; during epidemic typhoid; hot weather in autumn. Prone to become low typhoid. In typhus and yellow fever.

Time.—Every A. M. at 11. *Chill, fever, and sweat every afternoon.*

Prodrome.—Great languor; wants to lie down. General malaise; feels weak, tremulous, as after severe illness; sore, bruised (Arn., Pyr.).

Chill.—*Chilly all day; whole body feels sore, bruised* (**Arn.**). Chills; up and down the back (**Gels.**); over the back, and limbs; over the back while sitting by the fire; on going into the open air; with severe aching in muscles of whole body.

Heat.—Whole surface hot and dry, with occasional chills, mostly up and down the back (**Ars.**). Flushes of heat; from small of back in all directions (**Gels.**); over the face; over the whole body; 3 A. M. with feeling as if sweat would break out. Uncomfortable burning all over surface, especially face, as if sweat would break out; had to move to a cool part of the bed. Heat at night; burning in legs prevents sleep; limbs hot, but feel cold to touch.

Sweat.—Fetid, frequent, but not profuse.

Tongue.—White at first, with red edges and papillæ; brown streak down centre; later, dry, cracked, ulcerated. Taste flat or bitter; cannot digest food.

Pulse.—Small, thready, weak, variable, 120-160; temperature, rises rapidly to 103-106.

Apyrexia.—Indescribable sick feeling all over. Generally weak, restless, uneasy; can confine himself to nothing; wants to be continually moving from place to place.

Analysis.—Dark red, flushed face, with stupid, besotted expression.

The peculiar delirium and stupor.

The bruised soreness of parts lain upon.

The marked early prostration, and tendency to a low type of fever with decomposition.

BARYTA CARBONICA.

Characteristic.—Especially adapted to complaints of first and second childhood; scrofulous, dwarfish children who do not grow (children who grow too rapidly, Cal.); scrofulous ophthalmia, opaque cornea; attacks of colic; swollen abdomen; puffed face; general emaciation; mind and body weak; psoric or tubercular.

Memory deficient; forgetful, inattentive; child cannot be taught for it cannot remember; threatened idiocy.

Children both physically and mentally weak.

Apoplectic tendency in old people; complaints of old drunkards; headache of aged people, who are childish.

Persons subject to quinsy; take cold easily, or with every, even least cold, have an attack of tonsillitis prone to suppuration (Psor.).

Dwarfish hysterical women and old maids, with scanty menses; deficient vital heat, always cold and chilly.

Old cachectic people; scrofulous, *especially when fat;* or those who suffer from gouty complaints (Fluor. ac.).

Diseases of old men; hypertrophied prostate or indurated testes.

Swelling and indurations, or incipient suppuration of glands.

Offensive foot-sweat; toes and soles get sore; throat affections *after checked foot-sweat* (Graph., Psor., San., Sil.).

Great sensitiveness to cold (Cal., Con., Kali c., Psor.).

Aggravation.—While sitting; when thinking of his disease (Oxalic acid); lying on painful side; washing affected part.

Amelioration.—When walking in the open air.

Relation.—Frequently useful before or after Psor., Sulph. and Tub.

After Bar. c., Psor. will often eradicate the constitutional tendency to quinsy.

Incompatible: after Calc. in scrofulous affections.

Type.—Quotidian; tertian; continued.

Time.—8 P. M. Afternoon or evening.

Chill.—Without thirst.

Constant coldness, *as if cold water were dashed over her* (**Ant. t., Rhus**), relieved by warmth of stove (**Ign.**), but aggravated by exercise or the least draught of air. Chill begins in face and descends over the body; or shivering, beginning in the feet, *with bristling of the hairs.* Chills in pit of stomach (**Cal.**) alternate with warmth of body; *cold feet,* then chilliness comes on again. Sudden chill, with goose-skin, external coldness and *the hair standing on end. Icy coldness of the feet* from afternoon till evening; after lying down, heat in the whole body. Alternate chilliness and heat the whole night. Chill generally one (left) sided. Chill alternating with heat; evening and night. *Horripilation.*

Heat.—Without thirst. Skin hot and dry; *heat at night and anxiety. She cannot lie upon the left side on account of violent palpitation,* with a feeling of *soreness* in the heart, and great anxiety. Dry heat the whole night, with sleeplessness; *if she puts her hands out from under the cover of the bed, she feels cold, chilly and thirsty* (feels cold, **Hep.**); *next day, violent thirst,* drinks whole glasses of water. Frequent flushes of heat during the day; night attacks, with great anxiety and restlessness. Heat and redness, frequently of one cheek, with coldness of the other. *Very sensitive to cold air,* or *to change of temperature* (**Cal., Hep.**). Coldness of single parts.

Sweat.—Exhausting night-sweat; *anxious sweat. Sweat profuse, of the left side; offensive of one (the left) side;* returning *every other evening* (**Ant. c.**); < by eating, < in the presence of strangers. Sweat for several nights, after midnight. No thirst.

Tongue.—Very thick; white; fuzzy coating. Too weak to chew; too lazy to eat. Hungry, but cannot eat; sleepy, but cannot sleep. While at meals sudden disgust for food.

Apyrexia.—Excessive languor of all the limbs; prostration and inability to support one's self on the limbs. Constantly weak and weary, wishes to lean on something, or sit or lie down, and still feels weak and weary.

In fevers as sequellæ of scarlet fever or diphtheria; fevers occurring in young persons or old people of a psoric diathesis.

Analysis.—Extremely sensitive to cold air in every stage of the paroxysm.

Chilly from uncovering any part of body.

The constitutional cachexia of the patient.

BELLADONNA.

Characteristic.—Adapted to bilious, lymphatic, plethoric constitutions; persons who are jovial and entertaining when well, but violent and often delirious when sick.

Women and children, with light hair, blue eyes, fine complexion, delicate skin; sensitive, nervous, threatened with convulsions.

Great liability to take cold, sensitive to draft of air, especially when uncovering the head; from having the hair cut (Hep.); tonsils swell after riding in a cold wind (Acon., Hep., Rhus).

Over-excitability of all the senses; convulsions during dentition; spasms of single muscles or the whole body; chorea, epilepsy.

Quick sensation and motion; eyes snap and move quickly.

Convulsions during teething, with fever (without fever, Mag. p.); come on suddenly, head hot, feet cold.

Rush of blood to head and face (Amyl, Glon., Mel.).

Pains come on suddenly, last indefinitely, cease suddenly (Mag. p.).

Pains: usually in *short attacks; cause redness of face and eyes; with throbbing of carotids and fulness of head.*

Imagines he sees ghosts, hideous faces, and various insects (Stram.); black animals, dogs, wolves.

Fear of imaginary things, wants to run away from them; hallucinations.

Violent delirium; disposition to bite, spit, strike and tear things; breaks into fits of laughter and gnashes the teeth; wants to bite and strike the attendants (Stram.); tries to escape (Hell., Hyos.).

Head hot and painful; *face flushed;* eyes wild, staring, pupils dilated; pulse full and bounding, globules like buckshot striking the finger; mucous membrane of mouth dry; stool tardy; urine suppressed; sleepy but cannot sleep (Cham., Lach., Op.).

Vertigo: when stooping, or when rising after stooping (Bry.); on every change of position.

Headache: *congestive,* **with red face, throbbing of brain and carotids** (Mel.); < from slight noise, jar, motion, light, lying down, least exertion; > pressure, tight bandaging, wrapping up, during menses.

Boring the head into the pillow (Apis, Hell., Pod., Tub.).

Abdomen tender, distended < by least jar, even of the bed; obliged to walk with great care for fear of a jar.

Pain in r. ileo-cecal region. < by slightest touch, even the bed-cover.

The transverse colon protrudes like a pad.

Skin: of a uniform, smooth, shining, scarlet redness; dry, hot, burning; imparts a burning sensation to examining hand; the true Sydenham scarlet fever, where eruption is perfectly smooth and truly scarlet.

Pressing downwards as if the contents of abdomen would issue from the vulva; > standing and sitting erect; worse mornings (compare, Lil., Mur., Sep.).

Relations.—Complementary: Calcarea.

Belladonna is the acute of Calcarea and Tuberculinum which are often required to complete a cure.

Aggravation.—From touch, motion, noise, draught of air, looking at bright shining objects (**Lys., Stram.**); after 3 P. M. and midnight; while drinking; uncovering; hot sun; lying down.

Amelioration.—Rest; standing or sitting erect; warm room.

Type.—Quotidian, tertian. Sometimes the type is anticipating. Periodicity not marked. Continued; typhoid; yellow.

Time.—6 P. M. In evening, or at night.

Chill.—*Without thirst.* Chill, beginning in *both arms* at once, thence spreads all over the body (**Hell.**—begins in extremities, **Gel.**); a violent chill seized her *in scrobiculus cordis;* shivering running down the back, and terminating *in pit of stomach* (chill felt most severely in pit of stomach, **Arn.**—chill begins in pit of stomach with a *fixed cold, agonizing weight,* **Cal.**). Chill, *alternating* with *dry, burning heat.* Chill, with *violent, bursting, frontal headache, dilated pupils, dread of* *light and noise;* restlessness; *pale face when lying down; red face when sitting up* (the reverse of **Acon.**). *Congestive chill,* with red face, delirium and bursting headache. Chill internal, with external burning heat. *Feet ice-cold; can scarcely be warmed, while face is red and bloated* (**Arn.**). Chill after eating (**Kali c.**, **Mar. v.**—chill after eating and drinking, **Asar.**). Chilliness *in the arms,* with redness and heat of the ears and nose (with coldness of tip of nose during chill, **Ced.**). Chilliness not relieved by heat of stove. *Rarely any thirst;* if any, it is during the alternate burning heat of the chill.

Heat.—INTENSE, *with great thirst* and desire for cold water, yet everything he drinks *feels as if too cold.* Constant dry burning heat with sweat only on head. **Burning heat within and without;** *burning heat of the body, with extreme distention of the superficial blood-vessels,* the distended veins lie like cords on the skin (distention of veins and congestive headache, **Cinch.**). *Violent, bursting* headache, with strong pulsations of arteries, especially *throbbing of the carotids; dilated pupils; very red face;* delirium, restlessness. External coldness of the body, and internal burning heat. Head sometimes ice-cold, sometimes burning hot. Face hot, with extremities cold; forehead hot, with cold head and cold cheeks (**Rhus**). Heat the predominant stage of the paroxysm. *Averse to uncovering. Sensitive to light and noise.*

Sweat.—Beginning at the feet and rising up to head; during heat, or immediately after it, mostly on face and down the nose; on *covered parts only,* or *on covering parts ever so little* (**Cinch.**); sweat stains linen yellow or dark; empyreumatic, smoky odor; profuse sweat with diuresis; sweat of head, hands, face (which is very red) and feet, with burning heat; profuse sweat over whole body by the least exercise (**Bry.**, **Camp.**), sudden, evanescent; during sleep, day or night, with gradual relief of pain (Nat.); *may be entirely wanting.*

Tongue.—*Red* and *dry,* with red edges and white coating in the middle; papillæ bright and prominent, like scarlatina (**Acon., Ant. t.**). *Offensive, putrid taste in throat when eating or drinking, although food tastes natural.*

Pulse.—Strong, full, large and frequent; globular, like buckshot; or small, wiry and hard; the former in chill and heat, the latter as paroxysm passes off. Throbbing of arteries.

Aconite.	**Belladonna.**
Chill.—Ascends from feet to chest.	**Chill.**—Begins in both arms at once, thence over body.
One hot cheek; contracted pupils. Red face when lying down; pale face and fainting when sitting up.	Hot face, dilated pupils. Pale face when lying down; red face when sitting up.
Chilly from being touched, or even lifting bed clothes. Body chilly, forehead and ears hot.	Chill after eating, with redness of the face. Chilliness, with redness and heat of ears and nose.
Heat.—Redness and heat of one, coldness and paleness of the other cheek.	**Heat.**—Forehead hot, with cold face and cold cheeks.
Sensation of coldness in the blood-vessels.	Distended superficial blood-vessels, like whip-cords on the skin.
Likes to be uncovered.	Averse to uncovering.
Sweat.—Covered or affected parts sweat profusely.	**Sweat.**—On covered parts only, or on covering parts ever so little.
Sour smelling sweat all over the body.	Sweat stains the linen yellow. Sweat of empyreumatic odor.
Tongue.—Coated white "strawberry tongue." Everything but water tastes bitter; taste of rotten eggs.	**Tongue.**—Red, dry, "scarlatina-like," mouth and fauces dry. Food tastes salty: bread sour.

"Where there is a doubt whether Aconite or Belladonna should be given, I have always found that a disposition to perspire constitutes a valuable indication for Belladonna."—BAEHR.

It has been taught by some authors, and believed by many members of the homeopathic faith, that Aconite and Belladonna—except as incurrents during the congestive stage of heat—are useless in the treatment of intermittent fever. But the law of cure, as enunciated by Hahnemann, knows no such narrow restrictions, and is not bound by the *ipse dixit* of individual opinion.

If Aconite or Belladonna cover the totality of the patient's symptoms, it will as certainly cure this fever, as any other remedy. They are comparatively rarely indicated, but will effectually do their work when called for. The characteristic symptoms of the remedy must always be the guide.

Analysis.—Congested, red, hot face; head and carotids throbbing; pupils dilated; cold extremities.

Heat; intense, burning within and without, great thirst, distended blood-vessels, < uncovering.

Sweat; on covered parts only, or on covering slightly.

A typical Belladonna picture, irrespective of the paroxysm.

BENZINUM.

Neither the type, time, chill nor any stage of the paroxysm of Benzinum is marked or peculiar; there is *chill of single parts,* but the heat is often wanting.

Like Petroleum and its products, Benzinum has both profuse and partial sweat; **sweat of single parts** is very characteristic.

Chill.—*Of single parts;* from extremities of fingers and toes to chest, head and vertex.

Sweat.—At night, copious, general, warm and very exhausting (Cinnab.); followed toward morning by perspiration only on *the breast,* in *the axillæ* and **on the side not lain upon** (Sanicula—Rev. of Acon., Bry., Nit. ac.).

Analysis.—The profuse sweat of single parts, especially the side not laid upon, is very guiding.

Dear Dr. Allen:

I have your first edition, and have been able to do some good work in consequence. One symptom under Benzinum helped me to relieve a poor fellow who had been annoyed by one-sided sweating for several months, and I had searched in vain for the remedy that had that particular symptom: "Sweat on the side of the body not lain upon."

I had tried every remedy in the Materia Medica for "partial sweat," without any relief. In looking over your .book one day, I accidentally stumbled upon *Benzine,* and behold! my long-looked for symptom and remedy, and it was marvelous how quickly my patient was cured of his discomfort.

ST. CLAIR SMITH.

BOVISTA.

Characteristic.—Sensation as if head were enlarging, or very much enlarged (elongated, Hyp.); dull, bruised pain, deep in brain.

Stool; first hard and difficult; then thin, watery, with much pain in abdomen (Pod.).

Diarrhea before and during menses (cholera-like symptoms during the menses, Amm. c.).

Menses: flow mostly or *only at night,* not in the daytime (Mag. c.—only during day, cease lying, Cac., Caust., Lil.); diarrhea before and during menses (Amm. c.); occasional show every few days between periods (Bor.); every two weeks, dark and clotted; with painful bearing down (Sep.).

Intolerable itching at tip of coccyx; must scratch till parts become raw and sore.

Leucorrhea: a few days before or a few days after the menses (before, Sep.; after, Kreos.; both before and after, Graph.); acrid, thick, tough, tenacious, yellow-green, leaving green spots on linen, causing soreness.

Adapted to old maids, subject to palpitation, leucorrhea, tettery eruptions, chronic urticaria (when Rhus fails to cure).

Great weakness of all joints: as if the muscles of lower limbs were too short (Caust., Guai.). Drops things from the hands as from weakness (from awkwardness, Apis).

Discharge from nose and all mucous membranes *very tough, stringy, tenacious* (Kali bi.).

Sweat in axilla, smells like onions.

Hemorrhage: after extraction of teeth (Ham.); from wounds; epistaxis.

Unusually deep impression on finger from using blunt instruments (knives or scissors).

Stammering; in children (Stram.).

Intolerance of tight clothing around the waist (Cal., Lach., Sulph.).

Time.—5 to 8 A. M., or 7 to 10 P. M.

Paroxysm: *Without heat or sweat* (Aran.).

Chill.—Generally with thirst. Chill predominates, even near a warm stove; constantly chilly on the uncovered parts, the neck and chest. Chilly the whole day, although she sat by a warm stove; must get near the stove as soon as chill begins (**Ign.**, **Lach.**). Chill immediately after going to bed at night commencing in back. *Severe chill every evening from 7 to 10* P. M., commencing with chilliness in the back, the first day with thirst, *without subsequent heat or sweat* (without heat or thirst, **Aran.**, **Caust.**); with violent drawing pain in abdomen. *Chilliness the whole evening;* she could not get warm. Feet very cold at night; could not be warmed. Chill with the pains.

Heat.—In the evening, daily, at 7 P. M. Frequent heat and oppression of the chest, with thirst, anxiety, restlessness; relieved by uncovering. Flying heat, alternating with shuddering; thirst with the shuddering.

Sweat.—Especially upon the chest, every morning from 5 to 6 A. M. *Profuse sweat in axilla—smells like onions.*

Tongue.—Coated yellow. Taste putrid; bitter.

Analysis.—The chill predominates.

The characteristic of the Bovista fever is a well-defined chill or shuddering; remaining stages of paroxysm being wanting, or if other stages occur, they are so light as not to produce inconvenience. Compare with **Aran.**, **Camph.**, **Dros.**

BRYONIA ALBA.

Characteristic.—Suitable to the gouty or rheumatic diathesis; persons with bilious tendency, exceedingly irritable, inclined to be angry; black hair, dark complexion and firm muscular fibre; prone to so-called "bilious attacks;" dry, nervous, slender (Nux).

Hering says: "Indicated in light complexions but more in dark."

Complaints: when warm weather sets in after cold days; from cold drinks or ices in hot weather; *after taking cold or getting heated in summer;* from exposure to draft, cold wind (Acon., Hep.); suppressed discharges of menses, milk or eruption of acute exanthema.

The pains are stitching, tearing, worse at night, greatly < **by motion, > by rest** and lying on the painful side (Ptel., Puls.—Similar pain but < and > are opposite, Kali c.). The parts which are the seat of subjective pain become subsequently sensitive to external pressure, and then swollen and red.

Children dislike to be carried, or to be raised.

Ailments from chagrin, mortification, *anger* (Col., Staph.); violence, with chilliness and coldness; *after anger chilly,* but with head hot and face red (Aur.).

Constant motion of left arm and leg (Apoc., Hell.).

Excessive dryness of mucous membrane of entire body; lips and tongue dry, parched, cracked; stool, dry as if burnt; urine, dark, and scanty; great thirst; cough, dry, hard, racking, with scanty expectoration.

In delirium: talks constantly about his business; desires to get out of bed and go home (Act., Hyos.).

Headache: when stooping, as if brain would burst through forehead; from ironing; on coughing; in morning after rising, or when first opening the eyes; commencing in morning and gradually increasing till evening; from constipation; dull pain in forehead.

Headache: gastric, rheumatic, congestive; with vertigo, heaviness, pressure, and rush of blood to head.

Desires things immediately which are not to be had, or which when offered are refused.

Cannot sit up from nausea and faintness.

Pressure, as from a stone, at pit of stomach, relieved by eructation.

Constipation: inactive, no inclination; stool *large, hard, dark, dry as if burnt;* on going to sea (Plat.); *forerunner of* ***typhoid.***

Diarrhea: during *hot days in summer,* bilious, acrid; like dirty water; of undigested food; from cold drinks when overheated; from fruit or saur kraut; < *in morning;* < **on moving,** even hand or foot.

Vicarious menstruation; *nosebleed when menses should appear* (Phos.); blood spitting, or hemoptysis; during course of typhoid.

Mammæ heavy, of a stony hardness; pale, but hard; hot and painful; **must support the gland** (Phyt.).

Great thirst for *large quantities,* at *long intervals.*

Cough: dry, spasmodic, *with gagging and vomiting* (Kali c.); with stitches in side of chest (Ran.); with headache, as if head would fly to pieces; < after eating, drinking, entering *a warm room,* a deep inspiration.

Aggravation.—Motion; exertion; touch; cannot sit up, gets faint or sick or both; warmth, warm food; at night; suppressed discharges.

One of the chief characteristics of Bryonia is, < from any motion, and corresponding > from absolute rest, either mental or physical.

Amelioration.—Lying, especially on painful side (Ptel., Puls.); rest, cold, eating cold things; pressure, heat, *sweat.*

Complementary: Alumina, Rhus tox.

Type.—Quotidian, tertian or quartan fevers, periodical sweats on single parts; restless every other night. *Anticipating or postponing.* Typhoid; typhus; yellow fever.

Time.—All periods—time not characteristic. *Morning.*

Cause.—Fevers caused by getting wet (**Cal.**, **Rhus**—sleeping in damp room or bed, **Aran.**); *in dry weather, whether hot or cold.*

Prodrome.—*Great thirst* for large quantities of cold water. Stretching and drawing in the limbs; *violent headache, stitching, jerking, throbbing from before backwards as if the head would burst;* vertigo.

Chill.—With *great thirst* for large quantities of cold water, which affords relief (**Ign.**, **Nat.**—unquenchable thirst, drinks little and often, but drinking causes vomiting, **Ars.**); heat of the head and face, with flushed cheeks; **cough violent, dry, racking, with pleuritic stitching pains in chest and region of the spleen** (dry, teasing cough, *before and during chill,* without pain, **Rhus**). Stitching pain in right hypochondrium and abdomen; oppressed breathing; chill with external coldness of body and violent pains in the limbs; evening chill, frequently *only of the right side* (chill of right side, with heat of left, **Rhus**—one-sided chilliness, **Caust.**, **Lyc.**). Shaking chill all over; hot head (internal), red, hot face and cheeks, with intense desire for cold drinks (**Arn.**). Chill begins on *lips, tips of fingers and toes,* in abdomen or stomach; worse in a warm room than in the open air (**Apis**); worse from moving, lessened by sitting. *Desire to lie down,* in this stage.

Heat.—With *increased thirst, same cough* with *pleuritic stitches* as in chill (dry cough during heat, **Acon.** **Ipec.**); increased headache and vertigo; *pain in limbs aggravated by motion;* nausea and vomiting. Dry, burning, internal heat, *as if the blood in the veins was burning, or as if molten lead was running through the blood-vessels* (**Ars.**, **Rhus**). More fever in a warm room than in the open air; *aggravation of all the sufferings during the heat.* Heat: with desire to uncover; in face with red face; with bitter taste. **Wants to be quiet and not move about in any stage.** Paleness of face. Thirst *less than in cold stage.*

Sweat.—**Profuse, sour, oily** (as if mixed with oil, **Cinch.**). *Easily excited by exercise* in open air (**Am. m.**), even from slow walking, it runs in streams from his face. Sweat flowed in streams from whole body, even dropping from the hair (**Cinch.**—the least exertion puts him into a perspiration, **Psor.**). Sweat in short spells, and on single parts only (**Petr.**); profuse, at night and towards morning. Sweat on side on which he lies (on side not lain upon, Benz., San.). *Sweat relieves.*

Tongue.—Thick, yellow coating on the tongue; mouth and lips dry and peeling off (**Cinch.**, **Ipec.**); everything tastes bitter. *Mouth bitter when not eating. Desires things which are refused when offered.* Aversion to food or drink (aversion to meat, **Arn.**—to pork, **Dros.**).

Pulse.—Full, hard, rapid and tense, sometimes intermittent.

Apyrexia.—All symptoms of this stage are characteristic and should be carefully studied. Gastric symptoms predominate (**Ant. c.**, **Puls.**, **Nux**), but the general constitutional are almost always to be found and if present are guiding. Every spot in the body is painful to pressure. (Soreness of the part lain on, which compels him to move, although motion hurts, **Arn.**, **Bap.**, **Pyr.**). *Feels best when lying upon painful side.*

"When fever is caused by getting wet, occipital cephalalgia, preceded by rheumatic pains in muscles of whole body; loss of appetite, eating a mouthful suffices; rotatory vertigo; redness of face, and thirst in all stages of paroxysms."—DR. HIGGINS.

Analysis.—Bönninghausen's picture of the Bryonia fever:

"Pulse hard, frequent and tense.

Chill.—Chill and coldness predominate, often with heat of head, red cheeks and thirst. Chill with external coldness of the body. Chill and coldness most at evening or on the right side of body. Chill more in the room than in the open air.

Heat.—Dry, burning heat for the most part internal only, and as if the blood burned in the veins. All the symptoms are aggravated during the heat.

Sweat.—Much sweat: easy sweating, even from walking slowly in the cold open air. Copious night and morning sweats."

CLINICAL.

CASE I.—*Tertian;* the fever *anticipates* one or two hours every day. The paroxysms are preceded by vertigo, with headache, and stitching in the chest during an inspiration. Moderate chilliness, followed by great heat. Delirium. *Unquenchable thirst,* with *dry cough.* Lastly sweat. Bry. 18 two doses, after fever. Cured.—*Hom. Clinique. Pr. Com.;* I., p. 181.

CASE II.—*Tertian fever* (this man had received large doses of Quinia under allopathic treatment). Violent chilliness for half an hour every third day at noon, preceded by violent headache; after this the skin became warmer, the pulse full and frequent, but no heat properly so called, although there was violent thirst. Sweat considerable. The apyrexia was characterized by pricking and cutting in the chest, especially when coughing; the cough being dry and troublesome. Face pale; no gastric symptoms; pulse normal; sleep tranquil. Bry. 21 soon after attack. Two days after, a feeble paroxysm. No return.—DR. THORER, *Hom. Clinique. Pr. Com.,* I., p. 38.

CASE III.—*Intermittent fever.* Patient had "double legs" while taking Bryonia. The symptom disappeared after taking Petr. 200, one dose.—GILBERT.

CASE IV.—*Remittent fever.* The symptom of the whole body being "double" was present for several days, though the patient was improving under Arsenic; with it there was occipital headache and vertigo on sitting up. After a dose of Bryonia the "double" first disappeared, then the headache followed, and the next morning the vertigo was gone.—GILBERT.

These cases—two of them reported many years ago, 1834—illustrate the fact that *one* or *two* doses of the properly selected remedy, even in the low potencies, given *after severity of the paroxysm had passed,* as Hahnemann advised in the *Organon,* are sufficient to cure. The single dose treatment is not new.

CACTUS GRANDIFLORUS.

Characteristic.—Sanguineous congestions in persons of plethoric habit (Acon.); often resulting in hemorrhage.

Fear of death; believes the disease incurable (Ars.).

Hemorrhage: from nose, lungs, stomach, rectum, bladder (Crot., Kreos., Mill., Phos.).

Headache: pressing, *like a heavy weight on vertex;* climacteric; congestive, periodic, right-sided, severe throbbing pulsating pain.

Whole body feels as if caged, *each wire being twisted tighter and tighter.*

Constriction: of throat, chest, heart, bladder, rectum, uterus, vagina; often caused or brought on by the slightest contact.

Pains everywhere; darting, springing, like chain-lightning, and ending with a sharp, vise-like grip, only to be again renewed.

Oppression of chest, as from a great weight; as if an iron band prevented normal motion.

Sensation of a cord tightly tied around lower part of chest marking attachment of diaphragm.

Heart feels as if clasped and unclasped rapidly by **an iron hand**; as if bound, "had no room to beat."

Palpitation: day and night; worse when walking and lying on left side (Lach.); at approach of menses.

Menstrual flow *ceases when lying down* (Bov., Caust.).

Aggravation.—Motion; touch.

Amelioration.—In open air.

Type.—Quotidian. Periodicity well marked. Return at same hour each day: pains down thighs, chill, fever, pains in uterus and ovaries.

Time.—11 A. M., or 11 P. M.—Characteristic. *Returns at same hour every day* (**Aran., Ced., Gels., Sabad.**).

Cause.—After exposure to heat of sun.

Chill.—*Without thirst. Coldness in the back and icy cold hands* (after water in the cellar,—**Ars., Rhus**). *Chilliness which lasts three hours,* makes the teeth chatter, and does not go off although he lies down and covers himself up with many blankets. Chill not relieved *by anything, either covering* or *external heat* (**Aran.**).

Heat.—Burning heat of 24 hours' duration (succeeding a three hours' chill), with dyspnea and shortness of breath, and a smothering sensation so that he cannot remain quiet in bed. Great heat in the head and *flushes in the face* as if before a strong fire, which causes *horrible anxiety. Insupportable heat in abdomen; lancinating pain in heart,* suppressed urine, pains in bladder and pulsating pains in uterine region, vomiting, headache, coma, stupefaction, insensibility, terminating in very slight perspiration.

Some thirst at close of heat.

Heat sometimes wanting.

Sweat.—*With great thirst* (**Cinch.**). After burning heat, with shortness of breath, inability to remain lying on account of dyspnea, a profuse sweat breaks out attended with unquenchable thirst for large quantities of cold water (**Ars., Cinch.**). Violent vomiting when perspiration fails.

Tongue.—Clean; taste soapy; stomach deranged.

Apyrexia.—From 11 P. M. till 12 M. the next day, complete apyrexia. The regularity of attack is perfect; and all stages are clearly defined. The congestive symptoms of brain and chest predominate during the heat (**Bell., Cinch., Natr. m.**). Rarely indicated, but has no substitute; effectually and permanently cures. May be compared with Aranea, Cedron, or Cinchona.

Quotidian internittent; congestion to head; flushes in face; suppressed urine; pains in bladder; lancinating in heart; violent vomiting; sweat does not appear after exposure to sun's rays.

Analysis.—Clock-like regularity of paroxysm, 11 A. M. or 11 P. M.

Congestive and constrictive symptoms of head and chest predominate.

After exposure to intense heat of sun.

CADMIUM SULPHURICUM.

Characteristic.—Symptoms chiefly clinical, but have been verified in cholera infantum and malignant yellow fever.

Traumatic opacity of cornea; bluish maculæ; after a slow conjunctivitis and keratitis with blenorrhea.

Cicatrix on cornea.

Craves cold water which is immediately vomited (Ars.).

Belching: salty, rancid.

Nausea: in mouth, throat, chest, abdomen; intense gagging and retching of tough mucus; deathly, must lie quiet to ward off black vomit; so sensitive that the least touch of the lips will bring on vomiting.

Nausea or black vomit when other medicines though well selected fail.

Vomiting: of black, sour or yellow matter; of all food taken, bile and stringy mucus; with cold sweat on face and griping pains in stomach and umbilical region and great prostration.

Intense burning, cutting pains in stomach and esophagus.

Stool: Yellowish-green, semi-fluid, almost gelatinous.

Aggravation.—Cool or cold air; draft of air; cold land wind (Acon., Bry., Hep.); checked perspiration, in the sunshine.

Gastric symptoms: in drunkards; after drinking beer; during pregnancy; after cramps in stomach.

Type.—Malarial; yellow.

Dr. Hardenstein, of Vicksburg, used this remedy with great success in the malignant epidemic of yellow fever in 1878.

Time.—Fever, before midnight.

Cause.—Fevers prevailing during epidemic yellow fever.

Chill.—Icy coldness. Blueness of skin.

Coldness: even when near the fire; after drinking; after sleep; after walking; with hot hands. Horripilation.

Sweat.—Profuse and exhausting; while sleeping; in axillæ; staining yellow; acrid.

When sweat is checked and grave symptoms appear, after exposure to a draft of air during fever or convalescence.

Falls asleep during evening fever and wakes when it stops.

Analysis.—Yellow and malarial fevers with deathly nausea, intense gagging and retching, and vomiting of black, sour or yellow matter.

When the best selected remedies fail.

CALADIUM.

Very sensitive to noise; slight noise startles from sleep (Asar., Nux, Ther.).

Eructations, frequent, of very little wind, as if stomach were full of dry food.

Impotence: with mental depression; *relaxed penis, with sexual desire and excitement* (Lyc., Sel.).

No erection, even after caresses; no emission, no orgasm during an embrace (Cal., Sel.).

Pruritus vaginæ: induces onanism (Orig., Zinc.); during pregnancy; with mucous discharge.

Falls asleep during evening fever and wakes when it stops.

Sweet sweat attracts the flies (Puls., Sumb., Thuja).

Mosquito and insect bites burn and itch intensely.

Aversion to motion; dreads to move (Bry.).

Destroys craving for tobacco.

Type.—Intermittent; remittent; typhoid; typhus.

Time.—Evening fever, or exacerbation.

Chill.—Beginning in abdomen and extending to fingers and toes. Coldness of single parts, sometimes with crawling; fingers and feet are icy cold. Chilliness over entire body, with drawing pains in l. little finger, that feels as if full and gone to sleep, with a stretched sensation in whole body.

Heat.—With thirst; internal with throbbing; rises up to head; with drowsiness; disappears during sleep; heat before midnight, chill after; after midday sleep, then sweat, then chill in open air.

Heat of hands, face, abdomen, with cold feet before midnight; after midnight, cold abdomen, hot feet.

Sweat.—Towards evening, with prostration, yawning, sleepiness.

Sweat: scanty, easy, with sweet odor; gentle, with internal heat and prostration; cold, over entire body.

Sweat > all symptoms (Nat., Psor.).

Pulse.—Hard and full in intermittents; very rapid, scarcely perceptible in typhoid.

After Acon., Bry., Ipec., Nat., Op. and Stram. failed in typhoid, Caladium cured completely.

CALCAREA OSTREARUM.

Characteristic.—Adapted to the leucophlegmatic; blond hair, light complexion, fair skin and blue eyes.

Scrofulous constitutions; pale, weak, timid, easily tired when walking; vertigo on ascending a height, going upstairs, is out of breath, has to sit down (vertigo on descending, Borax); **disposed to grow fat,** corpulent, unwieldy.

Children: with red face, flabby muscles, who sweat easily and *take cold readily* in consequence; large heads and abdomens; **fontanelles and sutures open; head sweats profusely while sleeping; wetting pillow far around** (San., Sil.); diseases of dentition; during sickness or convalescence great *longing for eggs.*

Acidity of digestive tract; sour eructation, sour vomiting, sour stool; sour odor of the whole body (Hep., Rheum).

Girls who are *fleshy, plethoric,* **grow too rapidly**; who begin with *early, profuse, protracted* menstruation; subsequently have amenorrhea and chlorosis with menses scanty or suppressed.

Women: with menses too early and too profuse; feet constantly cold and damp, feel as if she had on *cold, damp stockings;* difficult to stop menstruating, the least mental excitement causes profuse return (Sul., Tub.).

Fears she will lose her reason, or that people will observe her mental confusion (Act.).

Aversion to cold air; least cold air seems to go through and through; very sensitive to damp cold air.

Lung diseases of tall, slender, rapidly growing youth; upper third of right lung (Ars.—upper third of left, Myr., Sul., Tub.). Oftener the guide to the true remedy than Phosphorus.

Disorders arising from *defective assimilation; imperfect ossification;* difficulty in learning to walk; have no disposition, will not try.

Longing for fresh air, which inspires, benefits, strengthens (Sul.).

Coldness: general; *of single parts* (Benz., Kali bi.); head, stomach, abdomen, feet and legs.

Sweat: of single parts; head, scalp wet, cold; nape of neck; chest; axillæ; sexual organs; hands; knees; feet (Sep., Tub.).

Pit of stomach swollen like *an inverted saucer,* and painful to pressure.

Uremic or other diseases brought on by standing on cold, damp pavements, or working while standing in cold water; modelers or workers in cold clay.

Constipation: inactivity of rectum; stool has to be removed mechanically (Aloe, Sanic., Sel., Sep., Sil.).

Painless hoarseness, < in the morning.

Feels better in every way when constipated.

Desire to be magnetized (Phos.).

Complementary: Belladonna, which is the acute of Calcarea and Tuberculinum.

According to Hahnemann, Calc. *must not be used before* Nit. ac. and Sulph.; may produce unnecessary complications.

Aggravation.—Cold air, damp winds; getting wet; ascending heights; exertion of mind or body, walking, talking, writing.

Amelioration.—In dry, warm weather; lying on painful side.

Type.—Tertian. Chronic intermittent or remittent fevers.

Time.—2 P. M.—Fever without chill at 11 A. M. and 6 to 7 P. M. (11 A. M. one day, 4 P. M. the next.—E. C. PRICE).

Cause.—Working while standing in cold water. Potters, brick-makers who work in wet clay; gardeners and fruit growers, handling cold vegetables and fruit (**Zinc., Val.**).

Prodrome.—Drawing in all the joints, and great heaviness of head and body.

Chill.—*With thirst. Begins in scrobiculus cordis, with spasms, or fixed, cold, agonizing weight, increasing with the chill and disappearing with it.* External coldness and internal heat, or internal coldness and external heat, or chill and heat alternating (**Ars.**). Coldness of single parts; of face, of hands, of feet, *of internal organs;* icy coldness in and on head; feels an inward coldness. Heat followed by chill and cold hands. Shaking chill at night. Chill in the evening in bed;

was unable to get warm, though covered warmly, as though he had no warmth in his body. He was cold and his teeth chattered though he sat over the fire. Chill with headache and drowsy fatigue of all the limbs.

Heat.—*Without thirst,* followed by chill and cold hands. Frequent flashes of heat. *Severe heat in the head and great orgasm of blood.* Nightly internal heat, especially in the feet and hands; anxiety and palpitation. Frequent attacks of sudden universal heat, as if she had been drenched with hot water, with despair of life.

Heat, with inclination to uncover (**Acon., Lyc., Sec., Sul.**).

Fever at 11 A. M. *without thirst* and without *previous chill,* she felt hot and was hot to the touch, with red face.

Sweat.—*No thirst. Hot sweat.* Sweats during the day from the least exertion, even in the cold air (**Am. m., Bry.**). *Profuse sweat in the morning on moderate exertion.* Sweat of palms of hands; of the feet; knees; over whole body, with severe cramp in stomach; chest; nape of neck; male organs. Clammy sweat only on the limbs. Often sleep after sweat.

Tongue.—Dry in the morning on awaking; coated white. Taste: bitter, sour, foul, offensive; "too fresh," like ink, like iron.

Apyrexia.—*Never clear.* Intermittents with spasmodic symptoms; after abuse of quinine; chronic forms with scrofula; cachectic constitutions; suppressed eruptions, or sweat; desire for eggs.

Analysis.—The constitutional symptoms existing or aroused by the fever, form the chief guide in selection of remedy. The psoric cachexia of the patient is guiding, and is generally found in the apyrexia.

Chill, heat and sweat of single parts. The cause often indicative.

CAMPHORA.*

Characteristic.—Blondes most affected; persons very irritable and mentally weak. Catarrhal and choleraic diseases.

Exceedingly sensitive to cold air (Hep., Kali m., Psor.). Surface **cold to the touch, yet cannot bear to be covered;** throws off all the covering (Med., Sec.).

Bad effects of shock from injury; surface of body *cold, face pale, blue, lips livid;* **profound prostration.**

Skin of the whole body painfully sensitive, slightest touch hurts.

Sudden attacks of diarrhea and vomiting; *nose cold and pointed;* sweating, vomiting, purging; anxiety and restlessness; *skin and breath cold.*

Long-lasting chill, great coldness of skin and sudden and complete prostration.

Great coldness of the surface with sudden and complete prostration of the vital force; often a remedy in congestive chill; pernicious intermittent (Ver.); pulse weak, extremely small, scarcely perceptible; yellow fever.

Antidotes many vegetable remedies; hence its use in the sick room in the crude form of tincture is not advisable.

In most other cases the smelling of Camphor is not antidotal, but palliative by producing the symptom, "pain better while thinking of it."

Aggravation.—Cold air; night; motion; lying covered.

Amelioration.—When *thinking of existing complaint;* warmth; warm air; drinking cold water.

Type.—Periodicity not marked. Pernicious fevers: the so-called sinking or congestive stage of intermittents (**Ver.**); yellow fever.

---

*Note for Thought.—All our progress as a school depends on the right view of the symptoms obtained by proving with Camphor or Opium.—Hering.

Time.—At any time. All periods.

Chill.—*Without thirst. Long-lasting, terrible chills; icy-coldness all over; extremities cold and blue, with death-like paleness of the face* (**Ver.**). *The body generally is quite cold; coldness of the skin.* **Excessively sensitive to cold air**; *great aversion to cold air;* he is obliged to wrap himself up warmly, and even then he *is chilled through and through.* Great chilliness; excessive chill; *shaking chill* and *chattering of the teeth,* with *cold arms, hands* and *feet.* The skin of the whole body is painfully sensitive and sore to the slightest touch (**Apis**). Coldness for an hour, with *deathly paleness of the face.* Coldness increased by walking. Hands and feet extremely cold, complains of freezing, worse when walking. Chill with anxiety; pale face; unconsciousness; clonic spasm; *skin cold as marble, yet the child cannot bear to be covered; hot breath* (cold breath, **Carbo v.**). Frequent chilliness of back and loins (**Caps.**). Paroxysm of fever; severe chill, with gnashing of the teeth and much thirst; he sleeps immediately after the chill, with frequent wakings, almost without the slightest heat. Chill the predominant stage. Congestive chill.

Heat.—*Without thirst; of the whole body, which becomes excessive when walking.* Heat with *distention of the veins, increased by every motion* (> by motion, **Caps.**). Glowing heat, with full rapid pulse. Heat in the head, face, occiput, back, legs, lobules of the ears; body hot and sweating, but averse to uncovering.

Sweat.—At first warm and profuse, which relieves; then profuse cold sweat over the whole body, very weakening. Sweat most profuse during sleep, and on slightest exertion (**Bry., Cinch.**). Excessive perspiration of hands and feet. Sweat profuse, shirt and clothes drenched, having penetrated to lower side of feather-bed (**Thuja**). Sweat often clammy and *always exhausting. Cold sweat* on face, when beginning to vomit (**Ver.**).

Tongue.—*Cold,* trembling, flabby, spongy, covered with a tough yellowish mucus.

Pulse.—Small, weak, slow, often imperceptible.

Apyrexia.—Great weakness and exhaustion; lassitude. Convulsions may occur in children. Weak, weary and great anxiety. Face *anxious, pale, livid, haggard* and *sunken.* Yellowish, *green,* red, brown, turbid urine, of a musty odor. Terrible sinking and exhaustion.

In 1829, on the approach of Asiatic Cholera to Western Europe, Hahnemann, from a description of the disease, published in advance of its approach, that Camphor would be the remedy in the state of collapse; and the clinical experience of each subsequent epidemic demonstrated his prediction. This power of *prevision;* the crowning glory of our school of medicine; the absolute proof that "similia" is a *"Law of Cure;"* the demonstration of the claim of Homeopathy to be ranked as *a medical science;* was first shown by Hahnemann in the fatal typhus which followed the terrible retreat of Napoleon from his Russian campaign in 1812. He published in advance that Rhus would be the principal remedy, and the recognition of Homeopathy by the Austrian Government was the reward of its successful administration.

There is probably no stage of any disease that bears so close a resemblance to the collapse of cholera as the true, "pernicious" "sinking," or "congestive" stage of intermittent fever. Hence, Camphor should deservedly be placed in the front rank with Apis, Carbo v., Gels., Lach., Nux, Ver., as one of our "sheet anchors" in this form of fever, instead of Quinine, often so indiscriminately and empirically used.

This abuse of Quinine is borrowed by the pseudo-homeopath from his allopathic brother, who has no "law of cure" upon which to rely, and is compelled to depend upon his theories (malarial and cryptogamic) to prevent the return of the paroxysm. Quinine may suppress it, as it will many simpler forms of the fever, but there are many cases *it will neither suppress nor cure,* and these are generally the fatal cases that so often occur in the practice of regular (?) medicine. The *fatal* "third paroxysm" is rarely known under the properly selected homeopathic remedy. It is a "bug-bear" of allopathic teaching and practice. No homeopath, surely, would think of giving Quinine in cholera collapse, for no better reason than it is given by the rational (?) school of medicine. The statistics of comparative mortality of each system of practice "in cholera" ought to be convincing.

A CASE.—Last summer I had two cases, one a boy the other a girl, which defied all my efforts. When I saw her she was in the sweating stage; face looked cold, pale blue, pinched, anxious, and was covered with a profuse sweat. When I looked at her I thought if you were suffering from cholera I would give you Camphor. Why should I not give Camphor in this sickness? I accordingly gave her the 2x trit., three or four powders per day. I was agreeably surprised to find that she did not have a recurrence of the chills; has remained free ever since.

Her fever was of the tertian type.—R. C. ALLEN, M. D., *Med. Investigator,* Sept., 1885.

Analysis.—Chill; severe, long, terrible; congestive, of pernicious fever. Sensitive to cold air. Face and extremities cold, blue, pinched; cannot bear to be covered.

Heat: light, without thirst; of single parts.

Sweat: cold, profuse, exhausting.

CANCHALAGUA.

Characteristic.—Pain and fulness in head and scalp; feels tight as if drawn together by a rubber band (Carb. ac.). Skin of fingers shrivelled like a washer-woman's.

Type.—Especially for vernal intermittents (Gels., Lach., Sul.).

Chill.—*Severe,* especially down the spine (Ver.); violent, with chattering of the teeth; with extreme paleness of the face, hands and lips; all over body, especially in bed at night; with nausea, vomiting of mucus colored with bile. Fingers shriveled.

Heat.—In whole body, better in open air.

Sweat.—Not profuse, but causes a shriveling of the fingers and toes, like a washer-woman's (Ant. c., Mer., Ver.). Face, lips and hands cold.

Apyrexia.—Excellent appetite as soon as paroxysm is over. Constipation, stool hard, dry, knotty.

CANTHARIS.

Characteristic.—Pain; raw, sore, *burning in every part of body,* both internally and externally; with excessive weakness.

Over-sensitiveness of all parts.

Disgust for everything; drink, food, tobacco.

Drinking, even small quantities of water, increases pain in the bladder.

Passage of white or pale-red tough mucus with stool, like scrapings from the intestines, with streaks of blood (Carb. ac., Colch.).

Constant desire to urinate, passing but a few drops at a time, which is mixed with blood (**Sudden desire,** itching in urethra, Petrol.).

Intolerable tenesmus vesicæ, before, during and after urination.

Burning, cutting pains in urethra during micturition; violent tenesmus and strangury.

Bloody, nocturnal emissions (Led., Mer., Petr.).

Sexual desire: increased, both sexes; preventing sleep; violent priapism, with excessive pain (Pic. ac.).

Skin: vesicular erysipelas; vesicles all over body which are sore and suppurating.

Erythema from exposure to sun's rays (sunburn).

Aggravation.—Oil and coffee; drinking, or even sight of cold water (**Lys., Stram.**); after midnight and during the day.

Amelioration.—Warmth; rubbing; lying down.

Type.—No periodicity of fever. Many conditions or symptoms appear every seventh day. Typhoid; yellow fever.

Time.—3 P. M. till 3 A. M.—*long-lasting chill* (**Aran.**, 24 hours).

At all hours in afternoon, from 1 to 10 P. M.

Chill.—*Without thirst,* in afternoon or evening, *not* > *by external warmth or covering* (**Ars., Ign., Kali c.**, are all relieved by external heat—worse from external heat, **Apis, Ipec.**). General coldness of the whole body, especially the limbs. Coldness and chills *as soon as she attempts to rise, or puts one limb out of bed. Shivering and chill down the spine; feeling of coldness in the vertebral column* (*pain all down the spine on pressure,* **Quinine**). Shaking chill beginning in, or running up the back (**Caps., Eup. purp.**). *Icy-coldness of hands and feet, with fearful pains in the urethra.* Chill followed by thirst, without heat. Children pass urine frequently during chill.

Heat.—*With thirst;* burning in the palms and soles; burning heat at night, *which she does not feel* (unbearable heat—extreme restlessness, **Ars.**). Burning on soles of feet, while hands are icy-cold. Burning, violent fever; great heat, with thirst, and redness all over the body. Great heat of abdomen (**Apis**).

Sweat.—Profuse, on waking at night; when walking; *from every movement* (**Bry., Camph.**); cold on the hands and feet; on the genitalia and external pelvic region; *smells like urine.*

Tongue.—Coated with thick, yellow fur; red at the edges. Taste lost; trembling tongue.

Disgust for everything. Canine hunger, especially for meat (see Arn.). Every paroxysm characterized by the Cantharis dysuria.

Apyrexia.—Irritation of the urinary organs, *difficult, frequent and painful urination.* Scanty and painful emission of blackish urine; then secretion of urine increased to four-fold the amount of liquids taken, with great thirst and **desire for meat** (aversion to meat, **Arn.**). *Very thirsty, but disgust for all kinds of drinks.* Heaviness of the feet, a paralytic immobility of the limbs; *must lie in bed.*

Hemorrhages: from nose, mouth, stomach, intestines, genital and urinary organs, especially in typhoid and yellow fever.

Analysis.—The violent tenesmus, the burning, cutting pains in bladder and urethra is the red strand of the remedy in fevers as in all diseases. Chill followed by thirst without heat; the < of pain in bladder from drinking, the craving for meat and urinal odor of sweat are peculiar.

CAPSICUM ANNUUM.

Characteristic.—Adapted to the phlegmatic diathesis; persons with light hair, blue eyes, nervous, but plethoric habit; lax fibre and weak muscles; *awkward, indolent, easily offended.*

Children, *dread the open air,* are *always chilly; refractory, clumsy, fat, unclean and disinclined to work or think.*

Homesickness (of the indolent, melancholic) with *red cheeks* and sleeplessness, hot sensation in fauces.

Lack of reactive force, especially with fat, indolent persons, who are constitutionally opposed to physical exertion.

Desires to be let alone; wants to lie down and sleep.

Constriction: in fauces; throat; nares; chest; bladder; urethra; rectum.

Burning and smarting sensation, as from cayenne pepper, in throat and other parts, not > by heat.

Every stool is *followed by thirst,* and every drink by *shuddering.*

Every chill is *attended with thirst* and every drink *with shuddering.*

Relations.—Cina follows well in intermittent fever.

The constricting, burning, smarting pains differentiate from Apis and Belladonna.

Compare: Carbo an., Ign.

Aggravation.—From eating; drinking; cold open air. Night, after midnight.

Amelioration.—Warmth; during the day.

Type.—Periodicity strongly marked. Quotidian; rarely tertian. Malarial fevers of the tropics.

Time.—Evening; 5 to 6 P. M.; 10.30 A. M.

Prodrome.—*Thirst some time before chill* (**Cinch.**—*thirst and bone pains* 1 to 6 hours before chill, **Eup., Nat.**).

Chill.—With great thirst. Chill begins in the back, *between the shoulder-blades* (**Polyp.**—in lumbar region, **Eup. purp.**); **worse after drinking. Shivering and chilliness after every drink.** *Chill, with pain in back* and tearing in limbs, extorting cries and causing patient to bend double; > by jugs of hot water or hot irons to the back; *lessened by walking out-of-doors;* with painful swelling of spleen; contracted pupils; contraction of the limbs (**Cimex**); anxiety, giddiness and headache; *intolerance of noise* (**Bell.**); ptyalism and mucous vomiting; in the open air, particularly in a draft, extremely sensitive to cold air (**Bar., Camph.**); inward burning and external chill.

Chill followed by sweat; or by heat with sweat and thirst (**Ant. c.**). Chill spreads gradually until extreme points are reached, then as gradually declines. During chill, coldness of chest, with a sensation of water dropping down the back.

"As the coldness of the body increases, so also does the ill-humor."—HAHNEMANN.

Heat.—*Without thirst; lessened by motion.* Sweat and heat simultaneously (**Ant. c.**); *face alternately pale and red;* internal heat with violent burning (**Ars.**) followed by chill *with thirst during chill.* Headache with pain in the back, relieved by walking about (**Rhus**). Glowing hot cheeks, with cold hands and feet. *Heat of the ears, and hot, red tip of the nose, towards evening.* General heat; anxiety; uneasiness; dullness of the mind and *intolerance of noise.*

Fever at 11 A. M. (following chill at 10.30 A. M.), lasting all night, without subsequent sweat. Fever (after very short chill at 11 A. M. or 12 M.) lasts all night with great thirst. Great sleepiness after fever (**Apis, Pod.**); especially after eating; could scarcely be prevented from going to sleep.

Sweat.—*Without thirst;* violent; copious; *lessened by motion.* Sweat with the heat, or *after the chill, without previous heat* (**Caust.**). Coming on soon after fever commences, and continuing with it. Sweat in axilla (**Bov.**). *Acrid sweat;* so acrid that it caused the hands of any person brought in contact with it to burn and tingle. Cold on thighs.

Tongue.—Burning blisters, and flat, lardaceous, spreading ulcers on the tongue. Taste sour; of putrid water. Desire for coffee, but it nauseates. Better while eating; worse after. Appetite unimpaired.

Apyrexia.—Clear comparatively; chill is predominant; in mucous, flabby constitutions; sometimes dysenteric diarrhea of slimy, burning stools, attended with qualmishness of the stomach, and fullness at the epigastrium.

Intermittents attended with painful enlargement of spleen and torpidity of abdominal nervous centres. Fevers from or after abuse of Quinine.

Capsicum.	Eup. purp.
Time.—5 to 6 P. M. every day. 10:30 A. M.	**Time.**—Different times of day. Every other day.
Prodrome.—Thirst, without bone pains. Thirst during chill with pain in back and limbs.	**Prodrome.**—Bone pains in arms and legs. Thirst for lemonade, and acid drinks—not water.

Capsicum.	Eup. purp.
Chill.—Commencing in back *between the shoulders;* worse after drinking, relieved by putting jugs of hot water to back; *must have something hot to back.*	**Chill.**—Commencing in back, *lumbar region,* passes up and down spine with bone pains, blue lips and nails. Nausea as chill is leaving.
Violent chill with *general coldness of body.*	Violent shaking, with comparatively *little coldness of body.*
Heat.—Light, transient, or mixed with sweat. *No thirst* in heat.	**Heat.**—Protracted and well marked, *with thirst.*
Headache; intolerance of noise; sleepiness after.	Head light, as if *falling to left side.*
Sweat.—General; copious, or alternating with heat.	**Sweat.**—Light, mostly on forehead and head.
Chill, heat and sweat, all relieved by motion.	Neither stage relieved by anything.

Capsicum is a valuable remedy in intermittents occurring in midsummer; its symptoms are clearly defined and ought not to be confounded with any other remedy. The chill beginning in the back *between the scapulæ;* relieved by *hot irons* or *jugs of hot water* and *lessened by motion,* is characteristic. It is oftener indicated than used—just the reverse of Quinia.

Capsicum, Cinchona, Eupatorium perf. and Natrum mur., have thirst some time before paroxysm begins; "knows the chill is coming, because he wants to drink." It is a chief symptom of the prodrome in each. Both Capsicum and Cinchona are wanting in the bone pains and backache so characteristic of Eupatorium and Natrum.

Analysis.—Thirst before the chill (Cinch., Eup., Nat.) but no bone pains.

Chill; with great thirst < after drinking. Shivering and chilliness after every drink, > by heat to back.

Heat; without thirst, > by motion. Sleepy after fever and after eating (Apis, Pod.).

Sweat; without thirst, acrid; or *after chill,* or heat with sweat (Ant. c.); > by motion.

Midsummer fevers.

CARBO ANIMALIS.

Characteristic.—Adapted to scrofulous subjects, especially the young; or the venous plethora of elderly persons, with blue cheeks, blue lips and great debility; circulation feeble, stagnated, and vital heat sinks to a minimum.

Glands indurated, swollen, painful; in neck, axillæ, inguinal region, mammæ; pains lancinating, cutting, burning (Con.).

Benignant suppurations change into ichorous conditions.

Easily strained from lifting even small weights; straining and overlifting easily produce great debility.

Joints weak; easily turned or sprained (Led., Psor.).

Headache at night; has to sit and hold head with both hands to prevent it from falling to pieces.

Aversion to open, dry, cold air.

After appearance of menses, *so weak she can hardly speak* (can hardly stand, Alum., Coc.); menses flow only in morning.

A stitching pain remains in chest after recovery from pleurisy (Ran. b.).

Menstruation, leucorrhea, diarrhea are all exhausting (Ars. —are all offensive, Psor.).

Aggravation.—After shaving (> after shaving, Brom.); slightest touch; after midnight.

Amelioration.—From warmth; eating.

Type.—Periodicity not marked.

Time.—Evening paroxysm 5 to 8, and 11 P. M.

Chill.—*Without thirst. Great chilliness during the day. Chill after eating* (**Bell.**—after drinking, **Caps.**—after eating and drinking, **Asar.**). Internal chill on beginning to eat; *chill awoke her at night;* commencing *in the chest* (**Apis**), with shivering down the back; with ice cold feet; chilly when a little air entered the room (**Camph., Canth.**). Could not bear being uncovered because she immediately became chilly (**Acon.,**

Nux). Chill with goose-flesh, from 5 till 8 in the evening, afterwards at 11 P. M., waking with profuse sweat lasting till 2 o'clock, during which she could not tolerate the bed-clothes. Great chilliness during day.

Heat.—Without thirst; with redness and burning of the cheeks in the evening; frequent flushes of heat in the cheeks, with redness. Heat always after a chill, mostly at night in bed. Head and upper part of the body were hot, with cold limbs; which only gradually became warm towards morning. Averse to uncovering during heat.

Sweat.—Offensive night-sweat; stains the linen yellow (flies trouble him very mucn on account ot the perspiration, **Calad.**). *At night* or towards morning. *Fetid; debilitating; exhausting; profuse sweat* (Psor.); *when walking;* slightest exertion even *when eating.* Sweat in *hollows of knees* (Bufo); profuse of the *feet and thighs.*

Symptoms of this stage always guiding and predominant. (Bry. and Cinch. have profuse, debilitating sweat, but lack the offensiveness of Carbo a.).

Relations.—Complementary: Calc. phos.

Tongue.—Blisters on the tongue and sides of the tongue (**Canth.**), which pain as if burnt. Burning on tip of the tongue and rawness of the mouth, relieved by eating. *Ravenous hunger* (Cina, Phos.).

Apyrexia.—Never clear. All the constitutional troubles are aroused, and every disease is extremely prostrating. *Leucorrhea stains linen yellow.*

Analysis.—The profuse, debilitating, offensive, exhausting sweat, is characteristic.

Carbo an. will rarely be indicated, unless the fever be developed after or upon some constitutional trouble. The sweating stage is very exhausting, and out of all proportion to the chill and heat.

The fever generally accompanies some dyscrasia, with glandular swellings or where benign tend to malignant diseases.

Compare: Caps., Carbo v.

CARBO VEGETABILIS.

Characteristic.—Best adapted to persons, young or old, who have suffered from exhausting diseases (exhausted from loss of vital fluids, Cinch., Phos. ac., Phos.). Cachectic, with weak vitality.

Persons who have never fully recovered from the exhausting effects of some previous illness; asthma dates from measles or pertussis of childhood; indigestion from a drunken debauch; bad effects of a long ago injury; has never recovered from effects of typhoid (Psor.).

Weakness of memory and slowness of thought.

Ailments: from Quinine, especially suppressed intermittents; abuse of mercury, salt, salt meats, or spoiled fish, meats, fats (Cepa); *getting overheated* (Ant. c.).

Diseases of venous system predominate (Sul.); symptoms of imperfect oxidation (Arg. nit.); deficient capillary circulation causes blueness of skin and coldness of extremities; vital powers nearly exhausted; **desires to be constantly fanned, must have more air.**

Patients crave things that make them sick; old topers crave whiskey or brandy; want clothing loose around abdomen.

Weak digestion; *the simplest food disagrees.* Excessive accumulation of gas in stomach and intestines; after eating or drinking, sensation as if stomach would burst. Eructations give temporary relief. Effects of a debauch, rich food, late suppers.

Bad effects from loss of vital fluids (Caust.); hemorrhage from any broken down condition of mucous membrane.

Hemorrhage from any mucous outlet; in systems broken

down, debilitated; blood oozes from weakened tissues; vital force exhausted.

Epistaxis in daily attacks, for weeks, worse from exertion; face pale before as well as after a hemorrhage.

Hippocratic face; very pale, grayish-yellow, greenish, *cold with cold sweat;* after hemorrhage.

Looseness of teeth, easily-bleeding gums.

Awakens often from cold limbs, *especially cold knees.*

In the last stages of disease, with copious *cold sweat, cold breath, cold tongue, voice lost,* this remedy may save a life.

Aggravation.—Generally worse in changes of weather, especially warm damp weather; or in protracted sultry heat of summer or autumn; butter, pork, fat food; abuse of quinine, bark, mercury; mornings.

Amelioration.—From being fanned; cool air; eructations.

Relations.—Complementary: Kali carb.

Want of susceptibility, lack of reaction to well selected remedies (Laur., Op., Val.).

Compare: Cinch., Plumb. in neglected pneumonia, especially in "old topers;" Ant. t. in threatened paralysis from inability to expectorate loosened mucus; Caps., Carbo v. in fevers.

Type.—Periodicity not marked. Quotidian, tertian or quartan. Hectic, septic, typhoid, typhus, pernicious yellow fever.*

Time.—10 or 11 A. M.—evening.

Yearly return of paroxysm (**Lach., Sul.**).

Cause.—Fevers from getting over-heated; from living in damp dwellings.

Prodrome.—Headache, throbbing in temples, backache, tearing toothache, and tearing pain in the limbs; cold feet; the two latter may attend the entire paroxysm.

*In Memphis during the epidemic of 1873, charcoal came much into favor as a prophylactic; out of more than fifty persons who took it and were constantly exposed to the fever, not one was attacked. The usual dose was half a teaspoonful of the crude powder two or three times a day.—DR. MORSE.

Chill.—*With thirst;* at times left sided; *begins in left hand and arm* (begins in right arm, **Merc. per.**). Chill with headache and unusual lassitude; *with icy-coldness of the body and cold breath* (*with terrible coldness as if lying on ice,* **Lyc.**—as if a piece of ice were lying on the back between the shoulders, **Lachn.**); shivering and chills in the evening, *mostly* only on left side (**Caust.**—right side, **Bry.**); evening chill with tired, weary feeling and flushes of heat. **Coldness of the knees, even in bed** (**Apis**); of **left arm** and *left leg; very cold hands and feet; finger nails blue.* Irregular paroxysm, sometimes *sweat first, followed by chill* (**Nux**).

Heat.—*Without thirst.* Sensation of heat with great anxiety in the evening, although she was cold to touch all over; flushes of burning heat in the evening, with *headache, flushed face, vertigo and nausea;* tired, aching pain in legs; pain in stomach, abdomen, spleen; oppressed breathing (**Apis, Ars.**). Heat and chill are distinct and independent; rarely heat and sweat commingled together or alternate (chill and heat are mingled, **Ars.**—heat and chill alternate, **Cal.**). Flushes of burning heat in evening, usually without thirst. Headache continues *after the heat* (continues *after the sweat,* **Ars., Eup.**). *Loquacity during hot stage* (**Lach.**—during chill and heat, **Pod.**).

"Chill with a marked degree of thirst; no thirst, or but slight during the fever, but to compensate for lack of thirst, *the patient wishes to be constantly fanned.*"—GUERNSEY.

Sweat.—Profuse, of a sour or putrid odor; at night; great disposition to sweat even *when eating* (**Carbo a.**). Moist on upper parts of body. Sour morning-sweat, which makes his person offensive; feet sweat when walking; sweats easily in a warm room, and is just as easily chilled. Tearing pain in the legs and teeth.

Tongue.—Coated with white, yellow fur; dry, fissured, lead-colored (**Ars.**); cold and contracted. Bitter taste before and after eating. Aversion to milk, which causes flatulence, to meat and fat things (longing for them, **Carbo a.**—longing for coffee, sweet and salt things, **Nitr. ac.**).

Pulse.—Weak, irregular, intermitting, indicative of rapid sinking.

Apyrexia.—Prostration, paleness, weakness of memory, melancholic disposition. *Gastric symptoms;* stomach and abdomen distended with gas after eating (least mouthful *fills* up to the chin, **Lyc.**). *Sensation as if stomach or abdomen would burst after eating or drinking.* Great foulness of the excretions (**Bap.**).

"In cachectic patients with profuse sour-smelling perspiration, *thirst only during the chill,* excitability of nervous symptoms. Patients debilitated from previous drugging, and frequent suppression of paroxysm by Quinia. *One-sided chill (left) during afternoon, great prostration; with icy coldness of the body; thirst and rapid sinking; small pulse, contracted, cold and cadaverous tongue and face, with cold breath.*"—T. D. Stowe.

This picture very closely resembles a so-called "pernicious" or "congestive fever."

Analysis.—In patients who have been exhausted by some deep-seated cachexia or exhausting disease, abuse of mercury, salt, quinine, vital powers low, great prostration.

Chill; with thirst; one-sided, l. hand and arm; icy coldness of the body, rapid sinking, cold breath.

Heat; without thirst; flushed face, loquacity; desire to be fanned.

Sweat; profuse, sour, offensive; sweats when eating (Carbo a.).

Persons who have never recovered from effects of some previous illness or injury; suppression by Quinine or drugging; typhoid or yellow fever.

CARBOLIC ACID.

Characteristic.—Pains are terrible; *come suddenly,* last a short time, disappear suddenly (Bell., Mag. p.).

Profound prostration, collapse; surface pale and bathed in cold sweat (Camph., Carbo v., Ver.).

"Physical exertion, even much walking, brings on abscess in some part, but generally in the r. ear."—R. T. COOPER.

Dull, heavy frontal headache, as if *a rubber band were stretched tightly over the forehead,* from temple to temple (Gels., Plat., Sul.).

When burns tend to ulceration and ichorous discharge (Ars., Carbo, Kreos.); rapid decubitus.

Putrid discharges from mouth, nose, throat, nostrils, rectum and vagina (Anthr., Psor., Pyr.).

Malignant scarlatina and variola (Am. c.).

Lacerated wounds with blunt instruments; bones bare, crushed; much sloughing of soft parts (Calend.).

Longing for whisky and tobacco (Asar., Carbo v.).

Vomiting: of drunkards, in pregnancy, sea-sickness, cancer; of dark, olive-green fluid (Pyr.).

Dysentery: fluid mucus, like scrapings of mucous membranes and great tenesmus (Canth.); diarrhea; stools thin, involuntary, black, of an intolerable odor.

Constipation, with **horribly offensive breath** (Op., Psor.).

Leucorrhea: acrid, copious, fetid, green.

Relations.—Compare: Ars., Kreos. in burns.

Carbolic acid is antidoted by dilute cider vinegar.

Type.—Intermittent, with hypertrophy of spleen; remittent, low miasmatic, in autumn; enteric typhoid; typhus; scarlet; yellow; septic. All fevers tend to collapse or malignancy.

Chill.—Chilly; in a warm room, or in open air. Chill followed by fever and slight sweat, with numb ache in arms and legs; pulse small and rapid; < about sundown and through night; felt as if he had taken a bad cold.

Heat.—High fever and frequent recurring chills alternating. Skin, hot, dry, with intense restlessness.

Sweat.—Profuse; at night bathed in perspiration. Sweat cold, clammy, acrid, offensive, exhausting.

Pulse.—Rapid, 120-130; feeble, small, flickering; intermittent and slow; irregular.

Tongue.—Burning and tingling as if a thousand needles were pricking it (Arum). Coated, white; red papillæ here and there (Ant. t., Bell.); dark brown; thick yellow-white fur down centre; dry, shiny, glassy (Mur. ac., Pyr.). Sordes. Breath fetid.

Analysis.—The fever is high at onset; temp. high; pulse rapid, feeble; the attack sudden, rapidly prostrating and tends to malignancy. Fevers with splenic hypertrophy.

CASCARILLA.

Characteristic.—Complaints from loss of blood or vital fluids (Carbo v., Caust., Cinch., Phos.).

The concussion of every step is painfully felt in region of stomach (Bry.).

Chill.—*With thirst for warm drinks* (Ced., Sabad.—for warm drinks in prodrome, Eup.); slight when walking in the open air, which immediately disappeared on standing still, but returned after walking again.

Heat.—*With thirst and desire for warm drinks* (Ced., Eup. purp.); anxious of the whole body, and a slight sweat followed by sleepiness.

Sweat.—Slight, on the back, when walking in the open air. Profuse at night, drenching the clothes, but not debilitating.

"Cannot drink anything but hot drinks during fever."—A. O. Hardenstein.

The thirst and desire for warm drinks is as marked as under *Cedron,* and both remedies have proved very efficacious in the treatment of intermittents occurring in the lower Mississippi valley. The late Dr. Hardenstein, of Vicksburg, relied upon *Cascarilla* when he found this symptom present, and says it rarely failed to cure.

CAUSTICUM.

Characteristic.—Adapted to persons with dark hair, rigid fibre; weakly, scrofulous persons, with *excessively yellow, sallow complexion,* subject to affections of respiratory and urinary tracts.

Children with dark hair and eyes, delicate, sensitive skin, prone to intertrigo during dentition (Lyc.); or convulsions with eruption of teeth (Stan.).

Ailments: from long-lasting grief and sorrow (Phos. ac.); from loss of sleep, night watching (Coc., Ign.); sudden emotions, fear, fright, joy (Cof., Gels.); anger or suppressed eruptions.

Soreness or rawness: of scalp, throat, respiratory tract, rectum, anus, vagina, uterus.

Melancholy, sad, hopeless; looks on the dark side of everything; with weeping, "the least thing makes the child cry."

Children slow in learning to walk (Cal. p.).

Unsteady walking and easy falling of little children.

Menses: too early; too feeble; flow *only or chiefly during the day;* cease on lying down.

Constipation; frequent, ineffectual efforts; *stool passes better when standing;* impeded by hemorrhoids; tough, shining.

Urination; involuntary, when coughing, sneezing, blowing the nose (Puls., Squil., Ver.); nocturnal, during first sleep (Sep., Tub.).

Cough: with inability to raise the sputa, must be swallowed;

> by a swallow of cold water; *on expiration;* after pertussis.

At night, cannot get an easy position, nor lie still a moment.

Cannot cover too warmly, but warmth does not relieve.

Cicatrices, especially burns and scalds freshen up, become sore again; patients say "they have never been well since that burn."

Whatever part she grasps, burns.

Paralysis of single parts; vocal organs, tongue, eyelids, face, extremities, bladder; *generally of right side;* onset gradual.

Disturbed functional activity of brain and spinal nerves, resulting in paralysis.

Intense sympathy for sufferings of others.

Rheumatic affections, with contraction of the flexors and stiffness of the joints; tension and shortening of muscles (Am. m., Cimex, Guaiac., Nat.).

Rawness or soreness: of scalp, throat, respiratory tract, rectum, anus, urethra, vagina, uterus (as if bruised, Arn.; as if sprained, Rhus).

Warts: large, jagged, often pedunculated; bleeding easily, exuding moisture; small, all over the body; on eyelids, face; on the nose.

Patient improves for a time then comes to a "stand-still."

Relations:—Complementary: Carbo v., Petros.

Incompatible: Phos. Must not be used before or after Phos., always disagrees; the acids; Coffea.

Aggravation.—In clear, fine weather; coming from the air into a warm room (**Bry.**); cold air; draught of cold air; on becoming cold; getting wet; from bathing.

Amelioration.—In damp, wet weather; warmth; warm air.

Type.—Not characteristic. Left-sided (**Carbo v.**).

Time.—4 P. M. or midnight, with sweat at 4 A. M.

Fever *without chill*, 6 to 8 P. M.

Chill, *without thirst,* **lessened in bed and by drinking** (**Graph.**—increased by drinking, **Caps.**). Chilliness and coldness of *the whole left side* (**Carbo v.**); of diseased parts. Shivering, *beginning in the face,* thence extending over the body. Internal chill, followed by *perspiration without intervening heat.* (See **Caps.**, **Cimex.**) At 4 P. M.: first, chilliness, with creeping in the legs up into the back, with weariness, lasting three hours, followed by sweat *without heat or thirst* (*without heat or sweat,* **Bov.**). *Shaking chill over the whole body; shivering chill over the whole body, without thirst or subsequent heat. He is always either chilly or in a sweat.* Shivering from the face, over the chest or along the back, down to the knees. Shivering and coldness *of single parts,* as arm, forearm, thigh, leg, abdomen, back (rest of body normal), without heat or sweat. Sensation of cold water in a small stream running across the body; of cold wind blowing upon spine between the shoulder-blades. Takes cold easily (**Bar.**, **Cal.**). Very sensitive to cold air, or to a draft (**Camph.**, **Canth.**); *cold feet. Chill passes downward.*

Flushes of heat, followed by chill.

Heat.—*Without thirst,* occurring toward morning or at night; not a clearly defined hot stage, but *mixed,* not *alternating,* with chilliness. Heat of head and face; warmth and redness of face and heat in face and eyes *after eating.* Heat from 6 to 8 P. M., which is not preceded by chill or shivering—heat descending—and appears to be a secondary paroxysm of fever.

Sweat.—Without thirst. *Immediately after the chill, without intervening heat* (**Ant. t.**). *Profuse sweat when walking in the open air; from motion* (**Bry.**—relieved by motion, **Caps.**); *during the day when sleeping. Sour smelling night-sweat all over* (**Hep.**). *Viscid sweat of strong urinous odor.* Moisture over whole body, without heat or thirst, with yawning and stretching. **Awoke at 4 A. M.,** with profuse sweat all over the body—without thirst—which continued 24 hours. Heaviness and roaring in the head.

"Chill predominates, much more marked than the other stages, and left-sided; followed by perspiration and later by heat; all occurring towards and during the evening."—T. D. STOWE.

Tongue.—Not coated, dry, with painful burning vesicles on sides and tip of tongue; or coated white on both sides, red in the middle.

Desire for smoked meat; for beer. **Aversion to sweet things, which disagree.**

Apyrexia.—Not marked, except by previously existing symptoms, upon which *the force of the chill* is frequently expended. Previously diseased organs or parts are prone to become painful during, or the pain is renewed, after the paroxysm.

Analysis.—Chronic cases with constitutional cachexia. One of the few remedies where sweat follows chill without intervening heat.

Left-sided chill, most pronounced of any remedy, and a "guiding" symptom of Causticum.

Chill without thirst > in bed and by drinking.

No thirst in heat or sweat.

Flushes of heat followed by chill.

Morning sweat is characteristic.

CEDRON.

Characteristic.—Especially adapted to wor   ; persons of nervous, excitable temperament, of a voluptuous disposition.

Nervous depression, and choreic attacks after coitus, more pronounced in women (debility after, more marked in male).

Sick headache every other day at 11 A. M. (Every day, Nat.)

Pains; tearing and twitching in limbs.

Menses: during, mouth and tongue very dry; great thirst; epilepsy, premonitory symptoms appear *precisely same day that flow begins. Convulsions occur regularly at every menstrual period.*

Before: leucorrhea every mouth regularly, *five or six days previous to catamenia* (Kali c.); leucorrhea instead of the menses (Coc.).

After: profuse ptyalism.

Removes roaring in ears, produced by Quinine.

Aggravation.—Movement renews chill; before a storm.

Amelioration.—Warm drinks; warm room.

Type.—Quotidian; tertian; tropical miasmatic; *periodicity marked;* attacks occur with clock-like regularity (**Aran.**). Intermittent headache, neuralgia, prosopalgia. At same period of pregnancy, tendency to miscarry.

Time.—*Evening at 6 or 6.30 P. M.; 4 A. M. and 4 P. M.* **(3 A. M., Thuja); 3 P. M. till evening (Apis).**

Prodrome.—At noon, *preceding feverish paroxysm,* depressed spirits, dullness of senses, and pressive headache. For 20 to 40 minutes mental excitement; exaltation of vital energy; florid, animated face and a sensation of general heat.

Chill.—*With thirst.* Regular paroxysms, commencing by chills in the back and limbs, coldness in the feet and hands. Chill severe; shakes the whole body. Mouth dry, great thirst for cold water. *General coldness,* shivering in the back, ice-cold feet, burning hands, sensation in the eyes as after much weeping. Shivering all over at 3 A. M., with malaise and inclination to lie down (**Thuja**); shiverings are *renewed by every movement* (**Nux, Cinch.**); coldness of the hands, feet and nose; flushes of heat in the face; toward 6 P. M. face constantly hot, with smarting in the eyes, especially when closing them. Chilliness of the back and legs; unusual paleness of the hands, red face, heaviness of the head; chilliness followed by severe frontal headache, red eyes, and itching of the eyelids internally and externally, icy-coldness of the hands and *of the tip of the nose,* rest of the face hot and burning hot. During chill, hands, feet and nose cold, with congestion of the head, palpitation and hurried respiration. Cramps and painful feeling, with tearing, twitching pains in upper extremities, feet and hands icy-cold. Chills and shivering of whole body. Chill predominates (**Petr.**).

Heat.—*With thirst* for warm drinks (**Cas., Chel., Sab.**). "Cannot drink anything but hot drinks during fever." Dry heat during the night; dry heat of entire body; animated face and profuse perspiration; chattering of the teeth and shaking of the whole body; great desire and longing for warm drinks (rarely wants cold drinks), and emission of large quantities of pale urine. Desire to sleep as heat passes off (**Apis**). "Numb, dead feeling in the legs; they feel enlarged. Entire body feels numb" (hands and feet feel dead, **Cimex**—fingers feel dead, **Sep.**).

Sweat.—*With thirst. Dry heat, followed by profuse perspiration* (**Cinch.**), preceded by cramps, these followed by contracting, tearing pains in upper and lower extremities, with a cold sensation in the hands and feet; mouth dry, great thirst and desire for cold water; chills and shivering, sometimes very strong shivering of the whole body; *palpitation and hurried respiration; urine scanty and high colored.*

Tongue.—Coated yellow even to the tip, on rising in the morning. At 5 P. M. intolerable pricking-itching of the tongue, she had to keep rubbing it against the palate. At 5.30 P. M. pricking of the tongue, half an hour later chilliness, with heat of the face, pale hands; *feet and tip of the nose cold.* Pricking of tongue early in the morning; goes off after eating.

Pulse.—Weak and depressed during chill, quick and full, with animated red face, in heat.

Apyrexia.—Lasted from 15 to 17 hours, after which, and

at about the same time as previous day, the paroxysm was repeated; restless; very nervous; cold and pale; weakness, yet return of appetite; transient pains are felt in the joints, principally in right elbow, which seems to perspire; general malaise; great debility; body heavy; mind depressed. Roaring in ears, deafness at night.

The debility is almost as marked as in Cinchona, but appears to be due more to the action of the brain and nervous system than to the effect of the profuse perspiration which is so characteristic of the latter. Said to be adapted to the intermittent fevers, occurring in *low, marshy regions,* particularly *in warm seasons* and *in tropical countries.* Ought to be the first remedy thought of in "Panama" fever.

The chill or chilliness predominates, but no stage of the paroxysm is "clear cut" or well marked, as in Cinchona, Eupatorium and some other remedies. *With the chill* there is chilliness and heat, or hot flushes, or hot hands, or red face and congestion of the head, particularly of the meninges. During heat, shivering, shaking, cold hands and nose. During sweat, coldness and heat, and heat and sweat irregularly intermingled.

Were it not for "its clock-like periodicity" Cedron would be much better adapted to remittent than intermittent fevers, if we were treating a name alone. Has been used with more success in Southern States and tropical climates than in higher latitudes, where it has fallen into disuse of late years from frequent failures, though apparently indicated.

Analysis.—Clock-like regularity of paroxysm (Aran.).

Craves warm drinks.

Profuse perspiration.

Miasmatic fevers of the low marshy regions in tropical countries. "Panama" or fevers of the Isthmus; in persons from tropical countries.

CHAMOMILLA.

Characteristic.—Adapted to persons, especially children—*new-born* and **during dentition**—with light or brown hair, excitable, nervous temperament; oversensitive from use or abuse of coffee or narcotics.

Peevish, irritable, oversensitive to pain, drives to despair (Cof.); cannot return a civil answer.

Child exceedingly *irritable, fretful;* **quiet only when carried**; impatient, wants this or that, becomes angry when refused, or when offered petulantly rejects it (Bry., Cina, Kreos.); "too ugly to live;" cross, spiteful.

Patient cannot endure anyone near him; cannot bear to be spoken to, answers snappishly; whining, moaning.

One cheek red and hot, the other pale and cold.

Oversensitive to open air, aversion to wind.

Complaints from anger, especially chill and fever.

Pains; spasmodic, distressing, wants to get away from them.

Toothache if anything warm is taken into the mouth (Bis., Bry., Cof.); on entering a warm room; in bed; from coffee; during menses or pregnancy.

Pain: seems unendurable, drives to despair; < by heat; < evening before midnight; with heat, thirst and fainting; with *numbness of affected part;* eructations <.

Convulsions of children from nursing, *after a fit of anger* in mother (Nux—after fright in mother, Op.).

Violent rheumatic pains drive him out of bed at night, compel him to walk about (Rhus).

Sleepy, but cannot sleep (Bell., Caust., Op.).

Burning of soles at night, puts feet out of bed (Med., Puls., Sang., San., Sulph.).

Relations.—Complementary: Bell. in diseases of children, cranial nerves; Cham., abdominal nerves.

In cases spoiled by use of opium or morphine. Mental calmness contra-indicates Chamomilla.

Aggravation.—Evening, before midnight; heat; anger; open air.

Amelioration.—From fasting; warm, wet weather; being carried.

Type.—*Quotidian;* regular stages in afternoon. Anticipates, usually two hours every day. Continued, typhoid, from anger, care, grief, taking cold.

Time.—11 A. M.—*4 P. M. lasting till 11 P. M.* Fever without chill, 9 A. M. to 12 M. *with redness of one cheek and paleness of the other.*

Cause.—Spring fevers (**Canch.**) in nervous, sensitive persons, especially residents of cities; from anger or abuse of coffee or opium; during dentition.

Prodrome.—"Very irritable, cross, peevish, irascible. Aching in all the joints."—E. V. Ross.

Chill.—*Without thirst;* slight shiverings frequently creep over the body, alternating with heat of face. *Shivers, when uncovering or undressing* (**Hepar**); in the cold air; in some portions, in the face, on the arms, over back and abdomen. Shivering of single parts and heat of others (sweat and heat of single parts, **Bry.**). Shivering and heat intermingled, **mostly with one red and one pale cheek.** *Chill only on posterior with heat of anterior portion of the body,* or vice versa; *returns in paroxysms.* Cold limbs, with burning heat of the face, in the eyes, and burning hot breath. Coldness over the whole body, with burning heat of the face, **which comes out of the eyes like fire.** Chill and coldness of the whole body, with burning heat of the face and hot breath.

Heat.—*With some thirst. Long-lasting heat, with violent thirst and frequent startings in sleep. Heat and shivering intermingled, with* **one cheek red, the other pale.** Burning heat in lightly covered parts, though almost cold when not covered. Heat and sweat of the face when eating and drinking (**Anac., Bell.**). *Great agitation, anxiety. Very irritable, can hardly answer one civilly* (**Bry.**—*exceedingly irritable, everything makes him angry,* **Anac.**).

Sweat.—*Hot perspiration, especially of the face and head;* sweats easily. *Profuse sweat on covered parts* (**Cinch.**—affected parts sweat profusely, **Ant. t.**). Profuse sweat at night; on waking the sweat ceases, and returns on falling asleep (**Sabad**). Sweat frequently of sour odor and with smarting of the skin (**Caps.**). Relief of pain, after sweat, not during.

Tongue.—Coated yellowish; or white at the sides and red in the middle (reverse of **Ant. t.**). Blisters on the tongue. Taste—bitter, sour, putrid.

Apyrexia.—Never clear; constitutional and mental symptoms of this stage are usually guiding. Patients suffer from bad digestion.

In consequence of anger or vexation, we often have instead of the usual fever paroxysm, violent colic, bilious bitter vomiting and diarrhea. Chamomilla vies with Cina and Arsenicum in the treatment of intermittents occurring in children.

Analysis.—Fevers of children; irritable, cross Fever attacks in spring, in nervous persons residing in cities; from anger, vexation.

Heat.—One cheek red and hot, the other pale and cold. Coldness of body with burning heat of face (Arn.).

Sweat: hot, of head and face; profuse on covered parts (Cinch.).

Instead of fever paroxysm, violent bilious colic with vomiting and diarrhea from anger or vexation.

CHELIDONIUM.

Characteristic.—Adapted to thin, spare, irritable persons; light complexion, blondes; subject to hepatic, gastric and abdominal complaints (Pod.).

Constant pain under the lower and inner angle of right scapula (Kali c., Mer.—under left, Chenop. g., Sang.).

Ailments brought on or renewed on change of weather (Mer.); > after dinner.

Periodic orbital neuralgia (right side) with excessive lachrymation, tears fairly gush out (Rhus).

Desire for *very hot drinks,* unless almost boiling stomach will not retain them (Ars., Casc., Ced., Eup. purp.).

Constipation; stool hard; round balls (Opium, Plumb., Sanic.).

Diarrhea: at night; slimy, grayish, yellowish, watery.

Debility and lassitude after eating, wants to lie down.

Face, forehead, nose, cheeks, remarkably yellow.

Yellow-gray color of the skin; wilted skin; of the palms of hands (Sep.).

Spasmodic cough; small lumps of mucus fly from mouth when coughing (Bad., Kali c.).

Affects right side most; r. eye, r. lung, r. hypochondria and abdomen, r. hip and leg; right foot cold as ice, left natural (Lyc.).

Relations.—Chel. antidotes the abuse of Bry., especially in hepatic complaints.

Ars., Lyc. and Sulph. follow well, and may often be required to complete the cure.

Aggravation.—Morning (**Bry., Nux**).

Amelioration.—Evenings (rev. of **Puls.**).

Type.—Variable. Periodicity not marked. Remittent, continued, bilious, malarial. Typhoid and hepatic complications.

Time.—*Hour,* not characteristic.

Afternoon and evening paroxysm.

Chill.—Without thirst, over whole body, *beginning in hands and feet* (**Gels.**), when walking in open air; passes off in the room. Shaking chill in the evening in bed. *Shaking chill, with shivering, chattering of the teeth, as if dashed with ice-*

cold water (**Am. m., Ant. t., Sabad.**). Shaking chill, with nausea; worse on hands and feet; *with distention of veins of hands and arms* (enlargement of veins of arms and legs during heat, **Chin. s.**). Right leg and foot as far as knee, icy-cold (coldness of right limb as if standing in cold water, **Sabad.**). Coldness of nose; face; cheeks; occiput; pit of stomach; abdomen; hands and feet; intestine, after drinking water; in open air; running down the back (**Meny., Petr.**).

Heat.—Burning heat of hands, face, cheeks, eye-lids, head, ears, tip of nose, forehead. Flushes of glowing heat of different single parts of body; on scapula; in hip-joints. Burning cheeks, of a dark red circumscribed color (**Sang.**—of a mahogany color, **Eup.**). Heat of the cheeks, with red swollen face (**Cact.**).

Sweat.—During sleep; towards morning; better after waking. Sweats when pains disappear (pains relieved by profuse sweat, **Arn., Nat., Eup.**).

Tongue.—Coated thickly, white or yellow, with red margin; shows imprint of teeth (**Mer., Pod.**). Taste: bitter; insipid; bitter saliva collects in mouth. *Desire for milk, which agrees now* (which causes flatulence, **Carbo v.**). Pain in stomach > *by eating* (**Anac., Petr.**).

Pulse.—During chill, small and quick; after paroxysm, slow.

Apyrexia.—Never clear; liable to run into a remittent or continuous fever. Stitching pains in region of liver, shooting toward the back. Left hypochondrium sensitive to pressure.

Analysis.—The shaking, shivering, chill, as if dashed with ice water; < in open air.

Chill; of right side and of single parts.

Heat; burning, of single parts; circumscribed dark red cheeks. Pain in liver or under right scapula.

Sweat; during sleep; when pain disappears.

CICUTA VIROSA.

Characteristic.—Adapted to persons of a highly nervous organization. Women subject to epileptic and choreic convulsions; spasms of teething children, or from worms.

Convulsions: violent, with *frightful distortions* of the limbs and whole body; renewed from touch, noise or jar.

Epilepsy: with swelling of the stomach as from violent spasms of the diaphragm; screaming; red face; trismus; hiccup; loss of consciousness and distortion of the limbs; frequent, during the night; recurring at first at short, then at long intervals.

Puerperal convulsions: frequent suspensions of breathing for a few moments; upper part of body most affected; *continue after delivery.*

During dentition, grinding of the teeth or gums; compression of the jaws as in lockjaw.

Abnormal appetite *for chalk and indigestible things;* for coal or charcoal; child eats them with apparent relish (Alum., Psor.).

Suffer violent shocks through head, stomach, arms, legs, which cause jerkings of the parts; head hot.

Injurious chronic effects from concussions of the brain and spine, especially spasms; trismus and tetanus from getting splinters into flesh (Hyp.).

Aggravation.—From tobacco smoke (**Ign.**); touch; jar.

Amelioration.—In open air.

Type.—Quotidian intermittent; periodicity not marked.

Time.—Afternoon (2 to 3.30 P. M.) paroxysm.

Chill.—And chilliness, with desire for warmth and to go to the warm stove (**Lach.**). The chilliness begins in the chest and extends down the legs and into the arms, *after which follows a disposition to stare at one point.* Icy coldness of the whole body; ears cold; cold sensation streams through lower legs, especially the right. The whole abdomen was cold. *They all long for a warm stove* (**Bov., Ign., Lach.**).

Heat.—Without thirst; general of whole body; of single parts and special organs; in the chest and abdomen; in both legs. Sensation of hot water in the chest, arms, legs and ears; hot internally and externally. Burning and redness of the face. Constant desire for open air.

Sweat.—*On the abdomen;* at night, and in the morning hours. Feels invigorated after.

Tongue.—Swelling of the tongue. Thirst, with inability to swallow (**Cimex**).

The conditions calling for Cicuta are liable to occur during or following epidemic spinal meningitis. The chief symptom is the chill and coldness beginning in chest and extending downward.

CIMEX.

Characteristic.—Affects the right side most. Violent headache during the chill, which almost deprives him of the power of thinking; *worse when he drinks.*

Pain in liver as if strained; painful when touched and coughing.

Constipation: stool dry, like small nuts, and only able to pass a small piece with each effort (Chel., Op., Plb., Thuja).

Cough: with *gagging, belching or vomiting* (Bry., Dros., Kali); with purulent sputa; in daily attacks with fever paroxysms.

Irresistible drowsiness and sleepiness (Ant. t., Nux m.).

Aggravation.—Drinking; every movement, especially extending a limb, produces pain in extensor tendons; suffers the thirst rather than move.

Amelioration.—By abstaining from drinking.

Type.—Tertian or quartan.

Time.—All periods, day or night.

Prodrome.—Thirst; *can drink before the paroxysm begins.* Heaviness in lower limbs five or six hours before chilly stage begins (thirst with pains in bones of limbs one to three hours before chill begins, **Eup.**).

Chill.—*Without thirst.* Chill commencing in the feet, which first become cold; clenching of hands; violent raging; cold shuddering, as if cold water were poured over her (**Cinch., Rhus**); stretching, yawning; great drowsiness during chilly stage, he is unable to resist sleep (**Op.**); hands and feet feel dead (fingers feel as if they were dead, **Sep.**—all the body feels numb, **Ced.**). During chill, pain in all the joints (pain in ankles and wrists, **Pod.**), *as if tendons were too short, contracted,* so that the legs cannot be stretched, *particularly the knee joints, which he is unable to extend.* Oppression of the chest; must take a long breath frequently (oppression of chest; he must be raised up in order to breathe, **Apis**). Chill terminates with a feeling in the legs as if tired by walking, obliging constant change of position of limbs. *After the chill* (instead of fever), *thirst; but when he drinks, violent headache, which almost deprives him of the power of thinking;* with tickling in the larynx, causing dry, uninterrupted cough; oppressed breathing; heaviness in the middle of chest and anxiety. *Tormented with thirst,* yet he abstains from drinking, because it makes head ache and all the above symptoms unbearable (see **Ars., Caps., Eup.**).

Heat.—*Without thirst,* but desire to drink nearly all day, on account of dryness of throat (Nux m.). When the dry heat sets in the uneasiness disappears, in place of which she feels *a pressure and gaging in the esophagus, affecting whole chest and impeding respiration;* when she drinks for the purpose of putting a stop to the gagging *the water can only be swallowed at intervals, as if the esophagus were constricted* (**Cic.**). The *gagging does not cease until hot stage terminates,* after which ravenous *hunger* (hunger before chill, **Cinch.**—hunger during entire paroxysms, **Cina**). If he drinks during heat is obliged to urinate soon after; urine hot and brown, depositing much sediment; continues hot even 24 hours after fever.

Sweat.—*Without thirst;* > all the other symptoms (**Nat.**, **Psor.**). Musty-smelling, sour sweat (**Stan.**); the odor is very offensive to him (**Carbo a.**). Light sweat, mostly on head and chest, *with continued hunger* (**Eup.**).

Tongue.—Coated white; saliva collects on middle of tongue and tastes of iron; tongue, gums and palate feel burnt and scalded. Throat dry, causing drinking.

Apyrexia.—A good deal of thirst in this stage, in which, as in the prodrome, he can satisfy his thirst without headache, gagging or esophageal constriction.

Analysis.—Thirst; can drink only during prodrome. Contraction of joints as if tendons were too short. Gagging, belching or vomiting. Drinking causes violent headache.

CINCHONA.

Characteristic.—Adapted to stout, "swarthy" persons; to systems once robust which have become debilitated, "broken down," from exhausting discharges.

Apathetic, indifferent, taciturn (Phos. ac.); despondent, gloomy, has no desire to live, but lacks courage to commit suicide.

Ailments: from **loss of vital fluids, especially hemorrhages,** *excessive lactation, diarrhea, suppuration* (Chin. s.); of malarial origin, with marked periodicity; return every other day.

After climacteric with profuse hemorrhage; acute diseases often result in dropsy.

Pains: are darting or drawing-tearing; in every joint, all the bones, periosteum as if strained, sore all over; obliged to move limbs frequently as motion gives relief (Eup., Rhus); renewed by contact, and then gradually increase to a great height; < slightest touch, > by hard pressure.

Great debility, trembling, aversion to exercise; nervous; **sensitive to touch,** *to pain, to drafts of air;* unrefreshing sleep < after 3 A. M.

One hand icy cold, the other warm (Dig., Ipec., Puls.).

Headache: *as if the skull would burst;* intense throbbing of head and carotids, face flushed; from occiput over whole head; < sitting or lying, must stand or walk; *after hemorrhage or sexual excesses.*

Face pale, hippocratic; eyes sunken and surrounded by blue margins; pale, sickly expression as after excesses; toothache while nursing the child.

Excessive flatulence of stomach and bowels; belching gives no relief (Lyc., Pod.—gives relief, Carbo v.); < after eating fruit.

Colic: at a certain hour each day; periodical, from gall-stone (Card. m.); < nights, after eating; > bending double.

Labor-pains cease from hemorrhage; cannot bear to be touched, not even her hands.

Hemorrhages: from mouth, nose, uterus or bowels; *long continued;* longing for sour things; blood dark, or dark and clotted, with ringing in the ears, fainting, loss of sight, general coldness and sometimes convulsions (Fer., Phos.).

Relations.—Complementary: Ferrum.

Aggravation.—From slightest touch; every other day; *draft of air;* milk; at night; after the chills; mental emotion.

Amelioration.—Warmth; during rest; pressure; bending double.

Type.—Variable. *Tertian* or double tertian; quotidian or double quotidian; double quartan; malarial; remittent.

Anticipates from two to three hours each attack (**Quinine**).

"Paroxysm every seventh day, anticipating about three hours each succeeding chill."—W. J. HAWKES.

Time.—Not characteristic; may begin at any hour of day; generally toward midday; *never at night.* 5 P. M., 5 A. M. *Paroxysms return every seven or every fourteen days* (**Ars., Puls.**).

Cause.—Paludal fevers have always been considered its special domain. A change of theory may revolutionize the cause to which Cinchona is now supposed to be especially adapted; but thanks to *similia* it will not in the least affect its homeopathic indications.

Prodrome.—Great thirst (**Caps., Eup., Puls.**—thirst and bone pains, **Eup.**); *canine hunger; nausea; anguish;* headache; debility; *palpitation of the heart,* with anxiety; sneezing when exposed to cold air; oppressive colic; and a general feeling of illness.

"Restless sleep night before the paroxysm."—HAHNEMANN.

Chill.—*Without thirst* * (with thirst, **Caps., Ign., Quin.**). *Thirst ceases as soon as chill begins.* **General shaking chill over whole body,** beginning in the legs below the knees, *increased by drinking. Shivering or chilliness, with goose-flesh, after every swallow of drink* (abstains from drinking because every swallow increases the chill, **Eup. perf.**—because drinking causes vomiting, **Ars.**—shuddering and chill after every drink, **Caps.**—drinking makes headache and all symptoms unbearable, **Cimex**). Thirst *before* or *after,* but *not during* the chill. *Coldness and shivering* when walking in the open air at 5 P. M., *disappearing in the room;* an hour afterwards, *great heat,* especially in the face, *increased on motion and on walking* (**Bry.**); *thirst follows an hour after* the disappearance of the

Observation by Hahnemann.*—In all my observations I have found that the Cinchona fever is characterized by the thirst not appearing during the cold stage, either shuddering or chilliness; that, on the contrary, thirst came after the cold stage, or, which is the same thing, that thirst came **shortly before the hot stage set in.

heat. Wants to be near the stove, but it increases the chill (**Ipec.**—relieved by heat of stove, **Ign.**—relieved by external heat, **Ars.**). *Internal and violent chill, with icy cold hands and feet,* and congestion of blood to the head. Chill with pain in the liver. Shaking chill and *internal coldness* for several hours; shivering over the whole body *without thirst; coldness of the hands and feet even in a warm room;* chill alternating with heat, skin cold and blue (**Camph., Carbo v.**—hands cold, nails blue, **Nux**). Sensation of internal coldness in upper abdomen, *after every swallow of drink,* and renewed on every inspiration. Coldness over whole body *as if dashed with cold water* (**Ant. t., Rhus**). Paleness and icy coldness of the hands and feet, aggravated by walking; vertigo and paleness of the face.

Heat.—*Without thirst.* General heat, with distended veins, congested headache, desire to uncover, but chilly when uncovered* (chilly when uncovered in any stage of paroxysm, **Nux**). *Canine hunger* or aversion to food, pain in the region of the liver, back, chest, limbs; dryness of mouth and dry, burning lips, with redness of face and often delirium. *Long-lasting heat, with sleep.* Cough dry, spasmodic, fatiguing, with pain in both hypochondria and at pit of stomach (with stitching pain in chest, **Bry.**). Heat of the whole body, *externally and internally, with swollen veins of the arms and hands,* without sweat or thirst. Heat of the whole body, aggravated by walking (relieved by walking, **Caps.**). Sensation of heat in abdomen as of hot water running down. The cheeks are red and hot *to the patient,* although *they are not warm. If he eats in*

**Observation by Hahnemann.*—There is likewise no thirst in the Cinchona fever during the hot stage, except some burning of the lips, or some dryness of the parts, which dryness accounts for the symptom; sensation of slight thirst during the hot stage; "the thirst accompanying flushes of heat." In the Cinchona fever thirst sets in after the hot, or, which is the same thing, during the sweating stage.

this stage, sleepy after eating. On the least movement an unpleasant sensation of heat in the head and stomach.

"Entire absence of thirst during height of paroxysm."—AD. LIPPE.

Sweat.—With great thirst. The first indication of its approach is the return of the thirst which preceded the chill, but which was absent during the cold and hot stages. Intense thirst during chill and especially during heat, positively contra-indicates **Cinchona.**

Sweating during sleep. On being covered *he sweats profusely all over;* this he cannot avoid, although very troublesome, he is so sleepy he cannot get up. Partial; cold; greasy, or as if mixed with oil; *profuse and debilitating* (profuse, but not debilitating, **Samb.**); sweat on the back or side on which he lies (sweat on the side not lain upon, **Benz.**). Profuse sweat over the whole body *when walking in the open air* (**Bry.**). Easily excited sweat during sleep and motion (excited by motion only, **Bry.**—relieved by motion, **Caps.**). *The sweat parboils the skin* (**Canch.**—parboils the fingers, **Ant. c.**). Often slow in becoming established, and frequently out of all proportion to the intensity of the cold and hot stages (see **Eup.**).

"The patient sweats profusely, especially on the back and neck, when he sleeps."—HAHNEMANN.

Tongue.—White or yellow; thick, dirty coating. Taste too acute. *Bitter taste in the mouth.* Indifference to all food, even when thinking of it. Toothache, especially when infant nurses (**Sil.**).

Pulse.—*Quick, hard* and *irregular* during chill and heat; slow, feeble in apyrexia, sometimes intermittent; more quiet after eating; great swelling of the veins.

Apyrexia.—*Sweats easily; great debility* and *exhausting* night-sweats continue, *followed by ringing in the ears,* and constricting sensation over vertex from ear to ear. A saffron yellowishness of the skin of scalp, face, neck, chest and abdomen (**Chel.**); with the characteristic anemic and cachectic appearance, once seen, never forgotten. There is swelling of both hypochondria, which are painful to pressure and worse by motion, bending, or coughing. Swelling, pain and pressure of epigastric region, with hypertrophy of spleen. Entire loss of appetite, with sinking feeling in stomach, or hunger easily satisfied. Bitter eructations and bitter vomiting (sour eructations and sour vomiting, **Lyc.**). The urine is scanty and turbid, with a yellow or brick-dust sediment; and general dropsical symptoms are often present. Bloated or tympanitic abdomen, and hard spleen or liver in nursing children, with profuse sweating and great weakness (without profuse sweating, **Ars.**).

This constitutes **the paroxysm** *of Cinchona.* But Cinchona has also another, an exception to the rule (probably a secondary reaction) which is often confounded with Arsenicum; hence its notice in this place. It has only two different stages—Chill and Heat.

Chill.—With thirst (*no thirst* in regular chill). *Febrile chill over the whole body from time to time during the day,* especially upon forehead, which has cold sweat upon it; *violent thirst a quarter of an hour after the first chill.* (No thirst during *chill* or *heat*—which is long-lasting—in first paroxysm.) Cold hands in the evening, with hot cheeks; one hand is icy cold, the other warm; ice-cold feet, with warmth of rest of body. (This alternate heat of one part and coldness of another at same time belongs only to this paroxysm.)

Heat.—*With thirst* (*no thirst in previous heat*). Heat over the whole body, with fine, needle-like stitches in the skin, especially of the throat, together with *great thirst for cold water.* Heat alternating with the chill; *some thirst for cold water* with the chill; heat follows half an hour or an hour after the chill. A very transient sensation of heat over the whole body, with *thirst for cold water.* Sensation of flushes of heat, *with thirst for cold drinks.* Warmth and redness of the face, while the rest of the body was cold. The right hand is warm, the left cold; the hands are now warm, now cold; heat, with *burning lips and thirst,* followed by sweat; chill, *with thirst;* then heat, *with thirst; the thirst continues even during the apyrexia. Violent desire for cold drinks,* accompanied with stinging in various parts of the skin.

"The fever heat, accompanied with stinging over the whole body, seems to form an exception."—HAHNEMANN.

The symptoms occurring *before the chill* and *during the sweat and apyrexia* are alike in both paroxysms. The *thirst during the chill,* with alternate warmth and coldness of different parts at same time; the *thirst during heat,* with stinging or fine, needle-like stitches in skin, with heat of one part and coldness of another, are the characteristics of this paroxysm.

Analysis.—The paroxysm *anticipates* from two to three hours each attack (Chin. s.); returns every seven or fourteen days; *never at night;* sweats profusely all over on being covered, or during sleep.

The thirst of Cinchona is guiding.

Prodrome; with thirst, intense, long before the chill (Caps., Eup.).

Chill; no thirst, or it disappears as chill increases.

Heat; no thirst, as chill passes into fever thirst begins; as fever increases thirst decreases, when fever declines the thirst begins.

Sweat; with great thirst. No thirst during the nervous tension of chill and heat; great thirst during relaxation of sweat and before chill begins.

Marsh intermittents, with pains in region of liver, vomiting of bile and great anguish.

During apyrexia: exhausting sweats, anemic and cachectic

appearance; sensitiveness in hypochondria; scanty urine; loss of appetite; bloated abdomen.

CHININUM SULPHURICUM.

Characteristic.—Adapted to persons of *dark complexion,* bilious temperament; cachectic, weakened from loss of blood.

Whirling in the head like a windmill.

Ringing in the ears, especially the left (especially the right, Cinch.).

Intermittent neuralgia, pains return with great regularity.

Weak and nervous, a little exercise produces palpitation.

Spine extremely sensitive and painful to pressure, especially in the cervico-dorsal region.

Great weakness, especially of lower extremities.

"It will change an intermittent or remittent into a continued fever, and I have known it to cause typhoid and pneumonia (by suppressing the original disease)."—HALE.

Aggravation.—Contact (dorsal vertebræ); when covered (sweats profusely).

Type.—*Tertian;* rarely quotidian. Every fourteen days. Each attack anticipating from one to three hours (**Ars., Bry., Cinch., Nat., Nux**). A perfect regularity both in the invasion and progress of the paroxysm, is always guiding.

Time.—10 or 11 A. M.; 3 and 10 P. M.

Cause.—Marsh miasm; malaria. Acute intermittents of supposed malarial origin.

Chill.—*With thirst.* **Decided shaking chill at 3 P. M.** (**Apis, Ced.**); chilliness, with paleness of the face, pain in the forehead and temples, and ringing in the ears at 11 A. M. *Violent shaking chill followed by heat, then sweat for several hours. Violent chill with trembling in the limbs,* so that she could scarcely walk; after going to bed she had *violent heat with frequent yawning* and sneezing, which was followed by a *copious sweat.* Violent paroxysm with *shaking chill* and *severe pain in left hypochondrium;* chilliness for an hour, with *blue lips and nails* (**Cinch.**, **Nux**), paleness of the face and **pain in the middle dorsal vertebræ**; increased hunger and constipation.

Heat.—*With excessive thirst.* Intense heat over the whole skin, with *redness of the face.* External heat, with dryness of the mouth and fauces, obstinate constipation. Heat which passes over into sweat; over whole body; *which gradually breaks into sweat,* **while perfectly quiet** (**Staph.**). *Delirium during heat.* Flushes of heat in the face, with thirst at 4 P. M. "Great enlargement of veins of arms and legs."

Sweat.—*With thirst.* Sweat breaks out over the whole body from time to time, even during perfect quiet. Profuse sweat on the least motion (**Bry.**). Sweat during the morning sleep, so profuse that the bed was soaked with it. Profuse, exhausting sweats; nightly diarrhea (nightly diarrhea before the paroxysm, **Puls.**). Sweat often begins in latter part of hot stage, and relieves all symptoms of head and chest. (**Nat.**—sweat relieves all symptoms but headache, which is increased, **Eup.**). Drinking is grateful and affords relief. Most perspiration on parts pressed by clothing, back, axillary and perineal regions.

Tongue.—Flabby; white or yellow coating in the centre, pale on the margin (reverse of **Ant. t.**). Taste bitter, with clean tongue.

Pulse.—Large; full during chill and heat. Weak and trembling at close of paroxysm, ranging from 50 to 60 per minute.

Apyrexia.—Constant excessive thirst during the entire apyrexia, which in daily fever is short, the paroxysm closely resembling a remittent or continuous fever. But whether it be short or long, always distinguished by great debility and prostration (**Ars.**); the perspiration is exhausting (all the discharges are debilitating and weakening, **Carbo a.**). Canine hunger more marked, if possible, than in Cinchona, even in nervous enfeebled patients. Light exercise readily produces palpitation. Obstructions of the portal system are especially marked, and the spleen swollen and painful. Ringing and burning in the ears, accompanied with vertigo and a sensation of enlargement of head. Hiccup may become a troublesome symptom in any stage, but especially in apyrexia. Urine fatty and deposits a straw-yellow, brick-dust sediment; urates in large quantities. *Spine painful on pressure in all stages of paroxysm.* The sensitiveness of the spinous processes of the dorsal vertebræ should be borne in mind, for Quinine acts specifically upon the spinal cord and the nerves proceeding from it.

Cinchona.	Chininum sul.
Time.—All periods, except night. Variable type. Every fourteen days. Anticipating one to three hours.	**Time.**—10 A. M., 3 and 10 P. M. Regular paroxysms, tertian type. Anticipates two and a half hours every day.
Prodrome.—*Great thirst* and canine hunger; headache and debility.	**Prodrome.**—Premonitory symptoms are wanting.
Chill.—*Without thirst.* Chill increased by drinking. External and internal coldness.	**Chill.**—*With thirst,* paleness of face, lips and nails blue. *Dorsal vertebræ painful on pressure.*
Heat.—*Without thirst.* General, with distended veins, congestive headache, desire to uncover, but chilly when uncovered.	**Heat.**—*With thirst,* hot, dry skin, dry mouth and fauces; flushed face; delirium. *Pain in spine on pressure.*
Sweat.—*With great thirst.* Sweats profusely on being covered. Night-sweat very profuse.	**Sweat.**—*With great thirst.* Sweats profusely during perfect quiet; morning sweat. *Pain in lumbar vertebræ* and sacrum on pressure.
Apyrexia.—With *no thirst.* Sweats easily. Pain and soreness of hypochondria, worse on pressure and motion. Hepatic region swollen and sensitive. Jaundiced.	**Apyrexia.**—With *great thirst.* Apyrexia short; sweat hardly ceases before chill begins again. *Pain all down the spinal column on pressure.* Spleen swollen and painful.
Different *stages* of paroxysm follow in regular succession.	Cold stage may be long, light, irregular, or wanting in acute cases.
Contra-indicated where there is much thirst during cold and hot stages. Perspiration *always profuse,* or Cinchona is contra-indicated.	*Contra-indicated where there is no thirst during cold or hot stages.* Perspiration must *succeed the heat,* or will be contra-indicated.

Where the indications for any remedy are not very clear, the paroxysm incomplete but regular, Chin. sul. 30th or 200th may clear up or cure the case. The highest potencies are often antidotal when the symptoms are similar.

"In recent intermittents, there may or may not be a chill, but there must be fever, and it *must be followed by sweat*—and it generally is profuse and exhausting—or Quinine will be utterly useless." "As a rule, chronic, long-lasting intermittents are only aggravated by Quinine."—Burt.

The *cachexia* produced by long continued massive doses of Chin. sul., such as rheumatism of the extremities, chronic diarrhea, ascites and organic disease of the liver and spleen, although now a constitutional malady, requires antidotal treatment. This may be most speedily removed by Arn., Ars., Carbo v., Fer.. Lach., Nat., Puls.. as indicated by symptoms of each individual case.

Samuel Swan, M. D., of New York, has reported some bad cases of quinine cachexia, cured with Chin. s. 10 m. and cm. potencies—See last paragraph *Hahnemann's Chronic Diseases,* Vol. I, p. 195-196, as authority.

Chin. s. is often indicated in intermittent fever, and when indicated will cure more promptly and more safely in the potencies than in the crude form. There is little doubt that it is *oftener prescribed* than *indicated,* and that it will, in a majority of cases, suppress the paroxysm—without reference to *time of appearance,* whether *with* or *without chill, heat, sweat, thirst,* etc., etc.—there is as little doubt. But Morphine will also suppress pain and diarrhea, quite as effectually as Quinine will the fever paroxysm, and the homeopathic physician, half-read or not read at all, in his Materia Medica, "borrows both the theory and the Quinine from his allopathic brother, for the same reason that he borrows his hypodermic syringe and Morphine," with which to relieve the pain and diarrhea, viz., it is a "short cut" to palliate the pain, relieve and thus retain his patient, and avoid the necessity of studying the case. There is a wide difference between *suppressing* and *curing* a fever paroxysm, or any other disease. The homeopath *can* and *ought to cure,* not "break up the chill," "suppress" or "cover up" the disease. Leave the "breaking up of the paroxysm" to the allopath who invented the phrase; "rational (?) medicine" can do it "scientifically."

John Ellis, M. D., when Professor of Practice in Cleveland College, in treatment of "congestive chill," advised: "That 25 or 30 grs of Chin. s. given during the intermission, will rarely fail to prevent a return, or to rescue the patient from death." "Not that Quinine *may be given* in such cases, but that it *must be given.*" Also, "That in recent cases of 'pernicious' fever, two-thirds of our patients will die in spite of any known homeopathic remedy or remedies in the ordinary doses."—*College Note Book.*

L. M. Jones, M. D., of Michigan, who has had an extensive experience in the treatment of "congestive chill," on the other hand says: "It has fallen to my lot to treat a number of cases of 'congestive chills,' first and last. In my early practice I treated a few cases with Quinine, but it was not satisfactory; and since then I have relied on the attenuated homeopathic remedy, and never lost a case. Nux has been more frequently indicated in the cases I have met with than any other remedy."—*Private Letter.*

Dr. Lippe says: "I lived for ten years in the country, where ague prevailed, and **never** resorted to Quinine. I **cured** my cases. I have always been of the opinion that a physician who professes to be a homeopath **must** cure **all** his cases of intermittent fever with homeopathic potentized remedies, under the law of the similars."

I am convinced that **every case of "congestive chill,"** like Asiatic cholera, can be cured more safely and speedily by the potentized remedy than in any other way, if it can be cured at all; and the mortality under homeopathic treatment will never approach 66 per cent.; the record of the dominant school.

CLINICAL.

"I have recently made several satisfactory cures with Chin. s. Two or three of them with one dose each of the 200th, and as many others with the 6th. I think this is an important remedy with us, and that it succeeds *better in attenuation* than in the crude form. *The crude drug never gave me such satisfaction.* Some of the indications in a number of recent cases were *clear intermissions, regular paroxysms, clean* or *tolerably clean tongue,* and *profuse sweats.*"—H. V. MILLER.

Analysis.—Regular paroxysm; clear apyrexia; anticipating from 1-3 hours; clean tongue; painful congestion of spine; thirst in all stages; profuse exhausting sweat.

As in Natrum and Arsenic the potencies will always cure when the remedy is indicated. We must not overlook the fact that it is in the psoric and tubercular patient that we find the obstinate and chronic types of fevers, and no amount of crude quinine or any other drug, will cure such cases, though it may suppress the paroxysm and irretrievably injure the patient.

CINA.

Characteristic.—Adapted to the child with dark hair; very cross, irritable, ill-humored; wants to be carried, but carrying gives no relief; does not want to be touched; cannot bear you to come near it; averse to caresses; desires many things but rejects everything offered (Ant. t., Bry., Cham., Staph.); uneasy, distressed; rubs or picks the nose all the time (Arum t.); pitiful weeping when awake; starts and screams during sleep; suffers from worms.

Face is pale; sickly appearance around mouth and eyes; dark rings around the eyes, one cheek red the other pale (Cham.).

Canine hunger; *hungry soon after a full meal; craves sweets,* and many different things.

Child is afraid to speak or move for fear of bringing on a paroxysm of cough (Bry.).

Urine: turbid when passed, turns milky and semi-solid after standing; white and turbid; involuntary.

Intermittents of nervous, weakly, scrofulous children.

Aggravation.—At night.

Type.—Quotidian; quartan; tertian; regular; periodicity pronounced; continued fevers of children.

Time.—1 P. M., afternoon or evening. *At same hour every day* (Aran., Ced.). *Evening;* fever lasting all night (nursing children).

Daily fever (without chill) at same hour.

Cause.—Intestinal worms; eating sweets and pastry.

Prodrome.—*Ravenous hunger,* nausea, vomiting of food, and diarrhea, and vomiting of bile (when the stomach is empty); pale face, with blue margins around the eyes.

Chill.—*Without thirst. Febrile shuddering over the whole body, with hot cheeks, without thirst.* Chill extends from upper part of body to head, *even by the warm stove. Shivering-creeping over the trunk, so that he trembles even by a warm stove, not > by external warmth* (chill < by external heat, **Ipec.**). *Coldness of the pale face,* with warm hands; *cold face; cold cheeks; cold sweat on forehead,* nose and hands. Evening paroxysm of nursing children, *heat with hunger and thirst continue all night. Chilliness down the spine.* Vomiting.

Chill, followed by convulsions and high fever.

"Predominance of coldness, with cold sweat and *continued hunger.*"—J. S. DOUGLAS.

Heat.—*With thirst;* mostly in face and head (with red face and bursting headache, **Bell.**); *face puffed, pale, especially around the mouth and nose, with red cheeks; picks and bores in the nose with the fingers; rubs the eyes; restless sleep; starts and screams as if frightened,* pupils dilated. **Rising heat and glowing redness of the cheeks, without thirst, after sleep.** *Burning heat over the whole face,* with *redness of the cheeks,* and *thirst for cold drinks.* Daily fever at same hour, with very short breath. Fever daily in the afternoon. Violent fever, with *vomiting and diarrhea* (**Ver.**—see **Elat.**). Fever; vomiting of food, followed by chill all over, and then heat with great thirst. *Canine hunger.* Heat worse at night; with thirst; with anxiety. *Picking finger ends.*

Sweat.—*Without thirst; generally light; cold sweat on the forehead,* around the *nose* and on the *hands.* After the sweat, *vomiting of food* and *canine hunger,* at the same time (hunger after paroxysm, **Eup.**).

Tongue.—Always clean (**Chin. s., Psor., Sul.**).

Apyrexia.—*Never clear. Hunger* even in this stage, though not so marked, or so constant. The child had a craving appetite for some time previous to fever, then loss of appetite and desire only for dainties, with vomiting and whitish diarrhea. General *"worm symptoms"* predominate; restless, frightened sleep; *urine turbid, turns milky and semi-solid after standing.*

The vomiting during prodrome, often during and always after the paroxysm, succeeded by canine hunger with *clean tongue,* should always call attention to Cina.

In Antimonium crud. the same condition may be present but the tongue is covered with a thick, whitish coating.

In Ipecacuanha the tongue is sometimes clean, but there is nausea, and the vomiting predominates over the diarrhea.

The prostration of Veratrum is wanting, and the mental symptoms are entirely different.

"The child is very whining, peevish and complaining; weeps piteously if one goes to handle or lead him. Great earnestness and sensitiveness; cannot take a joke. Indifference to all impressions. Restlessness. Greediness. *Cannot be composed by things at other times agreeable, or by caresses."*—CARROLL DUNHAM.

"Cina is frequently the epidemic remedy for children when adults require other drugs. Is always to be thought of in patients between two and ten years of age."—A. MCNEIL.

Analysis.—Canine hunger; the sickly bluish-white circles around mouth; the mental irritability; peevish, whining, complaining children; general "worm symptoms."

Craves sweets; too serious or sensitive for joking.

CLEMATIS.

Light complexion; torpid, cachectic conditions; glandular swellings and indurations; *sycotic or syphilitic taint.*

Herpetic eruptions, following suppressed gonorrhea.

Herpes and eczema; angry during increasing, dry during decreasing, moon; intense itching < washing in cold water, wet poultices, warmth of bed, at night.

Urethral stricture; *inflammatory or organic,* with serous infiltration and formation of submucous callosity (Petros.).

Sleepless; restless tossing about, sleepy but unable to sleep from internal dry heat.

Aggravation.—Washing in cold water; wet poultices.

Type.—Remittent; typhoid; continued.

Cause.—Often from diseases of genital organs, especially suppressed gonorrhea; from exposure, getting wet; bathing while warm.

Chill.—With shivering, followed by sweat, without intervening heat, < uncovering.

Heat.—Of one side only; dry, at night with a general hot sensation.

Sweat.—Profuse at night; after midnight.

Cannot bear to be uncovered.

While convalescing from typhoid, sudden stupor and look as if dying.

COCCULUS.

For women and children with light hair and eyes, who suffer severely during menstruation and pregnancy; unmarried and childless women.

Adapted to book-worms, sensitive, romantic girls with irregular menstruation; rakes, onanists and persons debilitated by sexual excesses.

Nausea or vomiting **from riding in carriage, boat or railroad car** (Arn., Nux m.), *or even looking at a boat in motion;* sea-sickness.

Headache: in nape and occiput; extending to the spine; as if tightly bound by a cord; with nausea, as if at sea; at each menstrual period; < by lying on back of head.

Sick headache from carriage, boat or train riding.

Diseases peculiar to drunkards.

Time passes too quickly (Ther.—too slowly, Arg. n., Can. I.).

Cannot bear contradiction; easily offended; every trifle makes him angry; speaks hastily (Anac.).

Great lassitude of the whole body; it requires exertion to stand firmly; feels too weak to talk loudly.

Bad effects: from **loss of sleep,** *mental excitement and night watching* (Colch.); feel weak if they lose but one hour's sleep; convulsions after loss of sleep; of anger and grief.

Vertigo: as if intoxicated, when rising in bed or from carriage riding; must lie down (Bry.—worse when sitting than walking, and extreme when lying down and closing the eyes, Apis).

Sensation: in abdomen of cutting and rubbing on every movement, as of sharp stones; of hollowness in head and other parts (Ign.).

During the effort to menstruate she is so weak she *is scarcely able to stand* from weakness of lower limbs (Alum., Carbo a.); after each period hemorrhoids.

Leucorrhea: in place of menses, or between periods (Iod., Xan.); like the washings of meat; like serum, ichorous, bloody; during pregnancy.

Aggravation.—Drinking, eating, sleeping, smoking, talking, riding in a carriage, cold air; motion of carriage, swing or ship.

Amelioration.—At night, after sweat.

Type.—Bilious and lingering gastric; insidious, "sneaking," low, typhoid, nervous; especially when produced by fits of anger or disposition to anger.

Prodrome.—Great dread of the coming paroxysm (Nat.).

Time.—8-11 A. M. Afternoon or evening.

Chill.—*Without thirst.* Chilliness alternating with heat. Shaking chill for half an hour at 8 A. M., without thirst and without subsequent heat (**Caust.**). Shaking chill over the whole body in the afternoon, or in the evening. Chill, **with severe colic,** *not relieved by a warm stove;* with lameness of the small of the back; chill more in the back and on the legs; in afternoon or evening; with shivering through the whole body; not > by external warmth. Continuous chilliness with hot skin. Chilliness at 11 A. M. with disgust for even smell of food. Shaking chill (upward and downward) ceases when diarrhea and vomiting set in. Nervous, spasmodic symptoms. The cold stage is predominant.

Heat.—Without thirst. Dry heat during the night. Flushes of heat, with burning cheeks and cold feet. *Intolerance of both cold and warm air* (of cold air, **Bar., Camph.**). Burning heat in the cheeks, which are *glowing hot,* with coldness of whole body, or only of the feet (**Caps.**). Now one hand, now the other, is alternately hot or cold (**Dig.**—see **Caust.**—one foot hot the other cold, **Lyc.**). Vertigo and nausea on raising the head. Stupor with consciousness.

Sweat.—Of the body from evening till morning, which is *cold only on the face.* Sweat in the morning, especially on the chest. Cold sweat, now on one, now on the other hand. *Sweat over the whole body during the slightest motion* (**Bry.**). Sweat of the affected parts (**Amb., Ant. t.**).

Tongue.—Coated white, edges dry. Loss of appetite, with metallic taste (Mer.). Tobacco tastes bitter. Aversion to sour things (desire for pickles, **Ant. c.**).

Apyrexia.—When the fever threatens to assume a slow, "sneaking," nervous form, attended with vertigo; dull pains in the head, general weakness and physical depression; anorexia, with a tongue comparatively clean, but a marked tendency to nausea—as if the stomach was always nauseated, Cocculus should be thought of.

COFFEA.

Characteristic.—Over-sensitiveness; all the senses more acute, sight, hearing, smell, taste, touch (Bell., Cham., Opium).

Ailments: the bad effects of sudden emotions or pleasurable surprises (Caust.—exciting or bad news, Gels.); weeping from delight; alternate laughing and weeping.

Pains are felt intensely; seem almost insupportable; driving to despair (Acon., Cham.).

Sleepless, *wide-awake condition;* ecstacy, full of ideas, no sleep in consequence; physical excitement through mental exaltation.

Headache: from over-mental exertion, thinking, talking; one-sided, as from a nail driven into the brain (Ign., Nux, Ver.); as if the brain were torn or dashed to pieces, < in open air.

Unusual activity of mind and body.

Intermittent, jerking toothache; relieved by holding ice water in the mouth, but returns when water becomes warm (Bry., Caust., Puls., Sep.).

Aggravation.—*Excessive joy;* cold open air; narcotics.

Amelioration.—Warmth; during rest; evening until midnight.

Type.—Simple; quartan (?).

Time.—3 and 8 P. M.; fever usually without chill.

Chill.—Without thirst. Coldness and chilliness running all through the limbs. *Chills running down the back.* Chilly feeling, with external and internal warmth (**Cinch.**). Internal shivering, with external heat of face or whole body. Chills ascend from the fingers and toes to nape of neck, thence to vertex; increased by exercise (relieved by exercise, **Caps.**). Great sensitiveness to cold (**Bar.**). Cold hands and feet. Flushes of heat, or currents of cold air down the back. *Ecstacy.*

Heat.—*With thirst.* External, dry heat of the skin. External heat, with thirst, and shivering in the back after lying down at night. Dry heat at night, with hot flushes to the face, hot cheeks, and delirium. *Dry warmth of the face.* Feeling of heat when in bed, yet avoids being uncovered (**Acon.**—must uncover, **Bell.**). One cheek hot and red, with constant shuddering (**Cham.**). *Ecstacy.*

Sweat.—*With thirst.* Morning sweat. General over whole body, most on palms of hands, and in the face, with internal shivering. Extremely sensitive and nervous.

COLCHICUM AUTUMNALE.

Characteristic.—Adapted to the rheumatic, gouty diathesis; persons of a robust vigorous constitution. Old people's diseases.

External impressions, such as bright light, strong odors, contact, grief, *misdeeds of others,* make him quite beside himself (Nux, Staph.).

Pains are drawing, tearing, pressing; superficial during warm weather; affect the bones and deeper tissues when air is cold. From left to right.

Smell very acute; *the odor of cooking food causes nausea* (Ars., Sep.).

Aversion to food; loathing even the sight or still more the smell of it.

The abdomen is immensely *distended with gas,* feeling as if it would burst.

Burning or icy coldness in stomach and abdomen.

Autumnal dysentery, discharges from bowels contain white shreddy particles in large quantities. "Scrapings of intestines" (Canth., Carb. ac.).

Affected parts very sensitive to motion and contact.

Aggravation.—At night; mental emotion or exertion.

Motion: if the patient lie perfectly still the disposition to vomit is less urgent. Every motion renews it (Bry.).

Type.—Not marked. Epidemic or autumnal fevers, intermittent and remittent.

Low fevers following epidemic dysentery.

Time.—Hour not marked.

Prodrome.—Thirst for cold water; drinking is followed by coldness in stomach and beginning of chill.

Chill.—And shivering, running down the back, through the limbs; even in a warm room. Nose, cheeks and **extremities cold.** Chilly shivering in stomach and abdomen. Coldness in evening > by warm covering, but returning on going to bed as a chilliness, with chattering of the teeth, disappearing after a short time while lying still; it threatened to return on motion.

Heat.—External dry heat the whole night, with violent, unquenchable thirst. Internal with attacks of flushes of heat, or short flushes of heat intermingled with chilliness, even near the warm stove. *Great heat of the face,* of the hands and feet.

Sweat.—Wanting or *suppressed;* or profuse, easily produced; *sour-smelling sweat.*

Tongue.—Heavy, stiff, insensible; bright red; covered with a **downy white fur** (milky white coating, Ant. c.). Desire for, or aversion to, food, with loathing when merely looking at it, *and still more when smelling it;* the smell of broth nauseates, and that of fish, eggs, or fat meat, almost makes him faint.

Nausea with great restlessness; on assuming the upright position, great inclination to vomit.

Apyrexia.—Never clear. The gastric symptoms which come to the surface during this stage are usually characteristic.

Analysis.—In Colchicum we frequently find the *genus epidemicus* for the intermittents so often met with late in autumn, when epidemic dysentery prevails. The gastric and abdominal symptoms are guiding; especially sensitive to odor of food.

A CASE.—In the autumn of 1866, L. C. æt. 30, was attacked with ague of the quotidian type. The case lasted some eighteen days, a chill every day, and every day alike. It began at 10 A. M. with violent thirst, intense headache, greatly aggravated by the slightest motion, so that the patient lay on his right side with his head almost down to his knees, and moved only when the distress was so intense he could not avoid it. Wanted to be covered, but no relief from the covering. Chill lasted about an hour, and was followed by intense heat lasting about two hours, with continuance of thirst and headache, when the sweat began, with immediate relief of all the symptoms. He received a single dose of *Bryonia* 200. The next day the chill returned and I got this additional symptom: *he could not bear the sight or smell of food.* This suggested *Colchicum,* but, careful not to spoil the case by too hasty prescriptions, I gave Sac. lac. I took time to study *Colchicum.* My attention being given almost wholly to the fever symptoms, I concluded *Colchicum* did not cover the case, and gave *Nat.* 200, one dose. The chill returned the next day; but Hering says *Natrum* is a slow acting remedy, and I thought we must give it time. I waited four days with just the same chill every day. Soon it appeared that every day the chill began with a desire for cold water, immediately after swallowing which he begins to be cold in the stomach, the coldness at once becoming general. It is not necessary for me to mention the various remedies he received, as I floundered day after day trying to cure intermittent fever, with that symptom of the appetite prominent before me all the time. At length a friend called, and I asked him to go with me to see the case. He did so, and making his examination, took copious notes of the symptoms, till he struck that symptom of the appetite, when he whispered to me *"Colchicum."* "Yes," I said, "but that is the only symptom of it in the case." He finished his examination, and we gave Sac. lac. The next morning my friend called at my office and said: "That is *Colchicum* or *Cocculus;* I am not sure which." "Well," I said, "if you say *Colchicum,* here goes;" and putting a vial of Fincke's 21 m. in my pocket, I went at once to see my patient. I found him in a chill, as usual. I gave him Sac. lac. in solution, once in two hours, and left a powder of *Colchicum* 21 m. to be taken as soon as the paroxysm was over. He never had another chill. Moral: Treat the patient, not the disease.—WM. A. HAWLEY, M. D.

CONIUM MACULATUM.

Characteristic.—Especially suitable for diseases of old men, old maids; women with rigid muscles; persons with light hair who are easily excited; strong persons of sedentary habits.

Debility of old people; complaints caused by a blow or fall; cancerous and scrofulous persons with enlarged glands; complaints during and after climacteric.

No inclination for business or study; indolent, indifferent, takes no interest in anything.

Memory weak, unable to sustain any mental effort.

Morose; easily vexed; domineering, quarrelsome, scolds, will not bear contradiction (Aur.); excitement of any kind causes mental depression.

Dreads being alone, but avoids society (Bis., Kali c., Lyc.).

Vertigo: particularly when **lying down or turning in bed.** Moving the head or the eyes even slightly; on turning the head to the left (Col.); of old people; with ovarian or uterine ailments.

Menses: *feeble, suppressed;* too late, scanty, of short duration; with rash of small red pimples over body which ceases with the flow (Dul.); stopped by taking cold; *by putting hands in cold water* (Lac d.).

Leucorrhea: *ten days after menses* (Bor., Bov.); acrid; bloody; milky; profuse; thick, intermits.

Bad effects: of **suppressed sexual desire,** or *suppressed menses;* non-gratification of sexual instinct, or from excessive indulgence.

Glandular indurations of *stony hardness;* of mammæ and testicles in persons of cancerous tendency; after injuries of glands (Ast. r.).

Breasts sore, hard and painful during menstrual period (Lac c.); hysterical symptoms and vertigo increased

Cough: in spasmodic paroxysms, caused by dry spot in larynx (dry spot in throat, Actea); itching in chest and throat (Iod.); worse at night; when lying down; during pregnancy (Caust., Kali br.).

Great difficulty in voiding urine; flow intermits, then flows again; prostatic or uterine affections.

Aggravation.—At night; lying down; cold air; rising in bed.

Amelioration.—In the dark; moving; when walking.

Type.—Quotidian; simple.

Time.—4 or 5 A. M.—3 to 5 P. M. Very ill humored from 5 to 6 P. M.

Chill.—With trembling in all the limbs, and *constant desire for warmth,* especially **for heat of sun** (for heat of stove, **Lach.**—relieved by covering up, **Nux, Rhus**—warm air seems cold, **Thuja.**). Chilliness in the back, with cold hands and blue nails. Internal chill in the morning; with shivering in the afternoon. Extremities and whole body were icy cold. Shivering over the whole body.

Heat.—With thirst, and redness of the face. *Great internal and external heat, with great nervousness. Heat, with* **profuse sweat at same time.** Uneasy sleep, great trembling, and short, rapid, snoring respiration.

Sweat.—*Day and night,* **as soon as he sleeps, even when closing the eyes** (*sweats when awake, dry heat when he sleeps,* **Samb.**). Sweat over whole body, with redness of face. Sweat while sitting in a chair and dozing. Night sweat with offensive odor; smarting the skin (**Canth.**). Profuse sweat on limbs, perineum, genitals (**Hep., Thuja**). "Eruption during sweat" (what kind?).

Tongue.—Stiff and painful; taste bitter; saliva thready; lips and tongue *dry and sticky* (**Nux m.**). Craves coffee, salt, or sour things.

Pulse: slow and full or small and quick; pulsation in blood vessels of the whole body.

Apyrexia.—Complete; sometimes with vertigo on lying down.

Analysis.—*Chill;* with desire for heat of sun.

Heat; with profuse sweat at same time.

Sweat; as soon as he sleeps (Cinch.), even closing the eyes.

If the mental, urinary, or menstrual symptoms or the vertigo be present, the case is clear.

CROCUS SATIVUS.

Frequent and extreme changes in sensations; *sudden, from the greatest hilarity to the deepest despondency* (Ign., Nux m.).

Excessively happy, affectionate, wants to kiss everybody; the next moment in a rage.

Hemorrhage from any part, blood black, viscid, clotted, forming into **long black strings hanging from the bleeding surface** (Elaps).

Headache: during climacteric, throbbing, pulsating, < *during two or three days of accustomed menstrual flow;* nervous or menstrual headache before, during or after the flow (Lach., Lil., Sep.).

Eyes: sensation, as if room were filled with smoke; as if had been weeping; as of cold wind blowing across the eyes; closing lids tightly gives >.

Nosebleed: **black, tenacious, stringy, every drop can be turned into a thread;** with cold sweat in large drops on forehead (cold sweat, but wants to be fanned; with bright red blood, Carbo v.); in children who develop too rapidly (Cal., Phos.).

Dysmenorrhea: flow black, stringy, clotted (Ust.).

Sensation as if something alive were moving in the stomach,

abdomen, uterus, arms or other parts of the body (Sab., Thuja, Sul.); with nausea and faintness.

Chorea and hysteria with great hilarity, singing and dancing (Tar.); alternating with melancholy and rage.

Spasmodic contractions and twitchings of single sets of muscles (Agar., Ign., Zinc.).

Relation.—Nux, Puls. or Sul. follows Crocus well in nearly all complaints; in menstrual derangements (Ust.).

Compare: Tub., Staph., which have many symptoms in common.

Aggravation.—Motion (hemorrhage).

Amelioration.—Open air (all symptoms).

Time.—Afternoon; < towards evening.

Chill.—With thirst (Dul.); in the afternoon, increasing towards evening; with shivering from the back down the legs (Dul., Staph.); < by drinking.

Heat.—With thirst (Staph.); internal flushes with pricking and crawling in the skin; of head and face, with pale cheeks. Violent heat over whole body, < in the head, with intense redness of face and distention of blood vessels (Cinch., Cham.); great thirst without much dryness of mouth.

Sweat.—Scanty; only on lower half of body; or only at night, then cold and debilitating.

Analysis.—"Croc., Dul. and Staph. may be compared.

All have chill beginning in back.

Croc. and Dul. have thirst with chill, Staph. has not.

Croc. and Staph. have great thirst with heat, which is slight or wanting with Dul.

Dul. and Staph. have frequent urination in chill, Croc. has not.

Dul. alone has nausea and involuntary urine during chill.

With Croc. alone the chill is < by drinking.

Dul. has chill < in a warm room."—Geo. H. Clark, M. D.

CROTALUS.

Characteristic.—Is indicated in strumous, debilitated hemorrhagic, broken down constitutions; during zymotic diseases; in inebriates; tendency to carbuncles or blood boils (Anthr.).

Diseases caused by a previous low state of the system; low septic, typhoid or malarial fever; chronic alcoholism; exhausted vital force; genuine collapse.

Apoplexy; apoplectic convulsions in inebriates, hemorrhagic or broken down constitutions.

Hemorrhagic diathesis; blood flows from eyes, ears, nose, and every orifice of the body; *bloody sweat.*

Yellow color of conjunctiva; clears up vision after keratitis or kerato-iritis.

Malignant jaundice; hematic rather than hepatic.

Purpura hemorrhagica; comes on suddenly from all orifices, skin, nails, gums.

Prostration of vital force; pulse scarcely felt; blood poisoning (Pyr.).

Vomiting: bilious, with anxiety and weak pulse; every month after menstruation; cannot lie on r. side or back without instantly producing dark, green vomiting; black or coffee ground, of yellow fever.

Diarrhea: stools black, thin, like coffee-grounds; offensive; from noxious effluvia or septic matters in food or drinks; from "high game" (Pyr.); during yellow fever, cholera, typhoid, typhus.

Intestinal hemorrhage when occurring in typical, septic or zymotic disease; blood dark, fluid, non-coagulable.

Dissecting wounds; insect stings; bad effects of vaccination,

Vicarious menstruation; in debilitated constitutions (Dig., Phos.).

Menopause: intense flushings and drenching perspirations;

faintness and sinking at stomach; prolonged metrorrhagia, dark, fluid, offensive; profound anemia.

Malignant diseases of uterus, great tendency to hemorrhage, blood dark, fluid offensive.

Type.—Every type, but low grades, and all tend to malignancy; yellow fever; low, septic, typhoid states; pernicious fevers.

Fevers with a hemorrhagic tendency.

Cause.—Previous low states of system; alcoholic, septic, zymotic, miasmatic; depraved blood supply; debilitated capillaries; exhausted vital powers; hemorrhagic diathesis; psoric, sycotic, syphilitic complications; bubonic plague.

Chill.—Light. Chilliness and crawling sensation for five or six hours in afternoon; creeping chills up and down the back, chilliness alternating with heat or sudden cold sweat; skin *dry and cold,* especially of extremities.

Heat.—In first onset intense, burning heat; skin hot and dry; pulse, 130-150; temp., 104-106; face red, flushed; epistaxis.

Hardenstein gives following in yellow fever. Delirium, eyes open; confused, disconnected answers with cold skin and rapid pulse; severe headache; face red, puffed, yellow or pale leaden hue; hemorrhage from every orifice of the body, even bloody sweat; acrid sour eructations; intense thirst; nausea and vomiting of bile, of blood, on least exertion; bloody, involuntary stool; abdomen tympanitic; swelling of inguinal glands; urine scanty or retained; pulse weak and slow, or rapid, intermittent and scarcely perceptible; intensely yellow skin; ecchymosis or purple spots; great prostration of vital force; spasms, convulsions, syncope, death.

Sweat.—Cold, in sudden attacks; dark colored axillæ; bloody sweat (Cur., Lach., Lyc.).

Tongue.—Fiery red, smooth and polished (Pyr.); intensely swollen; dry and cracked; dark brown streak down the centre with deep red edges; yellowish brown, dry in centre; protruded.

Breath fetid; mouldy odor. Hemorrhage.

Pulse.—Rapid, feeble and quick, then slow; feeble, fluttering, frequent, quick, small, thready, trembling, scarcely perceptible; in waves, irregular.

Analysis.—Hemorrhage from every outlet of the body; black, fluid, non-coagulable, offensive. Low types, septic, malignant.

Lachesis, the skin is cold and clammy.

Crotalus, the skin is cold and dry.

CYCLAMEN.

Characteristic.—Best suited for leuco-phlegmatic persons with anemic or chlorotic conditions; easily fatigued, and in consequence not inclined to any kind of labor; feeble or suspended functions of organs or special senses.

Pale, chlorotic, deranged menses (Fer., Puls.), accompanied by vertigo, headache, dim vision.

Pains; pressive, drawing or tearing of parts where bones lie near the surface.

Ailments: from suppressed grief and terrors of conscience; from duty not done or bad act committed.

Great sadness and peevishness; irritable, morose, ill-humored; inclined to weep; desire for solitude; *aversion to open air* (rev. of Puls.).

Headache in anemic patients, with flickering before eyes or dim vision, on rising in morning.

Flickering before eyes, fiery sparks, as of various colors, glittering needles; dim vision of fog or smoke.

Satiety after a few mouthfuls (Lyc.), food then becomes repugnant, causes nausea in throat and palate.

Saliva and all food has a salty taste.

Menses: too early; too profuse, black and clotted (too late, pale, scanty, Puls.); membranous; better during flow (worse during, Act., Puls.).

Burning sore pain in heels, when sitting, standing or walking in open air (Agar., Caust., Phyt., Val.).

Relations.—Compare: Puls., Cinch., Fer., in chlorosis and anemic affections; Croc., Thuja as if something alive in abdomen.

Aggravation.—Open air; cold water; cold bathing; menses < sitting and lying at night; fat food.

Amelioration.—In a warm room, in-doors; menses > walking (leucorrhea, < sitting, > walking, Cac., Coc.).

Chill.—Begins in tips of fingers, toes and ears. Chilliness, general, not > by covering. Evening chill, very sensitive to cold air and uncovering. Chill forenoon and evening.

Heat and chill alternately; without thirst: with very cold hands.

Heat: of single parts (except face); after eating; of whole body; with swelling of veins of hands.

Heat, principally of face, without thirst; hands remain cold a long time.

Heat: of various parts of face and hands, with swelling of veins of hands; after heating, general.

Sweat.—At night, in sleep, offensive; sometimes only on lower part of body.

Analysis.—Especially to be thought of for the fevers of the anemic during the puerperal state or early months of lactation. The constitutional symptoms are guiding.

CURARA.

Characteristic.—Debility of old age, great failure of strength. Nervous debility from loss of fluids, or exhausting illness.

Spinal lesions, idiopathic or traumatic; sensation acute, motion paralyzed; painless paralysis.

Aggravation.—*Dampness, damp weather, change of weather, cold wind,* or *the least movement.*

Amelioration.—After *the first mouthful of food.* (Compare with **Aran.**)

Type.—Quotidian. Type not marked.

Time.—*2* or *3* P. M., *every day, and continuing well into the night.*

Chill.—Without thirst. Coldness commencing on the abdomen and spreading all over. Sensation of shivering, starting from the stomach and spreading over the whole body. Constant chilliness.

Heat.—With thirst; especially in the head, on the back and legs; burning in the hips; great weakness and prostration, crampy pains on the least movement. Fever with thirst and *great hunger;* yawning and stretching, hot head and hands, convulsive paroxysms and fainting. Daily fever, commencing at 2 or 3 P. M., and continuing well into the night; burning heat, accompanied by partial and transient chills, incoherent speech, and often by paralysis of the extremities. Lips get blue and body purple; after fever very red face, hammering headache. *Pernicious fever, with constant chilliness* (**Petr.**); heat increased at night or in the open air; less in the morning.

Sweat.—*Cold and bloody,* especially at night.

Tongue.—Deep red, cracked and bleeding.

Neither our provings nor clinical experience of Curara are sufficient to define many characteristics.

DIGITALIS.

Characteristic.—Suitable for sudden flushes of heat, followed by great nervous weakness and irregular, intermitting pulse, occurring at climacteric; < by least motion.

Sensation as if heart would stop beating if she moved (Cocaine—fears that unless constantly on the move, heart will cease beating, Gels.—See Fer.). Weak heart without valvular complications.

Faintness or sinking at the stomach, feels as if he were dying.

Great weakness of chest, cannot bear to talk (Stan.).

At night frequent waking in a fright, as from a dream, as if he fell from a height or into the water.

Face pale, death-like appearance and bluish-red.

Blueness of skin, eyelids, lips, tongue; cyanosis.

Distended veins on lids, ears, lips and tongue.

Respiration irregular, difficult, deep sighing.

The fingers "go to sleep" frequently and easily.

Dropsy: post-scarlatinal; in Bright's disease; with suppression of urine; of internal and external parts; with fainting when there are organic affections of the heart (with soreness in uterine region, Conv.).

Fatal syncope may occur when being raised to upright position.

Aggravation.—Headache by lying down; motion; in a warm room; sitting, especially when sitting erect.

Time.—No periodicity. Generally in early morning.

Chill.—Commencing in the fingers; palms of the hands, soles of the feet, thence over the whole body. Coldness first of hands and arms (of extremities, **Gels.**—of arms, **Bell.**, **Hell.**—in fingers, toes and lips, **Bry.**, **Cic.**). *Great coldness of skin. Great sensitiveness to the cold* (**Bar. c.**, **Camph.**); chilliness and shivering over the whole back; internal chill with external heat; chill and heat in alternation; *cold extremities;* excessive coldness of the hands and feet, with cold sweat. Chilliness over the whole body with heat and redness of the face.

Heat.—Without thirst. Sudden flushes of heat followed by weakness of all parts. General violent heat, with swollen veins and rapid pulse. *One hand hot, the other cold* (**Lyc.**—one hand is burning hot and pale, the other cold and red, Mosch.). Heat of body, with cold sweat of face. **Heat in the** head, face and ears, hands, with redness of the cheeks.

Sweat.—Immediately after the chill (**Bov., Caust.**—heat with profuse sweat at same time, **Con.**). Night-sweat, generally cold and clammy. *Covered with a copious perspiration, without relief of heart* symptoms. Cold sweat on body, warm sweat on palms of hands. Sweat on upper parts of body; on the face.

Tongue.—Clean or coated white. Taste: desire for sour drinks and bitter food; bread tastes bitter; want of appetite, or hunger. Constant ptyalism.

Pulse.—Third, fifth or seventh beat intermits. *Extremely slow and weak* when at rest; *accelerated, full and hard from every motion.* Often characteristic.

Digitalis should not be followed by Cinchona in any form, as according to Hahnemann, Cinchona increases the anxiety caused by Digitalis to deadly anguish.

DROSERA.

Characteristic.—Whooping-cough; in violent paroxysms, which follow each other so rapidly he is scarcely able to get his breath.

Cough: < by warmth; drinking; singing; laughing; weeping; **lying down**; after midnight; spasmodic with gagging, retching and vomiting.

Clergymen's sore throat (Arg. n., Arum); with rough, scraping, dry sensation deep in the fauces.

Constriction and crawling in larynx, hoarseness and yellow or green sputa.

Aggravation.—After midnight; warmth; during rest.

Type.—Quotidian; tertian.

Time.—Before 9 A. M., *every morning.*

Cause.—Frequently called for where fevers occur during prevalence of epidemic pertussis, then it often becomes the genus epidemicus.

Chill.—*Without thirst.* Chill with *icy cold hands, blue nails, cold, pale face* (**Nux**), *and cold extremities;* must lie down. *Febrile shivers over the whole body, with heat of the face and icy coldness of the hands,* and sometimes bilious vomiting. He always feels too cold, he cannot get warm (**Cal.**); he feels cold at night in bed; shivering during rest, but not during motion (chill, heat and sweat all relieved by motion, **Caps.**); even in bed he is unable to keep from shivering and feeling cold, though body is warm to touch (**Bar.**). Spasmodic cough with violent pressing, pulsating pains in the head. After midnight, coldness of the *left half of the face,* with sticking pains in it; the right half hot and dry (see **Caust.**). Constant chilliness, *cannot get warm* (**Aran.**).

Heat.—*Without thirst. Heat at night, chilly during the day.* Heat *worse after midnight.* Heat almost exclusively on face and head. Increased warmth of upper body, evening. After chilliness, slight thirst, heaviness of head, throbbing pain in the occiput, and heat of face, usual warmth of rest of body, lasting till 3 P. M. Feels well in the evening.

Sweat.—Cold sweat on face, feet, *abdomen.* Warm sweat, particularly just after midnight; *most profuse on* **face and abdomen.** Sometimes genera' sweat, particularly *at night,* attended with a *spasmodic cough, which brought on retching and nausea.*

Tongue.—Clean (**Cina**). *Food has no taste* (**Eup.**). Bread tastes bitter.

"Profuse discharge of watery saliva during febrile stage." —HAHNEMANN.

"Intermittent fever, with sore throat and nausea."—LIPPE.

Apyrexia.—Usually clear, though gastric symptoms may be present at times (clear with good appetite, **Canch.**). *Coughs* *more than in sweating stage.* As in Aranea and Bovista, the chill predominates, the other stages being light, sometimes only partially developed.

DULCAMARA.

Characteristic.—Adapted to persons of phlegmatic, scrofulous constitutions; restless, irritable; subject to catarrhal, rheumatic or skin affections, brought on or aggravated by cold, damp, rainy weather, or sudden changes in hot weather (Bry.).

The skin is delicate, sensitive to cold, liable to eruptions, especially urticaria, every time patient takes cold, or is long exposed to the cold.

Anasarca; after ague, rheumatism, scarlatina, measles.

Dropsy after suppressed sweat, or suppressed skin diseases, from cold air or damp dwellings; working in a milk dairy (Aran., Ars., Nat. s.).

Diarrhea from taking cold, in damp places or damp weather.

Catarrhal ischuria in grown up children, with milky urine; from *wading with bare feet in cold water.*

Rash before the menses (Con.—during profuse menses, Bell., Graph.).

Urticaria over whole body, no fever; itching, burns after scratching; < in warmth, > in cold.

Warts, fleshy, large, smooth; on face or back of hands and fingers.

Cannot find the right word for anything. Mental confusion.

Relations.—Complementary: to Baryta carb., Kali s.

Aggravation.—Evening; during rest; cold, damp weather; suppressed menses, eruptions, sweat.

Amelioration.—From moving about (Fer.); warm, dry air.

Type.—Double quotidian; tertian; double tertian; double quartan. Continued; typhoid.

Time.—Irregular hours.

Cause.—Fevers occurring during cold, damp, rainy weather; worse when weather suddenly becomes colder; caused by exposure; living in damp rooms, sleeping in a damp bed.

Chill.—With violent thirst. Commencing in or spreading from the back; not relieved by warmth (relieved by hot applications, **Caps.**); shaking, with a feeling of coldness, or actual coldness over the whole body, so that he could not get warm near the hot stove, with shuddering from time to time. Chilliness of the back, without thirst, in the open air, but especially in a draught (**Canth.**). Chilliness mostly toward evening, over the back, nape of the neck, occiput, with a feeling as if the hair stood on end (**Bar.**). With nausea and frequent or involuntary urine.

Heat.—General, dry, burning heat all over. Dry heat over whole body; heat and burning in the back. Burning in the skin of the whole back as if he were sitting by a hot stove, with sweat in the face and moderate heat.

Sweat.—*Offensive sweat,* night and morning, over the whole body; during the day more over back, in axillæ, and palms of hands. *Badly smelling sweat,* with profuse discharge of transparent urine. Often wanting.

Tongue.—Dry; swollen, as if paralyzed with cold. Bitter taste. Ptyalism; the gums are loose and spongy; saliva tenacious, soap-like. *Great desire for cold drinks.*

Analysis.—Like Aranea, the fevers to which Dulcamara is adapted, are rare. They are caused by rheumatic exposure, living in damp rooms, sleeping in a damp bed; during cold, rainy, changeable weather; but the fever of Aranea comes on with great regularity, while that of Dulcamara has no reference to time. Compare Crocus and Staphysagria.

Typhoid fever, when patient distinctly remembers having taken cold; tongue clean, stools yellow, liquid, with rumbling, cutting, digging or griping pain in umbilical region or whole abdomen.

ELATERIUM.

Characteristic.—Cholera morbus-like attacks; copious, liquid, frothy dejections; profuse flow of watery serum from mucous membrane.

When chills were suppressed, urticaria appeared over the whole body. Unlike Apis, Hepar, Ign., Rhus, in which the urticaria appears during different stages of the paroxysm.

Relations.—Compare, Colch., Crot. t., Sec., Ver., in diarrheic and choleraic symptoms.

Type.—Quotidian; double quotidian; tertian; double tertian; quartan. When suppressed by Quinine or "ague cures," prone to appear under some other type, or even assume the double type. *Frequent change of type.* Bilious. Remittent.

Time.—12 M.—1 P. M.—*Twice a day,* every third day.

Prodrome.—Chilliness with continued gaping and quivering; headache and soreness of the limbs, and pains in the bowels.

Chill.—With thirst, increased pain in the head and limbs and continued gaping and stretching. Pain under shoulder-blades; in small of back, left side, and cramps in the legs and soles of the feet. Yawning and gaping, with a sound resembling the neighing of a horse; lachrymation and profuse coryza.

Heat.—With intense thirst; violent, tearing pains throughout the head, more especially on the vertex. Increased cutting pains in bowels, and pains in extremities; the pains *shooting to the very tips of the fingers and toes,* and then shooting back again into the body. *Nausea, vomiting and copious discharges from the bowels of a frothy character.*

Sweat.—Copious, with gradual relief of all the symptoms.

Tongue.—Coated with a dirty brown fur; taste bitter.

Apyrexia.—Urticaria; intolerable itching > by rubbing.

Analysis.—If urticaria appear all over the body after suppression of intermittent fever, Elaterium is the remedy. Cutting pains in bowels, shooting to tips of fingers and toes. Copious frothy discharges. When chills were suppressed urticaria developed over whole surface, with a disordered state of mind, characterized by an irresistible propensity to wander from home, even in the night, and range the woods.

ELAPS.

Characteristic.—Fearful and apprehensive of some fatal disease.

Fear of being left alone, as if something horrible might happen.

Angry about one's self; does not wish to be spoken to.

At the least contradiction, body shudders, blood boils (Aur., Coc., Con., Fer.).

Vertigo with tendency to fall forward.

Weight in the stomach after eating.

Canine hunger, yet unable to eat.

Fruits and drinks lie on the stomach like ice (see Ars., Verat.).

Type.—Quotidian.

Time.—8 and 10 P. M., every day.

Chill.—Without thirst, followed by dry heat and burning redness of the face. *Chilliness and heat alternately* (**Ars., Cal.**) at 8 P. M.; *chilly for a few minutes,* then *heat for a quarter of an hour. Shaking chill,* felt internally as if *in the bones,* followed in half an hour by *burning heat;* the skin is hot, with thirst, the fever lasted whole night until 10 A. M. next day. Coldness < *by drinking cold water* (**Caps.**); after a drink, shivering from head to foot with chattering of the teeth. Terrible coldness after drinking, and as if ice water were rising and falling through a cylindrical opening in left lung. Great sensitiveness to cold. Right leg up to knee, cold as ice. Arms cold by putting hand in cold water.

Heat.—With thirst, *alternating with chilliness. Dry heat* from 7 to 9 P. M., followed by *chill till 10 P. M.* Fever at 7 P. M., with less chill, more violent heat, but little sweat; sleep interrupted by heavy dreams (of dead people), with difficult breathing the whole night. *Flushes of heat, with redness of the face and ears.*

Sweat.—All over. Sweat cold and profuse. Sweat on forehead and nape of the neck.

Tongue.—Deep red, clean, or swollen and black.

EUCALYPTUS.

For many years this has been a popular remedy in Australia, Italy, Algiers, some places in Spain, and Provence, France. The leaves possess a very penetrating odor, which is diffused to a great distance, and it appears to possess the power of antidoting marsh miasm and thus exercising a preventive action. The Abbé Féles Charmatant, missionary priest to the African missions, Algiers, writes: "I will give you some facts about our *Eucalyptus* plantations at Maison-Carrée, which is now become our Mother-House. This estate was, six years ago, an immense territory covered with brush, dwarf-palms, and rendered very unhealthy by the neighborhood of the stagnant waters of Harach. In 1869 and 1870, as fast as the brush was destroyed, we planted a considerable quantity of *Eucalyptus* in groups, or beside paths the whole length of our fields and gardens, and the result was most marvellous; for the intermittent fever, which often stopped our orphans in their agricultural labor, has gradually disappeared, so that to-day this domain, formerly the most subject to fevers, is now one of the most healthy suburbs of Algiers."

Our pathogenesis of this remedy has not been sufficient to give us any definite indications for its use. It is used as a substitute for Quinine by the other school of practice.

Characteristic.—Excessive salivation.

Mental exhilaration; irresistible desire to move about, sensation of buoyancy and increased strength. Congestive headache in the anemic, > pain and induces sleep.

Vascular tumors of the urethra (Thuja).

Diuresis with enormous quantities of urea.

Type.—Intermittent, quotidian, tertian, double tertian; remittent, continued, malarial, typhoid; all fevers tend to low types with subnormal temperature. Relapsing fevers of tuberculous subjects; the so-called La Grippe, sporadic influenza.

Fevers of a **relapsing,** obstinate and prolonged character, of a miasmatic origin, in which the spleen becomes affected early in the disease. It is at first swollen and sensitive, then becomes more resistant, harder, bunchy on its surface. Vertigo is pronounced in all its stages. There is a dull congestive headache; malaise; rheumatic pains of a jerking, tearing, stitching character, < at night.

Sweat.—Profuse, offensive, exhausting.

When convalescing from malarial fevers; chronic malarial affections; quinine cachexia.

EUPATORIUM PERFOLIATUM.

Characteristic.—Adapted to diseases of old people; worn-out constitutions, especially from inebriety; cachexia, from prolonged or frequent attacks of bilious or intermittent fevers.

Bruised feeling, as if broken, all over the body (Arn., Lac can., Pyr.).

Bone pains; affecting the back, limbs, head, chest, particularly the wrists as if dislocated, the eyeballs; the more general and severe the better adapted. Like Bryonia, they are accompanied by headache, constipation and pain in hepatic region, but here the similitude ends.

In Bryonia, the perspiration is profuse, easily excited by motion, and the pains compel patient to lie still upon the painful side.

In Eupatorium the sweat is scanty or wanting, the pains cause restlessness without any relief from motion, and there is entire inability to lie on left side.

Pains as if broken; come quickly and go away as quickly (Bell., Mag. p., Eup. pur.—reverse of Stan.).

Vertigo: sensation as if falling to the left (cannot turn the head to the left for fear of falling, Col., Con.).

Cough: chronic; loose with hectic; chest sore, must support it with hands (Bry., Nat. c.); < at night; following measles or suppressed intermittents.

Painful soreness of eyeballs; coryza, *aching in every bone;* great prostration in epidemic influenza (Lac c.).

Relations.—Followed well by Natr. mur., Sepia and Tub.

Aggravation.—Motion; drinking; uncovering.

Type.—Tertian; double tertian; rarely double quartan, and then only when changed from original type by Quinine. All types may be cured by it. Anticipating, remittent, bilious, malarial; sporadic La Grippe.

Time.—7 A. M.; 7 to 9 P. M.; 7 to 9 A. M. one day, lighter chill at 12 M. next day; 10 A. M.; 12 to 2 P. M.; 5 P. M. Will cure without reference to time, when totality of symptoms is present.

Prodrome.—Insatiable thirst, *but drinking causes nausea and vomiting, and hastens the chill. Sick stomach and thirst night before the paroxysm.* **Thirst,** sometimes for warm drinks (Casc., Ced.), *one to three hours before the chill;* he knows the chill is coming because *"he cannot drink enough"* (knows chill is coming because she is thirsty, **Caps., Cinch., Nat.**); yawning, stretching, *pain in back, especially over right* *ilium, and the bones of extremities as if broken.* Colicky pain in the upper abdomen (**Coc.**); *painful soreness of the eyeballs. Must be covered,* before and during chill (covered during entire paroxysm, **Nux**). *Hungry* (Cina).

Chill.—*With intense thirst; but drinking water* increases the nausea, and *causes bitter vomiting* (drinking causes vomiting, **Ars.**—drinking increases the chill, **Caps.**). Chilliness with excessive trembling and nausea (from the least motion). *Chilliness in the morning, heat throughout the whole day,* **but no perspiration.** Chill may leave for a few minutes and return again, but *no heat in the interval* (reverse of **Ars.,** which has alternate chill and heat). Shivering increased by motion; intense, throbbing headache; pain in back and bones of extremities; moaning with pain; distressing pain in stomach and spleen. Yawning and stretching; more shivering than the degree of coldness warrants. Must be warmly covered (Nux). Begins in or *may spread from the back,* or *runs up the back* (begins in back between the shoulders, **Caps., Polyp.**—begins in lumbar region, **Eup. purp.**). *At close of chill, nausea and vomiting of bitter fluids and bile, aggravated by drinking,* or *after every draft vomiting* (Caps.—sour vomiting at close of chill, Lyc.). Chilly one day, colic the next.

Heat.—Preceded by *thirst,* which is often felt most between chill and heat (**Ars., Cinch.**), or there may be little thirst, when cephalalgia and bone pains are increased; trembling, faint from motion; great weakness; cannot raise the head while the fever lasts; cheeks mahogany red; throbbing headache; internal soreness from head to foot, all over the body (Arn.); sleep with moaning. Seldom any nausea during this stage, but bitter vomiting (sour vomiting, **Lyc.**) occurs at close of heat if absent at close of chill. Heat and lachrymation. Much shivering even during heat. *"A swallow of water will make him shiver"* (will make him shudder, Caps.). Pain in scrobiculus cordis. Fever in the forenoon, preceded by thirst early in the morning, but no chill; attended by fatiguing cough, and not followed by perspiration.

Sweat.—Generally scanty, or absent altogether, in which case *the headache continues for several hours after fever is gone* (**Ars.**). When there is much perspiration, *it brings relief of all pains except cephalalgia,* **which is increased** (sweat relieves all pains, **Nat.**). *Coldness during nocturnal sweat.* Perspiration; at night giving no relief; during sweat the slightest movement of patient, or jar of bed, will cause a transient chill to run through the frame, especially along the back on uncovering (Nux); not debilitating if profuse (reverse of **Cinch.** and **Carbo v.**). *When chill is severe, sweat is light or wanting* and *vice versa.*

Tongue.—Coated white or yellow. Taste, insipid, bitter; food has no taste (**Dros.**). Desire for ice cream; thirst. Paleness of mucous membrane of mouth (**Fer.**). Cracks at the commissures of the lips (**Nat.**). Canine hunger after Quinine.

Apyrexia.—*Imperfect; very little remission.* Jaundiced hue of skin and conjunctiva; *loose cough;* if any sweat, it is attended with chilliness and worse from motion and uncovering. *Bone pains are present in every stage, and only gradually disappear with disappearance of sweat.* Feels worse morning of one day, and afternoon of next. The severity of vomiting has relation to time of eating; the nearer the meals the surer to vomit; first of ingesta, afterwards of bile, which is usually bitter.

"Eupatorium has been a favorite remedy with the most successful practitioners where remittent and intermittent fevers have prevailed epidemically *in miasmatic districts, along rivers, at fisheries, on marshes,* and their several neighborhoods."—C. J. HEMPEL., *S. C.,* I., p. 696.

"*Eupatorium perf.,* both by its pathogenesis and clinical verification in practice, is one of the most valuable of the Materia

Medica in the treatment of western intermittents."—J. S. DOUGLAS.

To this statement I would add that its efficacy is not bounded by latitude. Sometimes it corresponds to the genus epidemicus, and will alone cure nearly every case, particularly if occurring in autumn. It vies with Arsenicum, Cinchona and Natrum mur. as one of our sheet anchors in this disease; its symptoms are "clear-cut" and well defined; its action prompt and decisive. It has cured in all potencies from the tincture to the cm.

Arsenicum.	Eupatorium.
Type.—Quotidian; tertian; quartan; double tertian and quartan. Anticipating. Every fourteen days. Irregular both in type and stage.	**Type.**—Tertian; double tertian, rarely double quartan. Anticipating. All types may be cured with Eupatorium.
Time.—Characteristic; 1 to 2 P. M., 12 to 2 A. M. Afternoon paroxysm predominates.	**Time.**—7 A. M. or 7 to 9 A. M.; 7 to 9 A. M. one day, lighter chill at 12 M. next day. Forenoon predominates.
Prodrome.—*No thirst.* Headache, with vertigo and pale face; pain in bowels and watery diarrhea. Debility; great weariness; must lie down. Malaise.	**Prodrome.**—*Insatiable thirst.* Drinking hastens chill and causes vomiting. Know chill is coming because "he cannot drink enough." Yawning, stretching, backache, and bone pains in extremities.
Chill.—Irregular; mingling of chilliness and heat; or chills and heat alternate; *ameliorated by external heat.* Thirst is not always present; if present, drinks little and often, but generally for hot drinks. Thirst, except for hot drinks, contraindicates.	**Chill.**—*With great thirst.* Begins in back; with *yawning, stretching, backache and bone pains.* May leave and return, but no heat in interval. Must be covered warmly (Nux v.). Bitter vomiting at close of chill. More shivering than coldness warrants.
Heat.—Intense, dry, burning, long-lasting heat, pungent to the touch, and *insatiable thirst for cold water. Great restlessness.* Must be uncovered. Heat as if hot water were coursing through the blood-vessels.	**Heat.**—Great weakness; cannot raise the head while the heat lasts. Rarely any thirst; cheeks mahogany red, and intense throbbing headache; a swallow of water produces shivering. Body sore from head to foot.

Arsenicum.

Sweat.—*With unquenchable thirst for large quantities of water,* which causes vomiting. Cold, clammy. Great weakness and prostration. Previous symptoms relieved during sweat.

Tongue.—Tip red, sides furred, with red streaks down middle; brown-blue. Desire for acids, brandy; water tastes bitter; *aversion to food.*

Apyrexia.—*Never clear. Great weakness and prostration.* Face pale, sallow, sunken or bloated. Debilitating, watery diarrhea. General anemic appearance.

Fevers contracted at sea-shore watering-places, appear in autumn, or "wintered over" and come on in spring.

Eupatorium.

Sweat.—Scanty or absent. If much, is more profuse at night and then cold. Relieves all pains except cephalalgia, *which is increased.* When chill is severe, sweat is light or wanting, and vice versa.

Tongue.—Coated white or yellow, pale; food tasteless, insipid, bitter. Desire for ice cream. Canine hunger after Quinine. Commissures of lips cracked (Nat.).

Apyrexia.—Imperfect, very little remission. Jaundiced hue of skin and conjunctiva; loose cough. Bone pains in every stage, unless relieved by sweat.

Fevers of miasmatic, marshy regions; autumnal; often the genus epidemicus. Apt to become remittent.

EUPATORIUM PURPUREUM.

Characteristic.—Has been praised as a preventive.

All symptoms worse on left side.

Sensation as if *falling to the left;* persistent, cannot get rid of it.

Weak, tired feeling in every organ of the body; cannot move without making a desperate effort.

Rheumatic pains go from below upward (Ledum—shoot downward, Kalmia); change places frequently (Kali bi., Lac c., Puls.).

Sleep, restless, disturbed with frightful dreams.

Mechanical dysuria; from displaced uterus; jolting ride during pregnancy.

Constant desire to urinate; no matter how often he voids urine, bladder still feels full.

Incontinence of urine in children.

Chronic cystitis: uneasy; deep aching; dull pain and soreness in bladder; smarting and burning in bladder, in urethra, on urinating.

Aggravation.—Motion; changing position; draft of air.

Type.—Double tertian; double quartan; malarial.

Time.—Different times of the day; hour not marked (3 to 5 P. M.). No regularity.

Prodrome.—Bone pains in arms and legs (bone pains with intense thirst, **Eup. perf.**). Dry, hacking cough in spells.

Chill.—*With thirst; begins in small of back—lumbar region* (interscapular region, **Caps., Polyp.**), passing up and down, thence extends over the body.

Chill begins between scapulæ, thence spreading over body like waves; craves heat to back, yet heat does not relieve (heat >, Caps.).

Longing for lemonade, cold acid drinks, with *violent bone pains, blue lips* and *nails* (**Nat., Nux**), extremities cold, and *frontal headache. Violent shaking, with comparatively little coldness* (Eup. perf.). *Nausea, but no vomiting,* as the chill is leaving (vomiting at close of chill, **Eup., Lyc.**). Nervous, restless, hysterical mood. Numbness of the legs *after* or *in conjunction with* the severe bone pains.

Slight movement while covered or draft of air produces a return of chill.

Heat.—*With thirst. Long-lasting heat,* with bone pains, nausea and vomiting. *Hunger,* with desire to eat immediately after the fever (hunger before chill and during sweat, **Cinch.**). Frightful dreams. *Longing for hot drinks* (**Ars., Casc., Ced.**).

Sweat.—Without thirst; slight, mostly about forehead and head; *of upper parts of body.* Chilly down the back, *when changing position ever so little.* Very rarely, sweat is profuse (same as its congener, **Eup. perf.**).

Tongue.—Heavily furred, brown along the centre; bitter, pappy taste with the chill.

Apyrexia.—Passes more urine than normal. with frequent desire; scalding on urinating. Profuse flow of clear, limpid urine; weak, tired and faint after urinary symptoms. Vertigo, with "a dizzy feeling" all over, and a persistent sensation of *falling to the left* (Col.—of falling, **Gels.**).

Eup. purp.	**Eup. perf.**
Type.—Double tertian.	**Type.**—Tertian.
Time.—Different times of day; 10 A. M. Every other day.	**Time.**—7 A. M., or 7 to 9 A. M. one day; 12 M. next day.
Prodrome.—Bone pains in arms and legs. Dry, hacking cough in spells.	**Prodrome.**—*Thirst* several hours before, with bone pains and pains in back.
Chill.—*No thirst,* or thirst for lemonade and acid drinks. Chill begins in lumbar region, thence extends over body. Nausea as the chill is leaving, but no vomiting.	**Chill.**—Great thirst for cold water. Chill, with bone pains, pains in back, gaping, stretching, throbbing headache. Bitter vomiting at close of chill. Drinking hastens chill and causes vomiting.
Heat.—Long-lasting; thirst, bone pains, and hunger as the heat is passing off (Cina, Cinch.).	**Heat.**—With sleep; moaning, increased headache. "A swallow of water will make him shiver" (Caps.).
Sweat.—Chilly when changing position ever so little during sweat.	**Sweat.**—Bone pains disappear with disappearance of sweat. Light chill and profuse sweat, or shaking chill, and light or wanting sweat.
Apyrexia.—Vertigo, with falling to the left. Urine, profuse, urging, scalding.	**Apyrexia.**—Jaundiced hue; great weakness; anemia.

EUPHORBIUM.

Characteristic.—In the terrible burning pain as if *a live coal were on or in the parts,* of cancer, carbuncle, or erysipelas, when Arsenicum or Anthracinum fails to relieve.

Burning in caries and necrosis of bones.

Erysipelas bulbosa, vesicles as large as peas filled with yellow liquid.

In gangrene or blood boils of old persons.

Old, torpid, indolent ulcers, with biting, lancinating, lacerating pains; < in morning, on becoming heated near the fire, lying down, changing position, beginning to move, from touch; > from motion and walking.

Aggravation.—On becoming heated; lying; beginning to move; changing position.

Time.—Usually a morning paroxysm.

Chill.—Of the whole body in the morning; while walking in the open air; when beginning to eat (Bell.—after eating, Kali c., Nux). The body is cold with internal burning heat. Constant chilliness, with constant sweat; chill with sweat. Shivering; over the whole body; over the back, with glowing cheeks and cold hands.

Heat.—Great, the whole day; all the clothes seemed burdensome, even his whole body was too heavy for him, as if he had carried a great load. Heat with aversion to dressing; clothing feels too heavy. Heat only on the head.

Sweat.—*In the morning* in bed; extending from the feet over the whole body; some thirst. Morning-sweat; on the neck, thighs and legs; sometimes cold on the legs; only on the thighs.

FERRUM.

Characteristic.—Adapted to persons of sanguine temperament; pettish, quarrelsome, disputative, easily excited, least contradiction angers (Anac., Coc., Elaps); women who are weak, delicate, chlorotic, yet have a very red face.

Hemorrhagic diathesis; blood bright red, coagulates easily (Fer. p., Ipec., Phos.)

Extreme paleness of the face, which becomes red and flushed on the least pain, motion or exertion; blushing (Amyl, Coc.).

Irritability: slight noises, like crackling of paper, drive him to despair (Asar., Ther.).

Always feels better *by walking slowly about,* although weakness obliges the patient to lie down.

Erethic chlorosis, worse in winter.

Red parts become white; lips, face, tongue.

Menses: early, profuse, protracted, *with fiery red face;* ringing in the ears; intermit two or three days and then return; *flow pale, watery, debilitating.*

Vertigo; with balancing sensation as if on the water; *on seeing flowing water;* when walking over water, as when crossing a bridge (Lys.); when descending (Bor., San.).

Headache: for two, three, or four days, every two or three weeks; hammering, beating, pulsating pains, must lie down in bed; with aversion to eating or drinking.

Regurgitation and eructation of food in mouthfuls (Alum.), without nausea.

Canine hunger, or loss of appetite, with extreme dislike for all food.

Vomiting: *immediately after midnight;* of ingesta, as soon as food is eaten; leaves table suddenly and with one effort vomits everything eaten, can sit down and eat again; sour, acid (Lyc., Sul. ac.).

Diarrhea: undigested stools at night, or **while eating or drinking** (Crot. t.); painless with a good appetite; of consumptives.

Constipation: from intestinal atony; ineffectual urging; stools hard, difficult, followed by backache or cramping pain in rectum; prolapsus recti of children; itching of anus at night.

Relations.—Complementary to: Alum., Cinch., the latter the vegetable analogue follows well in nearly all cases.

Aggravation.—While at rest; sitting still; night.

Amelioration.—Walking slowly about; in summer.

Type.—Tertian. *Morning chill. Afternoon chill.*

Time.—7 A. M.—12 M.—3 P. M.—4 A. M.—LIPPE.

Fever, without chill, 3 to 8 P. M.

Prodrome.—Vomiting of ingesta as the chill is coming on. Loose stool in early morning (**Sul.**).

Chill.—*With thirst.* Chilliness with headache in the morning. General coldness of the body, hands and feet very cold. Chilliness and trembling all over. Chilliness in frequent short attacks. In the afternoon, violent chill for half an hour, then thirst, must go to bed, followed by heat with perspiration. Cold sweat from the beginning of chill for 12 hours. *During the chill his face got glowing hot* (Arn.). *Hands and feet cold and numb* (**Ced., Cimex, Sep.**), chilly all over, does not go off by walking. Feet *cold* and *numb* all night, as after skating. *Feet very cold, toes cold as ice, fingers stiff.* Feet and ankles feel as if in snow.

Heat.—*Without thirst.* Heat in the body, with *red cheeks,* but the head is cool (but head aches, **Bell.**). Sensation of heat all over the body, *which was cold to the touch,* with sensation in the face and around the eyes, as if swollen and bloated (reverse of **Bar.,** coldness of body which was hot to the touch). Flushes over the whole body, as if perspiration would break out. Heat of head, feet cold. Great heat of *palms of hands* and *soles of feet.* Heat in the stomach (relieved by eating), vomiting of the ingesta. Dry heat, worse towards evening; inclination to uncover (Sec.); > by moving about, eating, speaking. *Face very red.*

Sweat.—*From early morn till noon every other day, preceded by headache.* Sweat *profuse, long-lasting,* whether by day at every motion, or night and morning in bed. *Strong-smelling, clammy, debilitating night-sweat.* Sweat *stains yellow,* and is fetid on going to sleep. Sweat > while speaking and after eating. All the symptoms *are* < while sweating (all the symptoms are > by sweating, **Nat., Psor.**). "Nausea during sweat."—C. PEARSON.

Tongue.—Coated white. *Lips, gums, tongue* and *mucous membrane* of entire buccal cavity *pale* and *bloodless* (**Sec.**). All food tastes bitter, dry, woody and insipid. Taste like rotten eggs (**Acon., Arn.**). Anorexia; extreme dislike to all food.

Pulse.—Hard and full at beginning of paroxysm; or weak, small and scarcely perceptible during apyrexia; great ebullition of blood.

Apyrexia.—*Prostration, debility* and *great loss of muscular power. Anemia.* Edema of feet and face, especially upper and lower eyelids (**Apis, Ars.**—of upper eyelids, **Kali c.**). Headache; vertigo; *swelling of the cutaneous veins;* splenic region swollen and sore on pressure (**Apis, Arn.**). *Vomiting of everything eaten without being digested.* Constipation or chronic diarrhea with lienteria. Cadaverous, jaundiced complexion. Yellow spots on the face (Sep.). Very weak and tired, but always better when *walking slowly* about (better from being perfectly still, **Bry.**). Cases maltreated by Quinine.

"Iron is evidently one of the most precious remedies against the cachectic condition; but I admit that its action is due to neither the chemical reasons that have been imagined and which have been current even on the lips of our school, nor the massive doses which naturally flow from these considerations; it is by its dynamic virtues that Ferrum acts and confers all its benefits.—A. Charge.

Intermittent fever after abuse of Quinine; congestions to head and face; veins distended; vomiting ingesta; swelling of spleen; anemia marked by pseudo-plethora; skin transparent when it is not earthy. The totality of the characteristic symptoms.

Analysis.—A history of anemia, chlorosis, and general constitutional weakness.

Pale face, flushed during chill or heat.

Feet cold, as if in snow.

Profuse, long-lasting, debilitating sweat; clammy and cold at night.

Maltreated by Quinine.

GAMBOGIA.

Characteristic.—The conditions calling for Gambogia are apt to occur especially toward evening or night.

Frightful vomiting and purging with fainting (Elat., Ver.).

Stool: profuse, watery, with colic and tenesmus; dark green mucus, offensive, corrosive, discharged with a single, somewhat prolonged effort; great relief after stool as if an irritating substance were removed from the bowels.

Aggravation.—Evening and night; while sitting.

Amelioration.—During motion in the open air.

Type.—*Quotidian,* tertian; double tertian; intermittent often becomes remittent. Postponing oftener than anticipating.

Time.—7 P. M.; EVENING 6 to 8 P. M., lasting all night (Lyc., Puls., Rhus, Sarac., last all night).

Chill.—With thirst. *Violent shaking at 7 P. M., beginning in the back,* with external coldness of whole body, *continues till 4 A. M.* (chill lasts 12 hours, **Canth.**—24 hours, **Aran.**). *Internal and external coldness,* at 6 to 8 P. M., lasting from a quarter to two hours, or the whole night to 5 A. M. Sensation of chilliness and elongation of incisor teeth. Chill for two hours with chattering of the teeth, with violent thirst; the skin is warm to the touch. Sudden shaking chill at night, waking him from sleep, and as suddenly disappearing. Eructations; yawning.

Heat.—Increased warmth, with anxiety and flushes of heat. Always slight, often wanting.

Sweat.—Over whole body on waking at 4 A. M. Early morning sweat.

Analysis.—The fevers of Gambogia occur while diarrhea is prevalent. The paroxysm consists almost wholly of the cold stage; the others being light or wanting. Frightful vomiting and purging (Elat., Ver.); evening paroxysm.

GELSEMIUM.

Characteristic.—Adapted to children; young people; women of a nervous, hysterical temperament (Croc., Ign.); irritable, sensitive, excitable; onanists, both sexes (Kali p.).

Desire to be quiet, to be let alone, does not wish to speak, nor have any one near her for company, even if the person be silent (Ign.).

Fear of death (Ars.); utter lack of courage.

Weakness and trembling; of tongue, hands, legs; of the entire body.

Complaints: from exciting or bad news (from pleasant surprises, Coff.); sudden emotions (Ign.); the anticipation of any unusual ordeal brings on diarrhea; stage fright, nervous dread of appearing in public (Arg. n.); general depression from *heat of sun or summer.*

Vertigo: *spreading from the occiput* (Sil.); with diplopia, dim vision, loss of sight; seems intoxicated when trying to move.

Children: fear of falling, seize the nurse, grasp the crib (Bor., San.).

Lack of muscular co-ordination (Kali br.); giddy, confused; muscles refuse to obey the will.

Headache: *beginning in cervical spine;* pains extend over the head, causing a bursting sensation in forehead and eyeballs (Sang., Sil., begin in same way, but are semi-lateral); worse from smoking; preceded by blindness (Iris, Kali bi., Lac d.), > by profuse urination.

Sensation of a band around the head above the eyes (Carb. ac., Plat., Sul.); scalp sore.

Slow pulse of old age.

Great heaviness of the eyelids; cannot keep them open (Caust., Graph., Sep.).

Fears that unless constantly on the move, the heart will cease beating (would cease beating if she moved, Dig.).

Aggravation.—Damp weather; before a thunder storm; sudden emotions; bad news; rest; smoking tobacco; thinking of his ailments; spoken to of his loss.

Amelioration.—In the cold, open air.

Type.—Quotidian; tertian; same hour of the day with every paroxysm (**Aran., Ced., Sabad.**). Periodicity extends throughout its entire pathogenesis; all its fevers are of a regular type, but characterized by disorders of innervation. *Simple uncomplicated cases.* When the remittent takes on the intermittent type (reverse of **Bap., Eup., Quin.**). Malarial, yellow, typhoid.

Time.—Afternoon and evening paroxysm 2, 4, 5 and 9 P. M. Fever without chill at 10 A. M. (**Bap., Nat.**). Daily, *at same hour.*

Prodrome.—Sudden mental emotions, the anticipation of any unusual ordeal, fright, grief, bad news, may hasten chill or produce diarrhea. Could tell when chill was about to return, as incontinence of urine would set in. Thirst, but does not drink much; hurts to swallow.

Chill.—*Without thirst.* Chill commences in the hands and feet (in recent cases—in old chronic cases, **Nat.**). Chill ascending from feet; *chill and chilliness, especially along the spine; running up the back* from *loins to nape of neck,* and following each other in rapid wave like succession from *sacrum to occiput* (running *up and down* the spine, **Eup. purp.**). Chilliness with cold hands and feet, headache, and heat of head and face. Chilliness with tired, languid feeling in back and limbs; wants to avoid all muscular exertion. Feet feel as if in very cold water. Coldness is so severe as to be painful. Sleepy as chill is leaving (**Apis**). Transient chilliness with profuse urination. Nervous chill, the skin is warm; wants to be held that he may not shake so much. Child wants to be held so that he will not shake so hard (**Lach.**).

Heat.—Without thirst; **intense burning.** General heat, mostly about the head and face. Warmth over the whole body, as if sweat would break out, then chilly down the back. Directly after the chill comes a flying heat and pricking in the skin, rapidly followed by perspiration, which at times is profuse, and lasting from twelve to twenty-four hours (**Caust.**). *Heat in the face, sleep or sleepy,* stupid, besotted; with half-waking, muttering delirium; tired, *wants to lie still* (**Bry.**), or great nervous restlessness; sensation of *falling, in children; child starts and grasps attendant or crib,* and *screams out for fear of falling.* Semi-stupor; cannot open his eyes or think correctly; vertigo, staggers as if intoxicated. Sensitive to light or noise (**Bell.**—intolerant of noise, **Caps.**). Long-lasting heat; far into night; pain in one leg; jerking of the limbs. Loquacity.

Sweat.—With thirst. Profuse, which > the pain. Sweat coming gradually and moderately, always > the pains (sweat > all the symptoms, **Nat.**). Sweats freely from slight exertion (**Psor.**). Perspiration, sometimes profuse and continuing from a few hours to twenty-four, with languor and prostration. Sweat most profuse on genitalia. Freely on slight exertion.

Tongue.—Coated yellowish-white, or nearly clean, or with white centre and red margins. If coated thickly, breath fetid. Taste: bitter, foul, with blood-colored saliva.

Pulse.—Irregular, intermitting, yet full (**Dig.**). Small, weak, feeble, almost imperceptible.

Apyrexia.—*Often wanting,* or *very short.* Heat and perspiration are so extended that many fevers are more remitting than intermitting. *Great prostration of whole muscular system* Headache < by smoking tobacco (Ign.—> by smoking, **Aran.**). Patient is nervous, irritable, easily angered (**Cham.** —very irritable, **Anac., Bry., Tub.**).

Analysis.—Patient wants to be held during the chill (Lach.); fear of falling; chills along the spine, running up and down the back; sleep throughout heat; thirst during sweat; muttering delirium when half awake; absence of all gastric and hepatic symptoms. Fever apt to end in remittent or typhoid. Convulsions in children; masked ague from abuse of quinine; choreaic symptoms. Must be covered in all stages of the paroxysm.

"For intermittents or remittents which are contracted at summer watering places and 'wintered over,' making their appearance in early spring, Gelsemium is a remedy of great value."—Ludlam. (Ars., Eup., Lach.)

Gelsemium is one of the few remedies that have the regular periodic fever, *without chill.* It divides the honors equally with Arsenicum in the treatment of children's intermittents, from which it is distinguished by the regularity of the paroxysm, absence of thirst, and the burning fever and restlessness. The child is neither so weak and prostrated nor pale and feeble as in the Arsenicum fever. Sensation of falling is a genuine symptom, often occurring in children. Gelsemium is always to be thought of in recent uncomplicated cases, where chill begins in extremities (in chronic cases, **Nat. mur.**). Also where a remittent takes on the intermittent type, or *vice versa.* Tendency to typhoid.

GRAPHITES.

Characteristic.—Adapted to women *inclined to obesity,* who suffer from habitual constipation, and whose history reveals a tendency to delaying menstruation.

"What Pulsatilla is at puberty, Graphites is at the climacteric."

Morning sickness during menstruation; very weak and prostrated (Alum., Carbo a., Coc.).

Hears better when in a noise; when riding in a carriage or car, when there is a rumbling sound (Nit. ac.).

Excessive cautiousness; timid, hesitates; unable to decide about anything (Puls.).

Fidgety while sitting at work (Zinc.).

Sad, despondent; *music makes her weep;* thinks of nothing but death (music is intolerable, Nat. c., Sab.).

Eczema of lids; eruption moist and fissured, lids red and margins covered with scales or crusts.

Sexual debility from sexual abuse.

Menses: too scanty, pale; late with violent colic; irregular; delayed from getting feet wet (Puls.).

Leucorrhea: acrid, excoriating; occurs in gushes day and night; before and after menses (before, Sepia; after, Kreos.).

Hard cicatrices remaining after mammary abscess, retarding flow of milk; cancer from old scars.

Unhealthy skin: every injury suppurates (Hep.); eruptions, behind the ears, on various parts, from which oozes a watery, transparent, sticky fluid; nails brittle, crumbling, deformed; painful and sore, as if ulcerated; old cicatrices re-open.

Cracks or fissures of ends of fingers and nipples, labial commissures, of anus, between the toes (Nit. ac.)

Burning round spot on vertex (Cal., Sul.—cold spot, Sep., Ver.).

Diarrhea: stools brown, fluid, mixed with undigested substances, and of an intolerable odor; often caused by suppressed eruptions (Psor.).

Chronic constipation: stool difficult, large, hard, knotty, with lumps united by mucous threads; *too large* (Sulph.); smarting sore pain in anus after stool.

Children; impudent, teasing, laugh at reprimands.

Sensation of cobweb on forehead, tries hard to brush it off (Bar., Bor., Brom., Ran. s.).

Phlegmonous erysipelas: of face, with burning, stinging pain; commencing on right side, going to left; after application of Iodine.

Decided aversion to coition (both sexes).

Cataleptic condition; conscious, but without power to move or speak.

Takes cold easily; sensitive to draught of air (Bor., Cal., Hep.); suffering parts emaciate.

Relations.—Complementary: Caust., Hep., Lyc.

Follows well after Lyc., Puls.; after Cal. in obesity of young women with large amount of unhealthy adipose tissue.

Aggravation.—Cold or becoming cold; night; during and after menstruation; after eating.

Amelioration.—Eructations (Carbo v.); while walking; open air.

Type.—Quotidian; double quotidian.

Time.—6 or 7 A. M.; morning in bed; 4, 5, 6, 7, 8 P. M.

Chill.—Without thirst, in the morning in bed; from 4 P. M. till evening; chilliness and coldness of whole body at 5 P. M., with icy cold feet. Violent febrile chilliness morning and evening, the heat followed by sweat. Shaking chill every day, in the evening; after an hour, hot face and cold feet *without subsequent heat.* Chill in evening, with headache and tearing in the limbs, great thirst, and profuse perspiration after midnight, lasting till morning. Chill < *after meals;* > *after drinking* (Caust.—< after drinking, **Ars., Caps., Cimex**); > *in open air* (**Apis, Ipec.**—< in open air, **Ign.**). Icy cold feet, alternating with burning.

Heat.—At night; with restlessness; unable to sleep, or remain in bed on account of it; when riding in a carriage. Dry heat every evening and night, lasting till morning, with headache on vertex and in nape of the neck till noon. Hands and soles of the feet hot and burning.

Sweat.—*Profuse at night;* from the slightest motion; on front of body and center of chest (sternum); stains yellow; is sour and offensive (**Hep.**, **Lyc.**). Profuse sweat on the feet; they swell and become sore (**Iod.**, **Sil.**). Entire inability to sweat (**Hep.**).

Tongue.—Coated white and sensitive. Taste sour, salty, bitter; like rotten eggs. Rotten odor from mouth. Breath smells like urine. Lips and nostrils sore and cracked, as from cold. Averse to meat, fish, cooked food, salt.

Apyrexia.—Excessive hunger, or no appetite, with great distention of abdomen, as from accumulation or incarceration of flatulence. Constipation. Urine turbid, and deposits white sediment.

Constitutional symptoms of apyrexia are the best guide for selection of remedy.

HEPAR SULPHUR.

Characteristic.—For torpid, lymphatic constitutions; persons with light hair and complexion, slow to act, muscles soft and flabby.

Like Sulphur, Hepar is adapted to the psoric, scrofulous diathesis.

In Sulphur the skin affections are dry, itching and not sensitive to touch, in fact, > by scratching and rubbing; while in Hepar the skin is unhealthy, suppurating, even **slight injuries cause suppuration; extremely sensitive to touch,** the pain often causing fainting.

Diseases when *suppuration seems inevitable;* where the system has been injured by the abuse of Mercury.

Patient is peevish; angry at the least trifle; hypochondriacal; unreasonably anxious; *oversensitive, physically and mentally;*

the slightest cause irritates; quick, hasty speech and hasty drinking.

Extremely sensitive to cold air, imagines he can feel the air if a door is opened in the next room; must be wrapped up to the face even in hot weather (Psor.); cannot bear to be uncovered (Nux—cannot bear to be covered, Camp., Sec.); takes cold from slightest exposure to fresh air (Tub.).

Urine: flow impeded; *voided slowly, without force, drops vertically;* is obliged to wait a while before it passes; bladder weak, is unable to finish, seems as if some urine always remains (Alum., Sil.).

Cough: *when any part of the body is uncovered* (Rhus); **croupy, choking, strangling**; *from exposure to dry west wind,* the land wind (Acon.).

Croup: after exposure *to dry cold wind* (Acon.); deep, rough, barking cough, with hoarseness and rattling of mucus; < cold air, cold drinks, before midnight or toward morning.

Sensation of a splinter, fish bone or plug in the throat (Arg. n., Nit. ac.); quinsy, when suppuration threatens; chronic hypertrophy, with hardness of hearing (Bar., Lyc., Plumb., Psor.).

Ulcers, herpes, surrounded by little pimples or pustules and spread by coalescing.

Middle of lower lip cracked (Amm. c., Nat.—cracks in commissures, Cund.).

Diarrhea: of children with sour smell (Cal., Mag. c.—child and stool have a sour smell, Rheum); clay-colored stool (Cal., Pod.).

Eyeballs: sore to touch, pain as if they would be drawn back into head (Olean., Paris).

Aggravation.—Lying on painful side (Kali c., Iod.); cold air; uncovering; eating or drinking cold things; touching affected parts; abuse of Mercury.

Amelioration.—Warmth in general (Ars.); wrapping up

warmly, especially the head (Psor., Sil.); *in damp, wet weather* (Caust., Nux,—rev. of Nat. s.).

Type.—*Simple.* Quotidian. Period the same every day.

Time.—Morning at 2, 6 or 7 o'clock. The evening paroxysm, like Graph., Lyc., Puls. and Rhus, is most severe. **6 or 7 P. M.**—4, 5, 6, 7 or 8 P. M.

Fever, without chill, 4 P. M., lasting all night. Morning fever preceded by bitter taste in mouth, returning twice a day.

Prodrome.—Itching, stinging, nettle-rash. Bitter taste in the mouth, for hours before chill.

Chill.—Without thirst. **Great chilliness in open air**; *must get to warm stove;* heat feels agreeable but does not relieve (must get to warm stove as soon *as chill begins,* **Bov.**—must get to warm stove, *and lie down,* **Lach.**). **Great sensitiveness to open air** *with chilliness* (excessively sensitive to open air, **Camph.**—chill < by least draft of air, **Bar.**). *Violent chill every morning, at 6 or 7 o'clock, without subsequent heat* (without subsequent *heat* or *sweat,* **Bov.**). *Violent chill,* with chattering of the teeth, lasting a quarter of an hour, with *coldness of the hands and feet,* followed by heat with sweat, especially on the chest and forehead, and slight thirst. *Violent shaking chill* with chattering of the teeth, *icy coldness* and *paleness of* the *face, hands* and *feet, unconsciousness* and *coma* (**Bell., Op.**). *Febrile chill,* from 4 to 8 P. M., or in the *night, could not get warm,* with < *of all complaints* (**Ars.**); *without subsequent heat.* Chill at 2 A. M., with febrile shivering and hot, dry skin. **Nettle-rash with violent itching** *and* **stinging,** *disappears as heat begins* (nettle-rash appears as the chill is passing off, **Apis**—during sweat, **Rhus**—during heat, **Ign.**).

Heat.—*With thirst. Burning, febrile heat, with almost unquenchable thirst, distressing headache* and *slight delirium, lasting from 4 P. M. all night,* without chilliness. Larynx much affected, hoarse, weak voice. *Hect light* in comparison with the chill, though he was obliged to uncover himself

(**Puls.**). Dry heat of body at night, with sweaty hands which cannot *tolerate being uncovered* (**Bar.**). Febrile paroxysm during the day, chilliness alternating with heat, *with photophobia.* Violent fever, with flushing heat in the face and head. **Fever blisters around the mouth (Ign., Nat., Nux, Rhus)**

Sweat.—*With flushes of heat.* **Sweats profusely day and night without relief. Perspires easily on every motion, however slight,** *mental exertion, even on writing a few lines* (**Psor., Sep.**); or, at first, no sweat at all, then sweats profusely. *Profuse, sour-smelling sweat at night* which is often clammy (**Lyc.**). *Sweat of perineum, groins, and inside of thighs* (sweat most profuse on the genitalia, **Gels.**). **Constant offensive exhalations from the body.** Sometimes thirst with night-sweat. After sweat, burning redness of face with heat and dryness of palms of hands.

Tongue.—*Tip painful and sore;* back of tongue coated *like dry clay* (Cal. s.). Taste: bitter; putrid; metallic; of rotten eggs. Offensive odor from the mouth, which he notices (which he does not notice, **Puls.**). Longing for acids, strong-tasting things. Aversion to fat. Stomach out of order.

Apyrexia.—Characteristic: never clear. Constitutional symptoms always present, and always guiding. Unhealthy skin, with itching, apt to be developed by the fever.

"Intermittent fever; first chills, then thirst, and an hour later, much heat with interrupted sleep. Violent chill at 8 P. M. with chattering of teeth; hands and feet cold; followed by heat with perspiration, especially on the chest and forehead, with slight thirst."—LIPPE.

Analysis.—Sensitive to open air.

Nettle-rash with the chill.

Hydroa around the mouth.

Sweat: profuse, offensive, sour; easy, **on every motion; day and night.**

Without relief; from mental exertion, even writing a few lines.

HYDRASTIS CANADENSIS.

For debilitated persons, with viscid mucous discharges.

Cachectic or malignant dyscrasia, with marked derangement of gastric and hepatic functions; broken down by excessive use of alcohol.

Cancer: hard, adherent; skin mottled, puckered; pains knife-like, sharp cutting; nipple retracted.

Nursing sore mouth; tongue large, shows imprint of teeth.

Leucorrhea: ropy, thick, viscid, yellow; hanging from os in long strings (Bov., Kali bi.); pruritus.

Profuse discharge of thick, yellow, stringy mucus from nasal passages (Cor. r.).

Hawks yellow, viscid mucus from posterior nares and fauces; ulceration, after mercury or chlorate of potash; syphilitic angina.

Type.—Intermittent, tertian, quotidian; bilious, typhoid, yellow.

Time.—11 A. M.; 10 P. M. fever without chill.

Cause.—Often depends upon organic disease.

Chill.—Morning or evening; in back or thighs with aching; around shoulders and chest; pulse slow.

Heat.—In flushes, over face, neck, hand. Great heat of whole body followed by great debility.

Sweat.—Profuse, offensive of genitals (Petr.).

Tongue.—Large, flabby, thickly coated white, shows imprint of teeth.

Apyrexia.—Cachectic; gastric or hepatic symptoms with jaundice, and bilious disturbances; bad effects of Mercury or Quinine.

For days before an attack sensation of entire goneness at epigastrium, with loss of appetite.

Vertex headaches in paroxysms every other day at 11 A. M. with excessive nausea, anguish and retching.

Typhoid; atony, torpor and retarded convalescence; insomnia, copious sweats, debility.

HYOSCYAMUS.

Characteristic.—Persons of sanguine temperament; who are irritable, excitable, nervous, hysterical.

Diseases with increased cerebral activity but of a *non-inflammatory type,* as in hysteria or delirium tremens.

Convulsions: of children from fright or the irritation of intestinal worms (Cina); during labor or the puerperal state; after eating, child vomits, sudden shriek then insensible.

Spasms: without consciousness, very restless; *every muscle in the body twitches, from the eyes to the toes* (with consciousness, Nux).

Delirium: with restlessness, jumps out of bed, tries to escape; makes irrelevant answers; thinks he is in the wrong place; talks of imaginary wrongs, but has no wants, makes no complaints.

In delirium, Hyoscyamus occupies a place midway between Belladonna and Stramonium; it lacks the constant cerebral congestion of the former, and the fierce rage and maniacal delirium of the latter.

Fears: being left alone; poisoned; bitten; sold; to eat; to take what is offered.

Bad effects of unfortunate love; with jealousy, rage, incoherent speech, or inclination to laugh at everything; followed by epilepsy.

Lascivious mania; immodesty, will not be covered, kicks off the clothes, exposes the person; sings obscene songs, lies naked in bed and chatters.

Cough: dry, nocturnal, spasmodic; < when lying down, relieved by sitting up (Dros.); < at night, after eating, drinking, talking, singing (Dros., Phos.—> when lying down, Mang. m.).

Paralysis of bladder; after labor, with retention or incontinence of urine; no desire to urinate in lying-in women (Arn., Op.).

Spasmodic affections are apt to be epileptoid in character.

Intense sleeplessness of irritable, excitable persons; from business embarrassments; often imaginary.

Relations.—Compare Bell., Stram. and Verat.

Phos. often cures lasciviousness when Hyos. fails.

Aggravation.—Evenings; night; during menses; mental affections; jealousy, unhappy love; when lying down.

Amelioration.—Stooping (head); sitting up (cough).

Type.—Tertian; quartan. Remittent, malarial, typhoid.

Time.—11 A. M.—alternate days.

Chill.—Without thirst. Commencing in *the feet* and running up the spine to nape of neck. Coldness runs from small of back to the nape of the neck (commencing in *hands and feet,* and running up the spine to nape of neck, **Gels.**). *Chill from feet upward.* Shivering over the whole body, with burning redness of face and cold hands. *Whole body cold,* with *burning redness of face; chill alternating with heat* (**Bell.**); **cannot bear to be talked to** (**Cina, Sil.**), or **hear the least noise** (**Caps., Gels.**). Sudden chilliness; coldness of spine; body cold and stiff, cannot get warm in bed; *congestive chills with cold extremities.*

Heat.—With thirst. *Burning heat all over, skin hot and dry to touch, with distended veins* (**Bell., Cinch.**). Heat over whole body; much thirst, lips sticky. Burning heat without external redness; *the blood burns in the veins* (**Ars., Rhus**). The skin burning hot to the examining hand, which leaves a burning in place touched (**Bell.**). Heat along the whole spine, which runs up the back. **Epileptiform convulsions** (**Stram.**).

Sleeplessness. Throw bed clothes off, not because they are warm, but will not remain covered. Heat: dry, nocturnal, disturbs sleep.

Sweat.—Profuse, general perspiration, mostly on legs. Sweats during sleep. Sweat on back and pit of the stomach. Sweat cold, sour.

Tongue.—Coated brown or red, partially paralyzed, protrudes it with difficulty (Lach.). Taste bad, putrid, offensive. Thirst, drinks but little at a time. Dread of water (Lys.).

Apyrexia.—Extreme weakness; illusions of vision, spots before the eyes; mouth dry, difficult to swallow liquids, hiccough, nausea; vertigo and pressure in the head. Short, dry hacking cough at night.

Analysis.—The mental symptoms and the delirium, in all fevers, are the peculiar guides.

Restless, sleepless, desire to escape.

Lascivious mania; jealousy; rage; fear.

Spasms and convulsions.

Fever: pneumonia, scarlatina, *rapidly becomes typhoid;* sensorium clouded, staring eyes, grasping at flocks or picking bed clothes, teeth covered with sordes, tongue dry and unwieldy, involuntary stool and urine; subsultus tendinum.

IGNATIA (Strychnos).

Characteristic.—Especially adapted to the nervous temperament; women of a sensitive, easily excited nature; dark hair and skin, but mild disposition; quick to perceive, to execute. In striking contrast with the fair-complexioned, yielding, lachrymose, but slow and indecisive Pulsatilla.

The remedy of great contradictions: the roaring in ears > by music; the piles > when walking; sore throat feels > when swallowing; empty feeling in stomach not > by eating; cough < the more he coughs; cough on standing still during a walk (Ast. fl.); spasmodic laughter from grief; sexual desire with impotency; *thirst during a chill,* no thirst in the fever; the color changes in the face when at rest.

Mental conditions rapidly, in an almost incredibly short time, change from joy to sorrow, laughing to weeping (Croc., Nux m.).

Persons mentally and physically exhausted by **long concentrated grief**; *involuntary sighing,* and a weak, empty feeling at pit of stomach, not > by eating.

Desire to be alone.

Finely sensitive mood, delicate conscientiousness.

Inconstant, impatient, irresolute, quarrelsome.

Amiable in disposition if feeling well, but easily disturbed by very slight emotion; *easily offended.*

The slightest fault finding or contradiction excites anger, and this makes him angry with himself.

Bad effects: of anger, grief, or disappointed love (Cal. p., Hyos.); from bad news, from vexation with reserved displeasure; from suppressed mental sufferings; of shame and mortification; broods over imaginary trouble in solitude.

Children: when reprimanded, scolded, sent to bed, get sick or have convulsions in sleep.

Headache, as if a nail were driven out through the side, relieved by lying on it (compare, Cof., Nux, Thuja).

Cannot bear tobacco; produces or < headache (Lob.).

In talking or chewing, bites inside of cheek.

Sweat on the face, of a small spot only, while eating.

Prolapsus ani from moderate straining at stool (Nit. ac., Pod., Ruta).

Constipation: from carriage riding; of a paralytic origin; *excessive urging, felt more in upper abdomen* (Ver.); with great pain, dreads to go to closet; women who are habitual coffee drinkers.

Hemorrhoids: prolapse with every stool, have to be replaced;

sharp *stitches up the rectum* (Nit ac.); < for hours after stool (Rat., Sul.).

Cough: dry, spasmodic; after warm drinks; every time he stands still during a walk; the longer he coughs the more the irritation to cough increases.

Twitchings, jerkings, even spasms of single limbs or whole body, when falling asleep.

Pain: in small circumscribed spots; *oversensitive to* (Cof., Hep.).

In most cases Ignatia should be given in the morning.

Relations.—Incompatible: Cof., Nux, Tab.

Ignatia bears the same relation to the diseases of women that Nux does to sanguine, bilious men.

"There are many more Ignatia persons in North America than Nux vomica persons."—HERING.

Aggravation.—Tobacco; coffee; brandy. Contact; motion; strong smells; mental emotions, grief, etc.; cold air.

Amelioration.—Warmth; hard pressure; lying on the back.

Type.—Quotidian; tertian; quartan. Irregular; continually changing, especially by the abuse of Quinine (Eup.).

Postponing or anticipating; the former the rule, the latter the exception (postpones or anticipates, Gamb.). Typhoid.

The attacks are irregular both in periodicity and evolution of stages. Return each spring after suppression by Quinine.

Time.—Irregularity of hour, *characteristic.* Paroxysm at sunset, late in the afternoon or evening; then fever heat nearly all night. **At all periods.**

Prodrome.—Violent yawning and stretching; sometimes terrible shuddering.

Chill.—*Always with* **great thirst** *for large quantities of water* (same, but in all stages, **Bry.**—before and during chill, **Caps., Carbo v., Eup.**), **only during chill** (if thirst in any other stage, it is light and in short spells). Chill commences in *upper arms* and spreads to back and chest (in both arms at once, **Bell.**—in hands and feet, **Gels.**—*chill begins in and spreads from arms;* goose-flesh; hot face; drowsy; motion; < by getting out of bed, Hell.). Chilly at sunset; chilly in cool air; very cold all over, with one-sided headache. **Shaking chill, with redness of the face,** *in the evening. Coldness and chilliness of whole body,* or *only of posterior portions,* > **at once in a warm room or by a warm stove** (**Kali c.**). Chilliness on the back, and over upper arms, with *heat of ears;* about the knees, which are cold externally; in the face and on the arms, with chattering of teeth and goose-flesh; feet and legs, thigh and forearm; *chill* of single parts *only* (*chill and heat* of single parts, **Bell., Rhus**); *proceeding from the abdomen* (most severe in abdomen, **Meny.**—from the stomach, **Cal.**—running to and terminating in the stomach, **Arn.**). During the chill: ill humor, colic, nausea, vomiting of food, mucus and bile (rare); great paleness of face; pain in back; lameness of lower limbs. Chill and coldness aggravate the pains. External coldness, internal heat, or internal chill with external heat.

"The febrile coldness relieved by external warmth is characteristic of Ignatia."—HAHNEMANN.

Heat.—*Without thirst.* **Heat of the whole body in the afternoon, without thirst, with sensation of dryness of the skin. External heat and redness, without internal heat.** Sudden flushes of heat over the whole body. *External warmth is intolerable* (**Puls.**); *must be uncovered* as soon as heat begins (**Acon., Sec.**). *One ear, one cheek, and side of the face* **red and burning** (*one cheek* red and hot the other cold and pale, **Cham.**); hot knees with cold nose; heat of the face, with coldness of the hands and feet; continuous quick alternations from heat to cold. Heat and coldness of single parts (**Apis, Bell.**). **Deep snoring sleep during heat** (**Apis, Op.**); **frequent sighing**; beating headache; vertigo, delirium; pain in stomach and bowels; vomiting of ingesta, with coldness of the feet and spasmodic twitching of the extremities. *Urticaria* *over the whole body, with violent itching,* **easily > by scratching,** which disappears with the sweat (itching, stinging, nettle-rash before and during chill, **Hep.**—during chill and heat, **Rhus**—see **Dul.**). Patient is hungry after the fever (**Eup.**).

"The heat of Ignatia is almost always *external;* also, there is very seldom thirst with this heat, even in intermittent fever; hence Ignatia is able to cure *homeopathically* and *permanently in the smallest dose, intermittent fever which presents thirst during chill but not during heat."*—HAHNEMANN.

Sweat.—*Without thirst;* warm perspiration of extremities; usually light, though general. *Fainting during sweat,* or as the heat passes into sweating stage. Sweat when eating. Sensation as if sweat would break out over the whole body, which, however, does not follow. Warm perspiration on the hands, or on the inner surface of the hands and fingers, in the evening; at times cold, but generally warm and sour-smelling.

Tongue.—Clean. Saliva has a sour taste. Food tasteless.

Apyrexia.—Complete. The face is pale; *eruption on the lips and in the corners of the mouth;* lips dry and chapped; hungry about 11 A. M. (Sul.), but little or no appetite at time of meals; aching pain in pit of stomach; colic, with hard stools and ineffectual urging; pain in back and limbs; languor, apathy, giving away of the knees, starting in sleep, or sound sleep with snoring. The sleep usually continues from the heat during and through sweating stage, into apyrexia. All pain and headache aggravated by tobacco and coffee.

"During the chill thirsty, seeks external warmth; during the fever heat, no thirst, external warmth very pleasant; sitting up relieves the chill."—HAHNEMANN.

Ignatia is adapted to recent mild cases, or long-lasting and complicated ones, particularly those occurring among women and young people of a highly nervous organization. No remedy has *thirst during chill* and in no other stage, chill relieved by external heat, and heat aggravated by external covering, so prominently marked as Ignatia. The Ignatia patient is able to resume his occupation as soon as paroxysm is over. Ignatia is indicated if the tertian type has become quartan after taking large doses of Quinine.

Gelsemium.	**Ignatia.**
Time.—*2* P. M., 4 to 5 P. M., and 9 P. M. Regular—every day at same hour.	**Time.**—Not characteristic, chill late in afternoon or evening. Irregular—anticipates or postpones.
Morning fever, without chill.	Morning fever, with chill.
Prodrome.—No symptoms.	**Prodrome.**—Yawning and stretching.
Chill.—*Without thirst;* commencing in hands and feet. Chills follow each other in wave-like rapid succession up the spine from sacrum to occiput.	**Chill.**—*With great thirst;* commencing in upper arms *and spreads* to back. Shaking chill with red face, *relieved at once in warm room or by heat of stove.*
Heat.—Without thirst. Flying heat and flushes followed by perspiration.	**Heat.**—Without thirst. External heat and redness, without internal heat.
Sweat.—Profuse, coming on gradually, relieving all the pains.	**Sweat.**—Light, warm, chiefly on extremities, or of the face only.
Tongue.—Yellowish-white, breath fetid. Saliva blood-colored.	**Tongue.**—Clean. Saliva has a sour taste. Food tasteless.
Apyrexia.—Often wanting or very short. Intermittents often become remittents.	**Apyrexia.**—Complete. Face is very pale. One type frequently changes to another.

Analysis.—Red face during chill (Fer.); chill, *with thirst during chill only;* < by external heat; heat *without thirst,* < by covering (> by covering, Nux).

IODUM.

Characteristic.—Persons of a scrofulous diathesis, with dark hair and eyes; a low cachectic condition with *profound debility and* **great emaciation** (Abrot.).

Great weakness and loss of breath on going up stairs (Cal.); during the menses (Alum., Carbo a., Coc.).

Empty eructations from morning till evening, as if every particle of food was turned into air (Kali c.).

Ravenous hunger; eats freely and well, yet **loses flesh all the time** (Abrot., Nat. m., Sanic., Tub.).

Suffers from hunger, must eat every few hours, anxious and worried if he does not eat (Cina, Sulph.); *feels > while eating or after eating,* when stomach is **full.**

Itching: low down in the lungs, behind the sternum; causing cough. Extends through bronchi to nasal cavity (Coc. c., Con., Phos.). Hypertrophy and induration of the glands —thyroid, mammæ, ovaries, testes, uterus, prostate or other glands—breasts may dwindle and become flabby.

Hard goitre, in dark-haired persons (light-haired, Brom.); feels > after eating.

Palpitation, worse from least exertion (from least motion, Dig.—from least mental emotion, Cal. ars., Lith. c.).

Sensation as if the heart were squeezed together; as if grasped with an iron hand (Cac., Sulph.).

Leucorrhea: acrid, corrosive, staining and corroding the linen; most abundant at time of menses.

Cançerous degeneration of the cervix; cutting pains in abdomen and hemorrhage at every stool.

Constipation, with ineffectual urging > by drinking cold milk.

Croup: membranous, hoarse, dry cough, < in warm wet weather; with wheezing and sawing respiration (Spong.); especially in overgrown psoric boys.

Child grasps the larynx (Cepa); face pale and cold, especially in fleshy children.

Relations.—Complementary to: Lycopodium.

Follows well: after Hep., Mer.; is followed by Kali bi. in croup.

"Acts best in goitre when given after full moon, or when the moon is waning."—LIPPE.

Aggravation.—Warmth; wrapping up the head; cannot bear hat on (rev. of Hep., Psor.).

Amelioration.—Cold air; washing in cold water.

Type.—Quartan; tertian. Sporadic La Grippe; tubercular.

Time.—Any hour; often at night.

Chill.—Shaking chill, or unusual chilliness, even when in a warm room. Hands, nose, feet icy cold; cold feet the whole night. Chill frequently alternating with heat.

Heat.—*Quartan fever,* **with a constant diarrhea on the days free from fever** (urticaria when fever has been suppressed, Elat.). Hot flushes of heat over the body (**Fer.**, **Sep.**). Internal heat, with coldness of the surface. Burning heat of the hands (burning heat of palms of hands and soles of feet, with cold feet, **Sul.**). Fever with dry skin, weak and rapid pulse, twitching of the muscles, and more coldness than heat of skin.

Sweat.—With thirst. Debilitating, sour sweat all over in the morning hours, with great weakness of the limbs. Profuse, cold, viscid sweat at night. Palms of hands sweat continually. Cold feet sweat easily; so acrid that it corrodes the skin (**Graph.**).

Tongue.—Thickly coated, brown in centre, white at the edges. Salivation; salty or sour.

Pulse.—Large, hard, with orgasm of blood and throbbing in vessels, especially in larger arterial trunks; weak, rapid, thready, irregular; accelerated by every slight exertion.

Apyrexia.—Countenance *sallow; distressed look;* **ravenous hunger, must eat every few hours; left hypochondriac region hard and acutely sensitive to pressure.** Emaciation, debility, restlessness. Gets anxious and worried if he does not eat, *yet loses flesh all the time while eating freely.*

Analysis.—The general characteristic symptoms are the only guides; symptoms of the paroxysm not marked. Fevers of

Iodine often occur in tubercular persons, and may be result of suppressed intermittent by Quinine.

IPECACUANHA.

Characteristic.—Adapted to cases where the gastric symptoms predominate (Ant. c., Nux, Puls.).

In all diseases the constant nausea is guiding.

Nausea: with *profuse saliva;* vomiting of white, glairy mucus in large quantities, *without relief;* with distended abdomen; sleepy afterwards; worse from stooping.

Stomach feels relaxed *as if hanging down* (Ign., Staph.).

Stool: grassy green; white mucus (Colch.); bloody; fermented; preceded by *griping, pinching pain about the umbilicus,* as from a hand, each finger seemingly pressing sharply into the intestines, aggravated by the slightest motion; cutting colic about umbilicus.

Hemorrhage: **bright red** *from all the orifices of the body* (Erig., Mill.); uterine, profuse, clotted, heavy oppressed breathing during; stitches from navel to uterus; cutting across from left to right (from right to left, Lyc.); large accumulation of mucus in the bronchi, difficult to raise (Ant. t.).

Cough: dry, spasmodic, constricted, asthmatic.

Difficult breathing from least exercise; violent dyspnea, with wheezing and anxiety about the stomach.

Whooping-cough: child loses breath, turns pale, stiff and blue; strangling, with gagging and vomiting of mucus; bleeding from nose or mouth (Ind.).

Cough, with rattling of mucus in bronchi when inspiring (Ant. t.); threatened suffocation from mucus.

Pains as if bones were all torn to pieces (Lac c., Tub.—as if broken, Eup.).

Intermittent dyspepsia, every day or every other day at same hour; fever with persistent nausea.

Oversensitive to heat and cold.

Relations.—Complementary: **Cuprum.** Nux and Puls. follow well when gastric symptoms correspond.

Aggravation.—Slightest motion; worse in winter and dry weather; warm, moist south winds (Eup.); warm room; night.

Amelioration.—Rest; closing the eyes.

Type.—Quotidian; tertian; quartan. Apt to postpone and become irregular; bilious; remittent; malarial; yellow.

Time.—9 or 11 A. M. (10 to 11 A. M., Nat.) and 4 P. M. Fever, without chill, at 4 P. M.

Cause.—Irregularities and indiscretions in diet. Cases drugged with Quinine and Arsenic.

Prodrome.—Violent retching; yawning, stretching, backache, headache, and profuse flow of saliva. *Nausea.*

Chill.—Without thirst. Chilliness; he is always *worse when in a warm place. External coldness with external heat. Chill* **worse in a warm room**; or **from external heat** (**Apis**—> by external heat, **Ars., Ign.**), *lessened by drinking and in the open air* (**Caust.**—< by drinking, Caps., **Cinch., Eup. Nux**). *Shivering; then chilliness, with coldness without thirst,* at 4 P. M. The hands and feet are icy cold, and wet with cold sweat, with *redness of one cheek* and *paleness of the other.* Chill short and usually not severe, with or without nausea and vomiting. Paroxysm begins by an internal chill, *made worse by external heat.* Oppression of the chest.

Heat.—*With thirst; usually long-lasting,* over whole body, with alternate *coldness* and *paleness of face; nausea* and *vomiting;* anxious, *oppressed breathing,* and *dry, hacking cough,* often exciting nausea and vomiting (cough with pleuritic stitches, **Acon.**—dry, teasing cough, before and during chill, **Rhus**—cough during chill and heat, **Bry.**); cold hands and feet. Sudden heat about 4 P. M., with sweat on arms and back; heat of entire body in the evening. External heat without internal heat (see **Ign.**). One hand cold, the other hot (Dig., Lyc.). Heat about head and face, sometimes with, often without, redness of cheeks, with dilated pupils and prostration of body and mind.

Sweat.—Sudden attacks of sweat in a room; on upper parts of body; increased by motion and in the open air (**Bry.**—> by motion, **Caps.**); by being out of doors; cold on the forehead; *sour sweat with turbid urine;* stains yellow. Nausea and vomiting may be present. Always *worse during sweat; better after it* (> by sweating, **Eup., Gels., Nat.**). *Light sweat* in uncomplicated cases, but *may be sour. Sweat becomes profuse* **only after abuse of Quinine.** May cough in sweating stage. Sweat may only amount to a cold, sticky, clammy feeling of the skin in some cases.

Tongue.—At first clean; then coated yellowish or white; pale in all cases. Taste bitter, sweetish, like rancid oil. Desire for sweets, dainties.

Apyrexia.—Never clear; disturbed by more or less gastric trouble (**Ant. c., Puls.**); loss of appetite, nausea and vomiting. *Stomach feels relaxed and seems to hang down loose* (Staph.). Aversion to food (aversion to meat, **Arn.**); bad taste in the mouth, languor and debility, with absence of sleep. Bitter taste of everything eaten (Bry.—everything tastes bitter except water, **Acon.**); profuse secretion of saliva, and vomiting after eating. Herpes labialis.

"*Short chills; long fever; cold hands and feet;* great *oppression* of the chest, he *can hardly breathe.* Always after previous *drugging with Quinine.*"—N. A. Roth.

"Intermittent fever; nausea and vomiting predominate; slight chills are followed by much heat, with thirst and no subsequent perspiration. Fever consequent upon abuse of Quinine; slight chilliness without thirst, afterwards violent heat, with thirst, nausea and vomiting, dyspnea, stitches in the chest, finally copious perspiration."—Lippe.

If paroxysm has been suppressed by Quinine, Ipecacuanha is all the more indicated.

Relapses from improprieties in diet always an additional indication for Ipecacuanha. This is a very common cause of a return of paroxysm and one frequently overlooked by physicians. In all forms and types of fever, reckless or over eating is perhaps the most frequent cause of relapse.

The persistent nausea, which does not always amount to vomiting, that is usually present in every stage, is the *"guiding symptom"* of Ipecac., although it may be and often is indicated when neither nausea nor vomiting is present. When fever returns in another form, after *suppression by Quinine,* and symptoms do not clearly point to any remedy, *if nausea or vomiting were present in first onset of disease,* Ipecac. will often cure.

In his "Forty Years' Practice," Jahr places Ipecacuanha at the head of the list of remedies in the treatment of intermittent fever, and recommends its administration in commencing the treatment of every case. He says: "I almost always commence the treatment with Ipecac.[30], unless some other remedy is distinctly indicated. I give a few globules in water, a teaspoonful every three hours, beginning immediately after the chill. By pursuing this course I have cured many cases of 'fever and ague' by the first prescription, thus saving myself a good deal of unnecessary seeking and comparing. If it does not help altogether, it changes the character of the fever so that Arn., Ars., Ign., Nux, etc., will complete the cure."

This advice is also given by J. S. Douglas in his work on Intermittent Fever, p. 80; and a number of our closest and most successful prescribers have adopted it, with apparent success. H. V. Miller says: "I am apt to give Ipecac. when I do not clearly see the indications for another remedy. Then it serves to clear up the case and prepare the way for some other remedy to complete the cure."

I cannot endorse the above indiscriminate use of Ipecac., *on principle;* it is empiric practice, and will certainly be attended with many mortifying failures. That it is infinitely superior to the more prevalent, empiric and indiscriminate use of Quinine, and attended with less failures and less constitutional derangements, I have no doubt at all. If the attack can be traced to dietetic irregularities, this advice of Jahr is undoubtedly sound; the best proof being its success at the bed side. A case like the following very often occurs in practice:

A messenger is sent many miles for some medicine for "ague;" and that is all the information we can obtain. If we do not prescribe some one else will; and rather than lose a patient and have it said that we cannot cure "so simple a thing as ague" we make a "chance shot," and, unless we have found the *"genus epidemicus"* of the season, are as apt to fail as to cure.

This is, in my opinion, the opportunity to follow Jahr's advice and exhibit Ipecac.; and it would be infinitely better for *our patient, our school of medicine,* and *our professional reputation,* if we did so instead of sending Quinine. Ipecac. covers a much larger range of symptoms than Quinine, and, in a case like the above, will cure more patients.

In regard to this routine habit of prescribing Ipecac., Dr. Chargé says: "I have known practitioners, highly commendable in other respects, who always began with Ipecac, under the pretense that, after it, the case was better outlined and the choice of the true specific was consequently easier. This is simply an encouragement to indolence. Ipecac. presents itself to us with so clearly defined features, that it is impossible with a little attention not to recognize at once the cases which call for it."

Analysis.—Persistent nausea. Indiscretions in diet may have caused the original attack, or the relapse. Chill < in a warm room and from external heat. **Suppressed by abuse of Quinine. When the paroxysm is changed and masked by drugging.**

Chill not marked and distinct, being either a chilliness up and down the back or a mingling of chills and heat; half an hour the longest. If thirst in chill, may continue during chill and heat, although rarely so severe in heat. *Great lassitude and weariness during chill.* Chill usually followed by nausea and vomiting, first of contents of stomach, afterwards of bile. *Hot stage* lasts four or five hours, and even all night. *Sweat* light, partial, on single parts (**Bry.**), sour. If mixed with Quinine cachexia, *profuse, sour, and soaking the bed through.*

In the irregularity of the different stages of the paroxysm, as well as the universality of its indication, Ipecacuanha resembles Arsenic, and should always be thought of where indiscretions in diet may have been the cause of original attack, or have produced a relapse. The *greatest prostration occurs during chill* (the prostration of Arsenic. is greatest after heat).

Always < during sweat.

KALI BICHROMICUM.

Characteristic.—Adapted to fat, light haired persons, who suffer from catarrhal, syphilitic, or scrofulous affections; fat, chubby, short-necked children, disposed to croup and croup affections.

Affections of the mucous membranes—eyes, nose, mouth, throat, bronchi, gastro-intestinal and genito-urinary tracts—**discharges of a tough, stringy mucus which adheres to the parts, and can be drawn out into long strings** (Hydr., Lys.).

Complaints in hot weather.

Pains: *in small spots* can be covered with point of finger (Ign.); *shift rapidly* from one part to another (Kali s., Lac c., Puls.); appear rapidly, disappear suddenly (Bell., Ign., Mag. p.); neuralgia every day at same hour (Aran., Chin. s.).

Headache: *blurred vision or blindness precedes the attack* (Gels., Lac d.); must lie down; aversion to light and noise; sight returns as headache increases (Iris, Nat., Lac d.).

Gastric complaints: bad effects of beer; loss of appetite; weight in pit of stomach; flatulence; < soon after eating; vomiting of ropy mucus and blood; round ulcer of stomach (Gym.).

Nose: *pressive pain in root of nose* (in forehead and root of nose, Sticta); **discharge of "clinkers," plugs**; mucus tough, ropy, green, bloody; in clear masses, and has violent pain from occiput to forehead if discharge ceases; ulcers and scabs on, or ulceration of, septum (Alum., Sep., Teucr.).

Diphtheria: pseudo-membranous deposit, firm, pearly, fibrinous, prone to extend downwards to larynx and trachea (Lac c.—from bronchi to throat, Brom.); *bladder-like appearance of uvula,* much swelling, but little redness (Rhus).

Deep-eating ulcers in fauces; often syphilitic.

Cough: *hoarse, metallic in croup* (membranous or diphtheritic), with expectoration of tough mucus or fibro-elastic casts; in morning on awakening, with dyspnea > by lying down (cough on awakening, with dyspnea **when** lying down, Aral., Lach.); sputa tenacious, expectorated but cannot be easily detached, sticks to throat, mouth, lips (tenacious, frothy, detached with great difficulty, but easily expectorated, Aral.).

Sexual desire absent, in fleshy people.

Prolapsus uteri, seemingly in hot weather.

Aggravation.—Morning; after eating; *heat of summer.*

Amelioration.—Skin symptoms in cold weather (rev. of Alum., Pet.).

Type.—Complaints appear periodically (dysentery every year in the beginning of summer; headache in the morning) at the same hour daily. Pains intermit. "Any type of fever."—LIPPE.

Time.—Afternoon or evening paroxysm.

Fever, without chill, 4 and 5 P. M.

Chill.—Without thirst. Coldness and shivering of arms, shoulders, back, with sleepiness; seeks a warm place. Shivering, alternating with flushes of heat. Chilliness commencing in feet and legs and extending upwards over whole body, with sensation *as if vertex or pericranium* were constricted (**Sil.**), occurring in frequent paroxysms; an hour after chill, heat and dryness of mouth and lips, had to be frequently moistened, followed by great thirst next morning, but no sweat. Ill-humor. Chilliness, especially on the extremities, and flushes of heat alternating with general sweat. Feet and hands cold.

Chilliness, with giddiness and nausea, followed by heat, with sensation of cold and trembling; periodical pains in the temples; no thirst.

Heat.—With thirst. General heat over whole body at night. Flushes of heat in the face. Face and hands glowing hot, while arms were cold and deep internal chilliness continued. Sudden flushes of heat in the face which came on at 4 and 5 P. M.

Sweat.—Profuse while sitting quietly (profuse on least motion, **Bry., Sep., Sil., Sul.**). Sweat on forehead; *rest of face dry*. Hands cold and *bathed in cold sweat* (Sec.). General sweat, alternating with flushes of heat.

Tongue.—Broad, with indented edges (Mer.). Thick, yellow coating, coppery taste; *saliva stringy, ropy;* desire for acids (**Ant. c.**), for beer. Aversion to meat (Arn.).

Analysis.—The general symptoms: Ropy, stringy, viscid saliva and mucus. Sweat profuse while sitting quiet.

KALI BROMATUM.

Adapted to large persons inclined to obesity; acts better in children than in adults.

Loss of sensibility, fauces, larynx, urethra, entire body; staggering, uncertain gait; feels as if legs were all over sidewalk.

Nervous, restless; cannot sit still, must move about or keep occupied; *hands and fingers in constant motion; fidgety hands* (fidgety feet, Zinc.); twitching of fingers.

Fits of uncontrollable weeping and profound melancholic delusions.

Loss of memory; *forgets how to talk;* absent-minded; had to be told the word before he could speak it (Anac.).

Depressed, low-spirited, anxious, "feel as if they would lose their minds."

Incoördination of muscles (Gels.); nervous weakness or paralysis of motion and numbness.

Restlessness and sleeplessness due to worry and grief, loss of property or reputation, from business embarrassments (Hyos.).

Night terrors of children (Kali p.); grinding teeth in sleep, screams, moans, cries; horrible dreams, cannot be comforted by friends. Somnambulism (Sil.).

Spasms: from fright, anger or emotional causes in nervous plethoric persons; during parturition, teething, whooping-cough, Bright's disease.

Epilepsy: congenital, syphilitic, tubercular; usually a day or two before menses; at new moon; headache follows attack. Cholera infantum, with reflex irritation of brain, before effusion; first stage of hydrocephaloid.

Daily colic in infants about 5 A. M. (at 4 P. M., Col., Lyc.).

Nervous cough during pregnancy; dry, hard, almost incessant, threatening abortion (Con.).

Stammering; slow, difficult speech (Bov., Stram.).

Acne: simplex, indurata, rosacea; bluish-red, pustular, on face, chest, shoulders; leaves unsightly scars (Carbo an.); in young fleshy persons of gross habits.

Type.—Intermittent; quotidian; continued typhoid.

Chill.—Body cold; skin corrugated and mottled. Chilliness and general coldness, < especially about extremities; shivering, with external coldness.

Heat.—In face with fugitive flushes here and there.

Head hot, feels as if in a furnace, with coldness and chills.

Sweat.—Profuse and viscid, all over body; long-lasting and exhausting.

KALI CARBONICUM.

Characteristic.—Adapted to diseases of old people, dropsies and paralyses; dark hair, lax fibre, inclined to obesity (Am. c., Graph.).

After loss of fluids or of vitality, particularly in the anemic (deficient vitality, lack of susceptibility to medicinal action, Carbo v.).

Pains: *stitching, darting,* < during rest and *lying on affected side* (stitching, darting, > during rest, and lying on painful side, Bry.).

Cannot bear to be touched; starts when touched ever so lightly, especially on the feet.

Great aversion to being alone (Ars., Bis., Lyc.—desire to be alone, Ign., Nux).

Bag like swellings between upper lids and eyebrows.

Weak eyes; *after coition,* abortion, measles.

Nosebleed when *washing the face* in the morning (Am. c., Arn.).

Toothache: *only when eating;* throbbing; < when touched by anything warm or cold.

Stomach: distended, sensitive; feels as if it would burst; excessive flatulency; everything she eats or drinks appears to be converted into gas (Carbo v., Iod.).

Backache, sweating, weakness; after abortion, labor, metrorrhagia; when eating; while walking feels as if she must give up and lie down.

Asthma, relieved when sitting up or bending forward or by rocking (Ars.); worse from 2 to 4 A. M.

Cough: dry, paroxysmal, loosens viscid mucus or pus which must be swallowed; spasmodic *with gagging or vomiting of ingesta;* hard, white or smoky masses fly from throat when coughing (Bad., Chel.).

Feels bad, week before menstruation; backache, before and during menses.

Labor pains insufficient; violent backache; wants the back pressed (Caust.).

"Will bring on the menses, when Natrum muriaticum, though indicated, fails."—HAHNEMANN.

"Persons suffering from ulceration of the lungs can scarcely get well without this antipsoric."—HAHNEMANN.

Relations.—Complementary to Carbo vegetabilis.

Aggravation.—From 2 to 4 A. M., nearly all ailments, especially those of throat and chest; cold air; becoming cold; rest, and lying on painful side.

Amelioration.—Warmth; getting warm; eructations.

Type.—Quotidian; same every day. Intermittent, remittent or continued fevers with whooping-cough (Dros.).

Time.—9 A. M., 12 M. 5 *to* 6 *P. M.*

Fever, without chill, 9 A. M.

Chill.—With thirst; *great chilliness* **after eating** (Mar. v.), and *towards evening* (**Nux**). Chilliness *on every motion, even in bed* (**Nux, Hep.**). Chilliness, then heat, then chilliness again. Chill towards evening, *relieved near the warm stove and after lying down* (relieved by external heat, **Ars., Ign.**—increased by external heat, **Apis, Ipec.**). Chill with the pains (**Puls.**—all symptoms worse during chill, **Ars.**); *increased out of doors* (increased while going from a warm room into the open air, **Puls.**). Constant chilliness, violent thirst from internal heat; hot hands; and aversion to food; with oppression of breathing; constriction of chest; pain in right hypochondrium. After the chill, nausea and vomiting of bile.

"Violent chill towards evening for some minutes; he must lie down; followed by nausea, vomiting and spasmodic pain in the chest through the whole night, with short breath and much internal anxiety and much perspiration."—HAHNEMANN.

Heat.—Without thirst, with *long yawning, stitching pains in head and chest, pulsations in abdomen. Internal heat, external chilliness* (**Arn., Cal., Thuja**—chills intermingled with *heat,* **Ars.**). *Chill and heat, with dyspnea.* Dry heat of the cheeks and hands, *with shortness of breath.* Redness and heat in the face, with icy coldness of the feet (**Sep.**).

Sweat.—All night without relief (**Hep.**—sweat relieves, **Lach.**). Sweat of *axilla and perineum;* of upper parts of body; after eating; *perspires easily on least exertion.* **Sweat on every mental exertion,** *reading, writing,* etc. (Hep., Psor., **Sep. Sul.**—on least physical exertion, **Bry.**). Profuse warm sweat, with much heat, from 12 to 3 A. M.

Tongue.—Coated white; tip of tongue sore, burns as if raw or covered with blisters. Taste bad; bitter; flat.

Pulse.—Rapid mornings, slower in evening, unequal, irregular, intermitting; throbbing in blood-vessels; tendency to fatty heart.

Apyrexia.—Chest feels constricted; *right hypochondrium painful and tender to touch.* Excessive aversion to food, especially bread. Intense thirst, morning, noon and night. In the morning bad taste in the mouth; want of appetite; aversion to food, especially bread. Agglutination of the eyelids.

Analysis.—*Chill;* after eating; from every motion; < in open air, > by warmth.

Heat; without thirst; yawning, stitching pains in head and chest; dyspnea; internal heat, external chilliness.

Sweat; on every mental exertion; all night without relief.

KALI IODATUM.

Characteristic.—Adapted to scrofulous persons of lymphatic temperament; victims of mercurial, syphilitic or lead poisoning.

Chronic periosteal rheumatism of a syphilitic or mercurial origin; the nocturnal bone pains become intolerable at night, driving the patient to despair (Mer., Phyt., Syph.).

Before menses; frequent urging to urinate; the menstrual pains are felt most acutely in the thighs as if squeezed (Con., Nux m.).

Glandular swellings; interstitial infiltration.

Aggravation.—At night, the bone pains become unbearable; cold air; rest.

Amelioration.—Motion.

Time.—4 to 8 P. M. (**Hep., Lyc., Mag. m.**); 10 P. M.

Type.—Simple. Any fever.

Chill.—With thirst. Chilliness from afternoon till next morning. *Chilliness* **with sleepiness,** beginning by creeping up the back and extending over the whole body, from 6 to 8 P. M. Chill from 4 to 7 P. M., with shaking; *was able to get warm in bed, but* **not by heat of stove** (**Pod.**—relieved by heat of stove, **Ign., Sabad.**). *Shaking chill at night,* sleepy with frequent waking; *so chilly at night that she could not get warm.* Shivering fit; feels frozen; cannot get warm with any amount of clothing. *Sleepy* and *drowsy.* Coldness of the feet with anasarcous swelling (**Apis, Ars.**).

Heat.—Great heat with thirst (as after exertion) followed by excessive coldness with trembling. Flushes of heat with dry skin; at times chilly, at others profuse sweat. Heat of head with burning redness of the face, alternating with coldness, languor, and sometimes sweat.

Sweat.—Scanty; or occurs during hot stage. Night sweats.

All the preparations of Kali have febrile conditions marked by **hot flushes,** particularly **Kali c.** (same as **Sep., Sul.,** etc.).

LACHESIS.

Characteristic.—Persons of a choleric, melancholy temperament, dark eyes and a disposition to low spirits and indolence.

Women of choleric temperament, with freckles and red hair.

Better adapted to thin and emaciated than to fleshy persons; to those who have been changed both mentally and physically by their illness.

Climacteric ailments: hemorrhoids, hemorrhages, **hot flushes, hot sweats;** burning vertex headaches; especially at or after the menopause (Sang.).

Ailments from long-lasting grief; sorrow, fright, vexation, jealousy or disappointed love (Aur., Ign., Phos. ac.).

Women who have not recovered from the change of life, "have never felt well since that time."

Headache: pressing or bursting pain in temple $<$ from motion, pressure, stooping, lying, after sleep; dreads to go to sleep because she wakens with such a headache.

Rush of blood to head: after alcohol; mental emotions; suppressed or irregular menses; at climaxis; left-sided apoplexy.

Weight and pressure on vertex (Sep.); like lead, in occiput (Petr.).

Drunkards: with congestive headaches or hemorrhoids; prone to erysipelas or apoplexy.

Left side principally affected; **diseases begin on the left and go to the right side**—ovary, testicle, chest, face, throat.

Great sensitiveness to touch, throat, stomach, abdomen; can bear nothing tight around the neck or waist; cannot bear bed-clothes or night-dress to touch throat or abdomen, not because sore or tender as in Apis or Belladonna, but the clothes *cause an uneasiness* (Agar.).

Extremes of heat and cold cause great debility.

All symptoms, especially the mental, *worse after sleep, or the aggravation wakes him from sleep; sleeps into the aggravation; unhappy,* distressed, anxious, *sad,* < *in morning on waking.*

Mental excitability: ecstacy, with almost prophetic perceptions; with a vivid imagination; *great loquacity* (Agar., Stram.); wants to talk all the time; jumps from one idea to another; *one word often leads into another story.*

Constipation: inactivity, stool lies in rectum, without urging; sensation of *constriction of sphincter* (Caust., Nit. ac.).

Menses **at regular time**; too short, scanty, feeble; *pains all relieved by the flow; always better during menses* (Zinc.).

Piles: with scanty menses; at climaxis; strangulated; with stitches shooting upward (Nit. ac.).

The least thing coming near mouth or nose interferes with breathing; wants to be fanned, *but slowly and at a distance* (rapidly, Carbo v.).

As soon as he falls asleep the breathing stops (Am. c., Grind., Lac c., Op.).

Great physical and mental exhaustion; trembling in whole body, would constantly sink from weakness; worse in the morning (Sulph., Tub.).

Epilepsy: comes on during sleep (Bufo); from loss of vital fluids, onanism, jealousy; during menses (Ced.).

Hemorrhagic diathesis; small wounds bleed easily and profusely (Crot., Kreos., Phos.); blood dark, non-coagulable (Crot., Sec.); typhoid, yellow fever, great prostration (Kreos.).

Boils, carbuncles, ulcers with intense pain (Tar.); malignant pustules; decubitus; *dark, bluish, purple appearance;* tend to malignancy.

Bad effects of poison wounds; post-mortem (Pyr.).

Relations.—Complementary: Lycopodium, Nitric acid.

Natrum mur. follows well when type of fever changes.

Aggravation.—After sleeping; from acids, alcohol, cinchona, mercury; contact; morning and evening; extremes of temperature; in the sun; spring; summer.

Amelioration.—Warmth.

Time.—Periodicity strongly marked. 12 M. to 2 P. M. Afternoon or evening chill; fever lasting all night.

Type.—Quotidian; tertian; quartan; malarial; typhoid, typhus, septic, yellow fever. Every fourteen days.

Annually returning paroxysm every spring (Carbo v., Ign., Sul.), after suppression by Quinine the previous autumn. This is guiding.

Cause.—Especially useful when paroxysms of fever are sure to return after taking acids, or in the spring after Quinine.

Prodrome.—Thirst, then shuddering (shuddering after drinking, Caps.).

Chill.—Without thirst; **commencing in the small of the back (Eup. purp.)**, runs up the back to the head (**Gels.**), lessened in a warm room. *Violent chill in the evening, with chattering of the teeth,* soreness of chest, and **longing for the fire. Wants to be near the fire and lie down;** *heat makes him feel better,* but *his chill continues as long as if he were in bed* (*heat of stove > the chill.* Chill does not amount to much; *if he can sit near a hot stove he gets warm,* **Ign.**). Pain in the limbs; pleuritic stitches, oppression of the chest; convulsive movements, and *in children, convulsions.* **Child must be held firm to relieve the pain in head and chest, and prevent shaking (Gels.). If held firm or pressed down, feels relieved.** "A lady wanted her daughter to lie with her full weight across her during chill; a boy wanted a sack of flour put on him to keep him from shaking." *Chill and heat alternating and changing from place to place.* Nausea and vomiting accompany paroxysm when severe, with some thirst. Coldness in one side of the head. Icy cold feet, with oppression of the chest. After icy cold calves, shaking chill with warm sweat; then strumming through the limbs, intermingled with flushes of heat.

Heat.—With thirst; *violent headache; livid complexion; oppression of the chest;* backache, *deep breathing and sleep;* or *great loquacity* (**Mar. v.**—during chill and heat, **Pod.**). Violent fever every evening, with loss of appetite and headache; internal chill, external heat; in the evening great febrile heat which lasted all night. Heat in the evening, with red spots on the cheeks. *Internal sensation of heat with cold feet.* Burning in the palms and soles, evening and night, *must be uncovered* (**Acon., Sec.**). Heat in ears, face, abdomen, pit of stomach, alternating with coldness, with shivering when lifting the bedclothes (**Nux**). Flushes of heat as from orgasm of the blood, with great sensitiveness of throat at night.

Sweat.—*Profuse sweat, which affords relief,* or light, warm, transient sweat. Perspiration *between* the paroxysms of fever; on the back which stains sulphur-yellow. *Strong-smelling* perspiration in axilla, *smelling like garlic* (*sweat in axilla, like onions,* **Bov.**). Sweat cold; *stains yellow;* or *bloody, staining red.*

Tongue.—*Trembles when protruded; or catches behind the teeth; mapped,* coated white, or dry, red tip and brown centre. Sour taste, everything turns sour (everything bitter, **Ipec.**).

Pulse.—Palpitation; *can bear no pressure on throat or chest.* Pulse weak and small, or full and small alternately, but accelerated; intermittent; unequal. The least movement causes feeling of suffocation around the heart.

Apyrexia.—Complete remission of all the symptoms; complexion livid, yellow, or ashy, often with vermillion redness of the cheeks; great weakness of the whole body in the morning on rising, especially of the extremities.

"*Intermittent fever:* the paroxysms come on every spring, or after the suppression of the fever in the previous fall by Quinine; occur in the afternoon; are accompanied by violent pain in the small of the back and limbs, oppression of the chest, violent headache, with a red face and cold feet; during the hot stage continuous talking; face yellow or ash-colored."—LIPPE.

Analysis.—*Chill;* commencing in the small of the back; longing for the fire, heat >; wants to be held firmly to > chill and prevent shaking.

Heat; headache, face livid, or vermillion red cheeks, oppressed breathing; great loquacity or sleep.

Sweat: profuse which >; cold, stains yellow, bloody.

Fever: septic, typhoid, typhus, yellow; stupor or muttering delirium, sunken countenance, falling of lower jaw; tongue dry, black, *trembles,* is protruded with difficulty or *catches on the teeth* when protruding; conjunctiva yellow or orange color; perspiration cold, stains yellow, bloody (Crot., Lyc.).

LACHNANTHES.

Characteristic.—Loquacious delirium, brilliant eyes, circumscribed red cheeks, < from 1 to 2 A. M. (Ars.).

Torticollis: neck stiff, head drawn to one side; pain in the nape as if dislocated, when turning the neck or bending the head backward.

Sensation: as if a piece of ice was lying on the back between the shoulders; of burning, in sacrum, in spine four inches above the small of back, of palms of hands and soles of feet.

Time.—Evening fever; < from 6-12 P. M.

Chill.—With thirst; body icy cold, relieved by hot flatirons, but not by external covering (Caps.); head burns like fire (Arn.). Flushes alternate with chilliness. Feels hot, but chills run all over her before heat can develop.

Sensation as if a piece of ice were lying on back between capulæ, then a shock followed by coldness over whole body with goose flesh; recur on moving.

Heat.—Dry, feet burn; restless tossing about with rumbling in abdomen. Burning heat, red face, worse on right side; after heat, circumscribed dark redness of face, also worse on right side (Chel., Sang.). Flushes of heat alternating with chilliness. Evening fever without chill, worse from 6 to 12 P. M., with red cheeks and red face (worse on upper part of face). Fever with somnolency (Apis).

Sweat.—After 12 P. M.; after a restless sleep. Morning sweat. Skin cold, damp, clammy and sticky. Sweat with vertigo, boiling and bubbling in chest and region of heart. Icy cold, chiefly on forehead.

LAUROCERASUS.

Characteristic.—Coldness on forehead as from draft of air.

Drink rolls audibly through esophagus and intestines.

Painlessness with most complaints (Stram.).

Diseases attended with rapid sinking of the vital forces (Camph., Ver.).

Deficient reaction, want of energy of vital forces, especially in affections of the chest; the well chosen remedy does not act.

Long lasting fainting spells.

Irresistible sleepiness; after dinner; in the evening.

Chill.—With thirst; in the afternoon or evening. Violent chill and coldness, with shivering, not relieved by external warmth; coldness and shaking chill, not relieved by heat of stove, alternating with burning heat. Deficient animal heat (Led.). Vertigo; stupor, and apoplectic symptoms (Opium).

Heat.—After the chill; from evening till midnight; descending the back (see Ver.).

Sweat.—During and after the heat; after eating; rarely profuse.

LEDUM.

Characteristic.—Adapted to the rheumatic gouty diathesis; constitutions abused by alcohol (Colch., Crot.).

Hemorrhage into anterior chamber after iridectomy.

Contusions of eye and lids especially if much extravasation of blood; ecchymosis of lids and conjunctiva.

Rheumatism and rheumatic gout; *begins in lower limbs and ascends* (descends, Kalmia); especially if brought to a low asthenic condition by abuse of Colchicum; joints become the seat of nodosities and "goutstones" which are painful; arthritis.

Affects left shoulder and right hip-joint (Agar., Ant. t., Stram.).

Emaciation of affected parts (Graph.).

Pains: are sticking, tearing, throbbing, and pains in joints are $<$ by motion; $<$ at night, by warmth of bed and bed-covering (Mer.), $>$ only when holding feet in ice water (Sec.).

Complaints of people who are *cold all the time; always feel cold and chilly;* lack of animal or vital heat (Sep., Sil.); the wounded parts especially are *cold to touch.*

Parts cold to touch, but not cold subjectively to patient.

In some affections, warmth of bed intolerable on account of heat and burning of limbs.

Swelling: of feet, up to knees; of ankle with unbearable pain when walking, as from a sprain or false step; ball of great toe swollen, painful; in heels as if bruised.

Intense itching of feet and ankles, $<$ from scratching and warmth of bed (Puls., Rhus).

Easy spraining of ankles and feet (Carbo an.).

Punctured wounds by sharp-pointed instruments, rat bites (Hyper.); as awls, nails, stings of insects, especially mosquitoes.

Red pimples or tubercles *on forehead and cheeks,* as in brandy drinkers, stinging when touched.

Long-remaining *discoloration after injuries;* "black and blue" places *become green.*

Aggravation.—*Heat;* cannot bear heat of bed; becomes intolerable by midnight, compelling to throw off the bedclothes (rev. of Sil.). Motion (joints only): misstep; alcohol.

Amelioration.—Uncovering relieves the terrible burning at night in the gouty nodosities of joints.

Type.—Double quotidian. Arthritic fever.

Time.—9.45 A. M., 2.30 P. M., same day. Generally only a forenoon paroxysm.

Cause.—Exposure to cold. Diseases arising from cold and debility.

Chill.—*With thirst.* Chilliness *of single parts, as if cold water were poured over the parts* (chill over whole body as if dashed with cold water, **Rhus**). Chilliness mornings and forenoons; want of natural heat (Mar. v.). Shaking all over, with little chilliness (**Eup. purp.**), without heat, but with thirst for cold water. *Shaking chill over the whole back, with hot cheeks and hot forehead, without redness of face or thirst, hands cold.* Shivering and chilliness with goose-flesh, without external coldness. Coldness of the back between the shoulders and in lumbar region. (See **Caps.**—sensation as if a piece of ice were lying on the back between the shoulders followed by coldness over the whole body with gooseflesh; relieved by hot irons, **Lachn.**) General coldness with heat and redness of the face. Chill, *with colic every evening.*

"Violent chills and horripilation with cold limbs."—HAHNEMANN.

Heat.—All over, *without thirst;* on waking the body is covered with perspiration, accompanied by itching of the whole body. **The warmth of the bed is intolerable** *on account of the heat and burning of the limbs (external warmth is unbear-*

able, **Puls.**). *Heat in the hands and feet in the evening,* with much **distended veins of hands** (veins of face and neck distended, **Bell.**, **Cinch.**—veins in forearms and hands, **Puls.**).

Sweat.—*Perspires, and cannot bear the bed covers* (must be uncovered as soon as sweat begins, **Acon.**). Slight sweat all over, with itching of the whole body, provoking scratching. Warm sweat on the hands and feet, long continuing. Sour, offensive sweat on the forehead if he perspires when walking.

Pulse.—Hard, full and rapid; often can be felt on one arm only.

"Intermittent fevers with malignant rheumatism or gouty complications."

"The fever consists almost entirely of coldness, shivering, here and there a little heat, of the cheeks or forehead, while the limbs are very cold, and a sour-smelling sweat especially on the forehead; the sweat is often interspersed with shivering." —DUNHAM.

Analysis.—*Chill;* severe; of single parts as if cold water were poured over them, with colic every evening.

Heat; warmth of bed is intolerable from heat and burning of limbs.

Sweat; sour-smelling on the forehead.

Fever with rheumatic and gouty ailments.

LOBELIA INFLATA.

Characteristic.—Best adapted to persons of light hair, blue eyes, fair complexion; inclined to be fleshy.

Gastric derangements, *extreme nausea and vomiting;* morning sickness; spasmodic asthma; *pertussis, with dyspnea threatening suffocation.*

Headaches: gastric, with nausea, vomiting and great prostration; following intoxication; < afternoon until midnight; sudden pallor with profuse sweat (Tab.); < by tobacco or tobacco smoke.

Vomiting: *face bathed with cold sweat;* of pregnancy, *profuse salivation* (Lac. ac.—at night, Merc.); **chronic with good appetite, with nausea, profuse sweat and marked prostration.**

Faintness, weakness and an indescribable feeling at epigastrium, from excessive use of tea or tobacco.

Urine: of a deep orange red color; copious red sediment.

Dyspnea: from constriction of middle of chest < with every labor pain, seems to neutralize the pains; < by exposure to cold or slightest exertion, going up or down stairs (Ipec.).

Sensation of congestion, pressure or weight in chest as if blood from extremities was filling it, > *by rapid walking.*

Sensation as if heart would stand still; deep-seated pain at base (at apex, Lil.).

Sacrum: **extreme sensitiveness;** *cannot bear the slightest touch, even of a soft pillow;* sits leaning forward to avoid contact with clothes.

For the bad effects of drunkenness in people with light hair, blue or grey eyes, florid complexion, corpulent, Lobelia bears the same relation that Nux vomica does to persons of the opposite temperament.

Aggravation.—Cold washing; cold bathing; cause dyspnea and increase or return of pain (**Ant. c.**); slight motion; touch.

Amelioration.—After drinking; evening; walking rapidly > chest pain.

Type.—Quotidian; remittent; continued.

Time.—10.30, 11 A. M., 12 M.

Prodrome.—Thirst (**Caps., Cinch., Eup.**).

Chill.—*With thirst;* severe, shaking, coldness, increased after drinking (**Caps.**); down the back with heat in stomach; general shivering alternating with flushes of heat.

Heat.—With thirst; with sweat or inclination to sweat, particularly in the face; heat alternating with slight chilliness from noon till evening. Respiration short, anxious, laborious and wheezing, with tightness of the chest. Tickling in the throat-pit, with frequent hacking cough, severe headache extending round the forehead from one temple to the other. Great debility.

Sweat.—With heat, or after the heat has lasted some time; with sleep (**Pod.**); profuse, at night; cold.

Tongue.—White or coated on the right side, clean on the left. Loss of appetite.

Pulse.—Frequent, but small and weak in the evening.

Apyrexia.—Attended with great debility; dyspnea and oppression at pit of stomach, with weakness and sensation as if stomach was too full, as from undigested food. Complete loss of appetite. Nausea relieved by drinking. The weak sensation in stomach may extend through whole chest or down to abdomen. The thirst is often found only during heat and prodrome and not in chill. The sweat resembles that of Podophyllum, coming on after the heat has continued for some time and is accompanied by sleep.

Analysis.—*Chill;* with thirst; severe shaking < by drinking.
Heat; short, anxious, labored breathing.
Sweat; with sleep or heat.
Nausea > by drinking.

LYCOPODIUM.

Characteristic.—Best suited to persons intellectually keen, but physically weak; upper part of body wasted, lower part semi-dropsical; lean and predisposed to lung and hepatic affections (Phos., Sul.); the extremes of life, children and old people.

Children: weak, emaciated; with well-developed heads but puny, sickly bodies.

Weeps all day, cannot calm herself; very sensitive, even cries when thanked.

Irritable; peevish and cross on waking; ugly, kick and scream; easily angered; cannot endure opposition or contradiction; seeks disputes; is beside himself.

Baby cries all day, sleeps all night (rev. of Jal., Psor.).

Avaricious, greedy, miserly, malicious, pusillanimous.

Ailment from fright, anger, mortification, or vexation with reserved displeasure (Staph.).

Catarrh: dry, nose *stopped at night,* must breathe through the mouth (Am. c., Nux, Samb.); snuffles, child starts from sleep rubbing its nose; of root of nose and frontal sinuses; *crusts and elastic plugs* (Kali bi., Teuc.).

Deep-seated, progressive chronic disease.

Pains, chiefly aching-pressure, drawing, right-sided, < **from 4 to 8 P. M.**

Dread of men; of solitude; *fear of being left alone* (Ars., Bis., Kali c.).

Red sand in urine; on child's diaper (Phos.); *child cries before urinating* (Bor.); pain in back > by urinating.

Gastric affections: excessive accumulation of flatulence; *constant sensation of satiety;* good appetite, but a few mouthfuls *fill up to the throat,* and he feels bloated; borborygmus.

Complexion; pale, dirty, unhealthy; *fan-like motion of alæ nasi* (see Ant. t.); sallow; looks older than he is.

Affects right side, or goes from right to left; throat, chest, abdomen, ovaries.

One foot hot and the other cold (Cinch., Dig., Ipec.).

Constipation: since puberty; since last confinement; when away from home; of infants; with ineffectual urging, rectum contracts and protrudes during stool, developing piles.

Impotence: of young men, from onanism or sexual excess; penis small, cold, relaxed; *old men, with strong desire but imperfect erections;* falls asleep during an embrace; premature emissions.

Dryness of vagina: burning in, during and after coition (Lys.); physometra; prevents coition.

Discharge of blood from genitals during every stool.

Fetus appears to be turning somersaults.

Pneumonia; neglected or maltreated, base of r. lung involved especially; to hasten absorption or expectoration.

Cough deep, hollow, even raising mucus in large quantities affords little relief.

Relations.—Complementary: Iodum.

Follows well: after Cal., Lach., Puls., Sul.

Aggravation.—From 4 to 8 P. M.; after eating; cold food or drinks; oysters; salt food.

Amelioration.—On getting cold; uncovering; warm food and drinks; loosening the garments.

Type.—Quotidian; tertian; double tertian; quartan; double quartan; every seventh day (**Cinch.**); typhoid; typhus.

Time.—Morning paroxysm, 8 or 9 A. M. Afternoon paroxysm, 3 or 4 P. M.

Evening paroxysm (the most severe), **6 or 7 P. M.**, and continues until morning.

Evening fever without chill, every day, **or every other** day, *at same hour.*

Prodrome.—Sometimes flushes of heat, and nausea and vomiting precede the chill, without thirst.

Chill.—Without thirst. First, she awoke *in the morning with chilliness,* followed by great heat. Violent chill at 8 A. M., lasting half an hour, and followed by little heat. Chilliness at 9 A. M., *over the whole body; she cannot get warm even by a stove.* Pernicious intermittents with a long-lasting chill coming on at 9 A. M. and finally passing off *without subsequent heat or sweat.* Febrile paroxysm every afternoon at 3 o'clock, lasting till late in the evening; a constantly increasing chilliness, without subsequent heat or sweat (**Bov.**). Evening paroxysm; slight chill, followed immediately by violent, long-continuing heat, weariness, prostration, and pains in the limbs (**Ars.**). Alternating chill and heat, with great redness and heat of the cheeks (**Bell.**). *Chilliness at 4 P. M., goose-flesh over the whole body, with incessant yawning, nausea, inclination to vomit,* chilliness *starting from the back* and extending over the whole body (**Caps., Gels.**), with numbness and coldness of the hands and feet; *no sweat, no thirst; but heat,* which was confined to the face; the chill lasted two hours and a half, and ended with excessive weakness and weariness of the feet, inclination to sleep, and slight drawings in the wrists and fingers of both hands; she slept well through the night and woke well the next morning.

Chilliness over the whole body in the evening at 6 P. M., starting from the back, with a feeling as if water were spurted upon the back (**Ant. t., Led., Rhus**); chilliness with stupefying sleep, followed by uneasy sleep, with dreams; chilliness over whole body lasting two hours, with stupefaction of the head, sleepiness, tearing in the limbs, no thirst, and no sweat. At 7 P. M., *shaking chill, commencing in the back,* with *numb, icy cold hands and feet* (**Ced., Sep.**); *she cannot get warm in bed for two hours,* the tearing in the limbs is worse, with uninterrupted yawning, nausea and inclination to vomit.

Febrile paroxysm at 7 P. M.; *shaking chill, with icy coldness even in bed,* **as if she were lying on ice,** lasting two hours, with drawings in all the limbs, back and whole body, on waking from sleep full of dreams, *perspiration all over,* with **great thirst after the sweat.** During chill it seems as if the blood ceased to be warm and everything internal would come to a stand-still. **Chill on left side of the body** (**Caust., Carbo v.**—right side, **Bry.**). Nausea and vomiting, then chill, *followed by sweat, without intervening heat* (**Caust.**); **sour vomiting between chill and heat** (*bitter, bilious vomiting,* **Eup., Ipec.**); *face and hands bloated* (**Apis, Ars.**). Shivering after drinking (**Ars., Caps., Eup.**) and while eating.

The first chills are usually one-sided; most frequently on the left.

Heat.—With thirst. Flushes of heat over the whole body in the evening, *with frequent drinking of small quantities at a time* (**Ars., Cinch.**). *After eating, heat of the head and a red spot on the left cheek.* Frequent rising of heat from the abdomen to the head, with burning in the cheeks. Great heat and redness of the face, with irresistible inclination to sleep (**Apis, Ign.**). Face, cheeks, ears, eyes, fingers and palms of hands hot and burning. *Nausea after cold drinks* (*nausea relieved by drinking, Lob.*); *warm drinks are grateful* (Casc., Ced.). Constipation; increased urination, which relieves the backache. *Sour vomiting often occurs in* or lasts during *entire hot stage.* **Must uncover (Lach.).**

Sweat.—Perspiration in the night, or in the morning after a restless night. *Profuse sour-smelling perspiration on the body,* but not on the lower legs. Night-sweat on body, not on the limbs. Morning-sweat only of the joints. Morning-sweat *cold, sour, offensive, bloody, or smelling like onions.* May be general over whole body. **Perspiration immediately after the chill,** ***without intervening heat*** **(Caust.). Thirst after sweating stage.**

Tongue.—Clean, but dry; red, trembling, stiff, vesicles on tip, or brown, or cracked. Taste: *sour;* bitter; fatty; *eructations sour.* Desire for sweets (Ipec.); for oysters, which disagree. Aversion to boiled warm food; tobacco smoke (Ign.).

Pulse.—Sensation as if the circulation stood still; accelerated in evening or after eating; ebullition with trembling (Mer.).

Apyrexia.—Not pronounced; but the concomitants are often guiding symptoms. Constant sense of fulness in the stomach and abdomen as if they would burst. Repletion after eating ever so little. Rumbling in the bowels; obstinate constipation. Cough, with thick, yellow, salty expectoration. *Red, sandy* *sediment in the urine* (**Natr.**). Patient cannot bear to be left alone (wants to be alone, **Cinch., Nux**).

This remedy is frequently rejected, when indicated, in intermittent fever, if the paroxysm does not occur at 4 P. M., and the *red, sandy sediment* is not present in the urine. The *sediment* rarely occurs in acute cases; and the most severe and most frequent paroxysm is the evening one at 6 or 7 P. M., which lasts all night. The *flatulence, sour eructations, sour taste, sour sweat,* **sour vomiting**, are much more reliable guides, because more often present. No single symptom, however guiding, is sufficient to warrant a prescription. If the totality corresponds, Lycopodium will cure, irrespective of time of paroxysm. The general symptoms of Lycopodium *are aggravated from 4 to 8 P. M.,* and if present, constitute an additional indication.

Analysis.—The time 4-8 P. M. or 6-7 P. M.

Sour eructations, sweet taste and vomiting.

Sour vomiting between chill and heat or, during heat.

Chill; severe, with icy coldness, as if lying on ice.

Heat; thirst for warm drinks; must uncover.

Sweat; immediately after chill; most thirst after sweat.

Gastric repletion after eating ever so little.

Red, sandy sediment in the urine.

MAGNESIA CARBONICA.

Characteristic.—For persons, especially children, of irritable disposition, nervous temperament (Cham.); sour smell of the whole body (Rheum).

The whole body feels tired and painful, especially the legs and feet.

Pains: neuralgic, lightning-like, worse left side (Col.—worse right side, Mag. p.); insupportable during repose, must get up and walk about; toothache *during pregnancy < at night.*

Pain on vertex as if the hair were pulled (Kali n., Phos.).

All the symptoms are aggravated every third week (feels badly week before menstruation, Kali c.).

Menses: preceded by sore throat (Lac c.), labor-like pains, cutting colic, backache, weakness, chilliness; **flow only at night or when lying,** and in absence of uterine pains, cease when walking (Am. c., Kreos.—rev. of Lil.); acrid, dark, pitch-like; difficult to wash off.

Inordinate *craving for meat* in children of tuberculous parentage.

Diarrhea: preceded by cutting colic; occurs regularly every three weeks; *stools, green, frothy,* **like scum of a frog pond;** white, tallow-like masses are found floating in stool; milk *passes undigested in nursing children.*

Unrefreshing sleep, more tired on rising than when retiring (Bry., Con., Hep., Op., Sulph., Tub.).

Relations.—Complementary: Chamomilla.

Aggravation.—Cold; draft; change of temperature; contact; every third week; rest; milk during menses.

Amelioration.—Warm air, but worse in warmth of bed (**Led., Mur.**—> in warmth of bed, Ars.).

Type.—Periodicity not marked. Quotidian generally.

Symptoms return periodically every three weeks.

Time.—9 A. M., and 5, 7, 8, 9 and 10 P. M.

Chill.—Chilliness in bed, *as if dashed with cold water* (**Ant. t., Led., Sab.**). Shaking chill beginning in the feet, going off in bed. Shaking chill at 9 P. M.; even in bed she was unable to get warm for an hour. Shivering at 10 P. M. in bed without subsequent heat, sweat or thirst (without subsequent heat or sweat, **Bov., Sul.**). Coldness of feet, as if wading in cold water (as if standing in cold water up to the ankles, **Sep.**). *Chill running down the back; lessened by out-door exercise.*

Heat.—A feeling of warmth streams through her whole body (as if vapors rise up to the brain, **Lyssin., Sarac.**—as of hot water running through the veins **Ars., Bry., Rhus**).

Great internal heat at night, could scarcely remain in bed, yet dreads the slightest exposure (**Bar., Nux**). *Great aversion to uncovering* (**Bell.**—cannot move in the least or be uncovered without feeling chilly, **Nux**). Heat of the *head, face, hands;* one-sided (right), mostly in forenoon; *redness, burning* and *thirst* for half an hour; often with sweat on the head.

Sweat.—Profuse, with thirst; *from 12 P. M. till morning;* on slight motion; offensive night sweat. *Sour-smelling, oily perspiration, difficult to wash off;* stains yellow.

Tongue.—Clean or white-coated; taste sour, bitter. *Desire for meats, acid drinks.*

Analysis.—The constitutional symptoms are the chief guides.

MAGNESIA MURIATICA.

Characteristic.—Especially suitable to diseases of women; spasmodic and hysterical complaints complicated with uterine diseases; who have suffered for years from attacks of indigestion or biliousness.

Children: during difficult dentition are **unable to digest milk**; it causes pain in stomach and passes undigested; crave sweets.

Sensation of soreness, with great sensitiveness to noise (Ign., Nux, Ther.).

Headache: every six weeks; in forehead and around the eyes; as if it would burst; < from motion and in open air; > lying down, *strong pressure,* wrapping up warmly (Sil., Stron.).

Tendency of head to sweat (Cal., Sanic., Sil.).

Continual rising of white froth into the mouth.

Toothache; unbearable when food touches the teeth.

Eructations; tasting like onions (breath smells of onions, Sinap.).

Constipation: stool large, hard; knotty, like sheep dung; difficult to pass; **crumbling at verge of anus** (Am. m., Nat. m.); *of infants during dentition.*

Urine: pale yellow; can only be passed by bearing down with abdominal muscles; weakness of bladder.

Menses: with great excitement at every period; flow black, clotted; spasms and pain extend into thighs; metrorrhagia, < at night in bed, causing hysteria (Act., Caul., Xan.).

Leucorrhea: after exercise; with every stool; with uterine spasm; followed by metrorrhagia; *two weeks after menses* (Bar., Bov.).

Great tendency to foot-sweat (Sil., Sanic.).

Aggravation.—At night; when riding on horseback; sea bathing (great weakness); cold.

Amelioration.—Warmth; in bed; exercise.

Type.—Quotidian. Same time every day. Headache every six weeks.

Time.—4, 6, 7, 8 P. M.—4 to 8 P. M. worse (**Hep.**, **Lyc.**, **Sab.**—pains commencing at 4 or 5 P. M., worse until midnight, diminishing after, and ceasing at daylight, **Syph.**).

Chill.—With shaking, not relieved by warmth of stove; lessened in the open air and in bed. Shivering over the whole body, with icy cold feet. Chilliness, with goose flesh, frequent yawning, cutting in abdomen and constant desire for stool. Chilliness in the evening, that disappears after lying down, followed before midnight by heat, and after midnight, sweat, with thirst lasting till morning.

Heat.—With thirst, in the evening; averse to uncovering. Flushes of heat, with vertigo. Heat of head, with redness of face, without external warmth, with internal shivering and desire for stool.

Sweat.—Without thirst, after midnight, till morning; averse to uncovering. Early morning with thirst and dryness of the mouth.

Tongue.—Coated white in morning, or tip and edges clean. Taste sour at night. Desire for sweets.

MALARIA OFFICINALIS.

To Dr. G. W. Bowen, Fort Wayne, Indiana, we are indebted for this valuable remedy. It is the product of dried, peat-like, decomposed vegetable matter from a marsh, placed in closed jars, covered with water and allowed to stand from one to three weeks at a temperature of 90° F. The longer it was allowed to stand the more intensely offensive it became. This was in 1862. Fragmentary provings only have been made. First by paid laboring men, under Dr. Bowen, from the crude drug, by inhalation of the gases evolved during the process of re-decomposition, presumably similar in modus operandi to the infection from marsh malaria, with which the author had to contend in disease met with in daily practice during the summer and autumn. Many patients were suffering from malarial affections—the so-called dumb ague—which were very intractable, as this type of autumnal fevers generally is in the West. It was to find a remedy for this nondescript type that the experiments were undertaken, and it is to be regretted that the symptoms elicited from inhaling the fumes in the various stages of decay were not expressed in the original language of the provers. Provings also with 30 potency by Yingling:

After first week: Headache, nausea, white-coated tongue, gastric distress, continuing two or three days.

After second week: Increased headache, nausea, aversion to food, distress in stomach, liver, spleen, and on the third day chills, which would have continued indefinitely if not antidoted.

After third week: To the above symptoms were added extreme lassitude, nausea, loss of appetite, continued fever with aches almost unbearable, and profound weakness with typhoid condition.

Type.—Quotidian, tertian, remittent, continued, malarial, typhoid.

"Dumb-ague;" of every type; from drug suppression; from "ague cures."

Time.—No marked periodicity. All hours, both day and night.

Cause.—Malarial exposure, especially during summer and autumn drought; suppression of fever paroxysms by Quinine and "ague cures;" cases spoiled by drugging. Rheumatic, psoric, tubercular diathesis.

Prodrome.—Aching in the hands, wrists, elbows; feet, ankles, knees.

A tired aching in the wrists and thighs, abdomen and chest. A general sense of weariness.

Chill.—Chilly sensation in left forearm, followed by chilly feelings in hands and fingers; feet cold with sensation as if chilliness would creep up the legs. A few moments later knees feel cold.

A sense of coldness ascending over body from the legs.

Backache; lumbar region feels tired.

General sense of weariness from a short walk, especially through pelvis, sacral region and upper thighs; inclined to lie down to rest.

"At times I felt as if I should become cold or chilly; then again I felt as if I should become feverish or hot, though neither is very marked."

Gaping, yawning and desire to stretch.

Legs restless, fidgety; must stretch and move them.

"Felt as I did before having ague twenty-five years ago."

Face and head feel warm as if flushed; becomes general over body, feverish.

Analysis.—Malaria officinalis seems to bear the same relation to chronic malarial affections that Ipecac., Natrum, Cinchona and its alkaloids do to acute. It is especially effective in "spoiled cases" coming from the tropics and the suppressive treatment of the dominant school, where the type has been changed and it is impossible to distinguish the symptoms of the original disease from drug effects.

The following cures by Dr. W. A. Yingling, Emporia, Kansas, reported in Trans. I. H. A., 1900, may aid, in absence of verified provings, in ascertaining its range of action:

Case I. October, 1898. Mr. C. F.—, 28, a Kansas volunteer. After a week of wet and chilling weather in camp he came home sick. Had a chill followed by fever. Aching over entire body. Nausea, retching and vomiting of bile. Wants cold drinks. Cannot eat; vomits everything, except once could eat raw tomatoes. Craves acids. Tongue, thickly coated white. Lips dry and parched. Urine high colored, like strong tea. Retching and gagging from hawking mucus. Face, eyes and skin very sallow; skin very dry. Mouth dry subjectively, but really moist. Very weak and tottering.

Malaria off. m.

Case II. Mrs. S. A. H., 63, has been sick several days. Vertigo on rising. Head feels badly; threatens to ache. Bitter taste; mouth parched; tongue white. Thirst for lemonade; not so much for water. Ravenous appetite for some days; none now. Shooting pains in the muscles all over body; bones ache. High fever during the night. Restless tossing about. Restlessness most marked in the arms. Stretching and yawning this morning. Diarrhea, painless; five or six stools this morning; watery, yellowish, somewhat foul; tenderness in right iliac region; weakness in bowels. Skin hot and dry.

Malaria off. m.

Case III. M. H., 16. "Dumb ague" a year ago; slight chills and fever; no sweat. Aching through forehead and temples. Little appetite; thirst all the time. Bowels loose yesterday, but no stool to-day. Feels well on rising in morning, < after being about for a time; > toward evening. Backache in lumbar region, pains shoot up the back; < when first lying down, then gets better; < after walking; lying on abdomen. Last four days has been weary and languid; yawning; "malarious feeling."

Malaria off. 6m.

Case IV. M. B., 13. Every evening, at twilight, anticipating daily, chilly with flushes of heat, great desire for fresh air, cannot breathe on account of pain in the liver; < lying, > from hard pressure on region of liver; during the day has no pain or tenderness. Seems entirely well, except is getting weaker. Slight fever for a couple of hours in the evening; raves, sings, talks all night; restless sleep. Tongue clean. Appetite variable; craves potatoes, apples, beefsteak.

Malaria off. m.

CASE V. G. C., 28. Ague every other day; chill over whole body; icy cold from hips down; heat < about the trunk; sweat general, but slight. Begins about noon. Had frequent severe attacks of ague when living in Missouri, also on the Pacific coast, and is now run down. Feels languid, weak and drowsy during apyrexia; unable to be up. Little appetite, great thirst, breath foul. Pulse weak; flashes of heat all the time. Has taken much Quinine and "salts for costiveness." Stool hard, and at times bleeding after stool. Intense headache as if it would burst.

Malaria off. m.

Dr. George Hering, of London, hints at its use in tuberculosis, quoting from notes of Dr. Casanova, made nearly forty years ago:

"I know several localities in South America, Africa and Spain where the marsh miasma has unquestionably arrested and cured that fatal scourge of the human race, phthisis pulmonalis, without any other treatment or restriction in food or drink."

"Miasmatic places are the most healthy places—for some of us at least. Now, I can give some support to this statement of Dr. Casanova. I was once on board a Liverpool steamer which put into Aspinwall, on the swampy Isthmus of Panama, for nine days. Upon our return home several of the sailors, otherwise healthy fellows, were prostrated by Panama fever, whilst I myself, who had formerly suffered from tubercular disease of the lungs, was totally unaffected."

MENYANTHES.

Characteristic.—Adapted to complaints from abuse of Cinchona and Quinine.

Fevers in which the cold stage predominates; coldness felt most acutely in abdomen and extremities (Ver.).

Anxiety about the heart, as if something evil were going to happen, precedes or attends many attacks.

Headache: *pressing in vertex* from above downwards, > *during hard pressure with hand* (Ver.); as of *a heavy weight* pressing upon the head at every step (Cac., Glon., Lach.); < ascending (Cal.); often with icy coldness of hands and feet (Cal., Sep.).

Tension: in root of nose; in arms, hands, fingers; in skin, as if several sizes too small and was crowded into it by force.

Aggravation.—Evening; during rest: lying down.

Amelioration.—Motion; pressing on the affected part.

Type.—*Quartan.* Irregular.

Time.—Irregular time.

Chill.—Without thirst. *Chilliness, especially of the fingers and toes.* Chill over whole body, most severe in back, relieved by heat of stove; or chilliness, disappearing by warmth of stove and returning soon as he leaves the stove or remaining in the back only (not relieved by external warmth, **Ver.**—increased by external heat, **Ipec.**). Chilliness and cold creepings externally, without internal chilliness. Horripilation over the back, as if the parts had long been exposed to cold air, without chilliness. **Coldness in the abdomen** (Cal.), *especially on pressure with the hand;* on rising from bed in the morning, creeping coldness over abdomen, back and sides. *Coldness of the spine,* with shaking. **Feet cold as far up as the knees,** *as if they were in cold water* (coldness *as far up as the ankles,* **Mag., Sep.**). **Icy coldness of the hands and feet, with warmth of the rest of the body.** *Coldness of the dorsal spine, with shaking* (see **Quinia**). Coldness of the feet lasting till night, could not get them warm in bed. *Shivering over the upper part of the body, with yawning,* immediately. Febrile shivering over the whole back as if he had been uncovered for a long time in the open air. *Veins of lower arms and hands distended, while the feet are icy cold* (**Puls.**—of hands, **Led.**).

Chill the predominant stage.

Heat.—Without thirst; especially in the face, followed by chilly feeling. Great heat over the whole body, without sweat or thirst, with cold feet. Flushes of heat on trunk and back, with redness of face, mingled with sensation of coldness. *Flushes of heat,* with *hot ears and cheeks.* Increase of heat, with delirium.

Sweat.—From evening till morning. Sweat at night immediately after lying down, continuing all night.

Tongue.—Bitter-sweetish taste in the mouth. *Ravenous hunger;* **great desire for meat** (great aversion to meat, Arn.).

Pulse.—Slow during the cold stage (Dig.); only slightly accelerated during heat.

"It is a very efficient remedy in irregular intermittent fever, when paroxysm consists chiefly of cold stage, which is incompletely developed, the hands or ends of fingers, and the toes or feet, and the end of the nose, becoming very cold."—DUNHAM.

"*Quartan Intermittents* were the pest of my life until I struck Menyanthes. The symptoms in 'Lippe' (No. 60 to 66, inclusive) and the *excessive coldness of legs* (not thighs) have been the leading symptoms."—A. L. FISHER.

"Intermittent fever, with chilliness in the abdomen, lasting six hours, then a disagreeable feeling of heat comes on, alternating or intermingled with chilliness, with cold feet and legs, and slow pulse."—J. S. DOUGLAS.

Analysis.—Quartan fever; icy coldness of the extremities, of legs especially, rest of body warm; coldness in the abdomen, and end of nose; slow pulse. Craving for meat.

MERCURIALIS.

Time.—Afternoon; 9 P. M.

Chill.—Chilliness over the whole body, with heat of the face; she could only get warm by lying down and covering herself up, then fell asleep, because warm, and afterwards perspired. *Chilliness over the whole body,* **commencing in the right arm and right side of chest** (left hand and left arm, **Carbo v.**—of the whole left side of body, **Caust.**), with shivering, great exhaustion, weakness, weariness, pains in the limbs, and constant desire to sleep; pain in stomach and abdomen aggravated by touch; dyspnea; *cutis anserina on* **the cold right arm,** *which extends over the whole body;* after midnight *offensive perspiration on both sides, worse on arms.* Cold and chilly, with dark red cheeks. Chill in stomach at 9 P. M., which extends to *right arm, right side of chest, abdomen* and *right hip,* with difficulty of breathing; at 4 A. M., heat, thirst, and sweat of right side of body, with heat of face and redness of cheeks.

Heat.—With thirst; of head and dark redness of cheeks. Great heat of head and hands, face red, *veins of hands distended* (**Puls., Led.**), and feet hot. Violent and burning heat of head, face, hands and afterwards of feet, with *distended veins of hands.* Heat without preceding chill, rarely followed by perspiration.

Sweat.—Over the whole body from 3 A. M. till towards morning; after sleep. Great thirst.

MERCURIUS.

Characteristic.—Indicated in bone diseases, **pains worse at night**; glandular swellings, with or without suppuration, but especially if suppuration be too profuse (Hep., Sil.).

Affects light-haired persons most.

Hurried and rapid talking (Hep.).

Breath and body smell foul (Psor.).

Cold swellings; abscesses, slow to suppurate.

Great weakness and trembling from least exertion.

Profuse perspiration attends nearly every complaint, *but does not relieve* and may even increase the suffering (profuse perspiration relieves, Nat., Psor., Ver.).

Ptyalism: *profuse, fetid, metallic-tasting saliva;* soapy, stringy.

Crowns of teeth decay, roots remain (crowns intact, roots decay, Mez.).

Dysentery: **stools slimy, bloody,** *colic, fainting;* **great tenesmus** *during* and **after,** followed by chilliness, and a "cannot finish sensation." The more blood and pain the better indicated.

Morning sickness; *profuse salivation* wets pillow in sleep (Lac. ac.).

Mammæ painful, as if they would ulcerate, *at every menstrual period* (Con., Lac c.); milk in breasts instead of the menses.

Leucorrhea: acrid, burning, itching, with rawness; *always worse at night;* pruritus, < from contact of urine, must be washed off (Sul.).

Cough: dry, fatiguing, racking; in two paroxysms; *worse at night, from warmth of bed,* with utter impossibility of lying on right side.

Affects lower lobe of r. lung; stitches through to back (Chel., Kali c.).

Suppuration of lungs, after hemorrhages of pneumonia (Kali c.).

Tongue: **large, flabby, shows imprint of teeth** (Chel., Pod., Rhus); painful, with ulcers; red, or white.

Intense thirst, although the tongue looks moist and the saliva is profuse (dry mouth, but no thirst, Puls.).

Quantity of urine voided is larger than the amount of water drank; frequent urging to urinate.

Nocturnal emissions stained with blood (Led., Sars.).

Trembling extremities, especially hands; paralysis agitans.

"Ulcers appear on the gums, tongue, throat, inside the cheek, with salivation; irregular in shape; undefined edges; have a dirty, unhealthy look; lardaceous base surrounded with a dark halo; apt to run together. The syphilitic ulcers are circular, attack posterior parts of mouth and throat; have well-defined edges; surrounded with a coppery hue, and do not extend from their primary seat."—DUNHAM.

Relations.—Follows Hep., Lach. and Sul. well, but should not be given before or after Silica; in low potencies hastens rather than aborts suppuration.

Compare: Mezereum, its vegetable analogue, for bad effects of large doses or of too frequent repetition.

Aggravation.—At night; wet, damp, cool air especially in evening; in autumn, warm days and cold, damp nights; uncovering, cold air coming in contact with exposed parts (Bar., Hep.); lying on the right side; perspiring; heat of bed.

Amelioration.—In open air; active motion, during work; rest in bed. Both Arsenic and Mercury have aggravation and amelioration in bed.

Mercury is < by heat of bed, but > by rest in bed.

Arsenic is < by rest in bed, but > by heat of bed.

Type.—Periodicity not marked. Tertian rarely; anticipating occasionally. Bilious forms of typhoid or typhus.

Time.—No certain hour. Midday; 12 M., 1 P. M., evening; night.

Cause.—Atmospheric variations; exposure to cold, to damp places, to cold wet weather.

Chill.—Without thirst; in the morning when rising; more generally in the evening after lying down, or in bed at night. Chilliness *on going into the open air* (**Rhus**—reverse of **Puls.**). Chilliness all over, with ice cold hands; *as from cold water poured over one* (**Mag. c., Rhus**). More chilly in the open air than in the house, same temperature. Violent shaking chill in evening, in bed; she could not get warm. *Chilliness in the abdomen* (coldness of abdomen, **Meny.**). Chill; not relieved by warmth of stove; alternating with heat; of single parts only; internal with hot face. Sensation in soles of feet as if put in cold water, simultaneously with burning in them. *Hands and feet constantly cold.*

Heat.—With thirst. *Alternate sensation of heat and chilliness;* not perceptible to external touch. *Heat in bed; chilly when not in bed.* Heat alternating with chill, often of single parts. Aversion to uncover (**Mag. c.**). Heat and redness of face, and palms; then shaking chill far into the night, and thirst towards morning.

Sweat.—Profuse on every motion (Bry., Samb.). Profuse sweat at night; same in the morning. Unusually profuse sweat that is sour and offensive and makes the fingers look *softened, spongy, wrinkled, like a washerwoman's* (**Ant. c., Canch.**). *Profuse,* **fatty and oily perspiration at night (Thuja, Sabad.)**, makes linen yellow and stiff. *Profuse, offensive perspiration, soaking through the bed-clothes; the linen was stained saffron yellow and could not be removed by washing* (**Carbo a., Cinch., Bry.**). Sweat that causes a burning sensation in the skin (**Caps.**). Profuse sweat on single parts not over six inches large, while other parts are dry. *Worse while sweating; weakness aggravated* (**Rhus**). *Sweat towards morning, with palpitation and nausea.*

Apyrexia.—Great weakness, trembling from least exertion; vertigo when sitting down; gums inflamed and painful; thick, salty saliva; throat sore, painful when swallowing.

Analysis.—The constitutional symptoms are guiding. *Sweat;* profuse on every motion; at night and in early morning; oily, greasy; fingers wrinkled like a washerwoman's; offensive, wetting the bed, stains saffron yellow.

MEZEREUM.

Characteristic.—For light-haired, irresolute persons of a phlegmatic temperament.

Hypochondriacal and despondent; indifferent to everything and everybody; angry at trifles and perfectly harmless things, but is soon sorry for it.

Eczema: intolerable itching, < in bed and from touch; copious, serous exudation; itching eruptions *after vaccination.*

Child scratches face continually, which is covered with blood; eruptions moist; itching < at night; inflammatory redness of face.

Violent headache, after slight vexation; it was painful on the slightest touch; generally right side.

The head is covered with **a thick, leather-like crust**, under which thick and white pus collects here and there; hair is glued together; pus after a time is ichorous, becomes offensive, breeds vermin.

Toothache: in carious teeth (Kreos.); feel elongated, dull pain when biting on them and when touched with tongue, < at night; > with mouth open and drawing in air.

Ulcers covered with thick, whitish-yellow scabs, under which thick yellow pus collects.

Linen or charpie sticks to the ulcers, when it is torn away they bleed.

Vesicles appear around the ulcers, itch violently, burn like fire (Hep.); fiery-red, shining areola around.

Bones, especially long bones, inflamed, swollen; nightly pains going from above downwards; after abuse of Merc., after venereal diseases; caries; exostoses, tumors soften from within out.

Pain in periosteum of long bones < at night in bed, least touch, in damp weather (Mer., Phyt.).

Neuralgic burning pains, after zona.

Aggravation.—Cold air; cold washing; night; contact, motion; one side (right) is usually affected; bad effects of mercury or alcohol.

Type.—Fevers tend to remittent or typhoid. Epidemics occurring in January and February often call for Mezereum.

Chill.—With thirst, *with dry mouth posteriorly,* and *much saliva anteriorly;* predominates even in a warm room, with sleepiness; from upper arms extending to back and legs (Mer.). Chilliness out of bed; heat in bed (same during heat, **Mer.**). *Asthmatic constriction and oppression of chest* (oppression of chest as if the patient would smother, **Apis**). Chilliness, *of single parts, as if dashed with cold water,* especially over *arms, abdomen, hips, feet,* with yawning, while face and hands are warm (**Led.**). *Great chilliness over the whole body, hands and feet very cold,* with *blue nails,* with small hot spot on top of the head. *External coldness for 36 hours, with great thirst, without desire for warmth or dread of open air, and without subsequent heat* (chill 24 hours, **Aran.**—12 hours, **Canth.**). Chill > *by heat* (**Ars., Ign.**—> by drinking, **Ipec., Caust.**). Very sensitive to cold air—less so in hot stage.

Heat.—Burning of internal parts with external chilliness. **Heat of left side of body** (of right side, **Meny.**). *Following the chill,* **intense heat with sleep, sweat breaking out during sleep** (deep sleep as chill passes off and breaks out with urticaria, **Apis**—falls asleep at climax of hot stage, and sweats profusely, **Pod.**).

Sweat.—Skin dripping with cold perspiration.

Tongue.—Thick, white coating on the tongue, with large, red, elevated papillæ (**Acon., Bell.**).

Pulse.—Full and hard; accelerated in the evening; intermittent at times; morning frequent, evening slow.

Apyrexia.—Headache; pale face; hardness and swelling of the spleen, with pressive pain in left hypochondrium; loss of appetite; sensitiveness to cold air. General weakness. Great tendency to run into remittent or typhoid, particularly the latter.

Analysis.—*Chill;* severe, long-lasting; of single parts; great thirst, no desire for heat or dread of open air, no subsequent fever.

Heat; intense, with sleep, sweat breaking out during sleep.

Sweat; drenching, cold.

MURIATIC ACID.

Characteristic.—Adapted to persons with black hair, dark eyes, dark complexion.

Irritable, peevish, disposed to anger and chagrin (Nux); restlessness and vertigo.

Diseases of an asthenic type, with moaning, unconsciousness, fretfulness.

Ulceration with fungus-like growths and pseudo-like membranous deposits of intestinal tract.

Great debility: as soon as he sits down his eyes close; **lower jaw hangs down; slides down in bed.**

Mouth and anus are chiefly affected; the tongue and sphincter ani are paralyzed.

Malignant affections of mouth: studded with ulcers, deep, perforating; having a black or dark base; offensive, foul breath; intense prostration; diphtheria, scarlatina, cancer.

Cannot bear the thought or sight of meat (Nit. ac.).

If the anus be very sensitive either with or without hemorrhoids; anus sore during menses.

Hemorrhoids: *swollen, blue;* **sensitive and painful to touch**; appear *suddenly in children;* too sore to bear least touch, even the sheet is uncomfortable. *Prolapse while urinating* (Bar. c.).

Diarrhea: stool involuntary *while urinating; on passing wind* (Aloe); cannot urinate *without having the bowels move at the same time* (Alum.).

Urine passes slowly; bladder weak, must wait a long time; has to press so that anus protrudes.

Cannot bear *least touch,* not even of sheet on genitals (Mur., Plat.).

Palpitation of heart is felt in the face.

Freckles; eczema solaris.

Relations.—Follows well: after, Bry., Mer., Rhus.

Cures the muscular weakness following excessive use of opium and tobacco.

Type.—Continued, typhoid, typhus, yellow; depraved, scorbutic, hemorrhagic; low forms of intermittent and malarial fevers.

Chill.—Awakens in the morning; coldness in back in evening; general shivering with hot cheeks and cold hands; burning face. Extremities cold; cold sweat on feet; periosteal pains.

Heat.—Without thirst; at night with palpitation; internal, wants to uncover. Burning of palms and soles.

Sweat.—During first sleep, until 12 P. M., < on head and back; night and morning; < when sweating; taciturn; wants to uncover. Great prostration.

Tongue.—Heavy, hinders talking; lame, sore, bluish; deep ulcers with black bases; almost whole mouth covered with a grayish white fur; blisters and vesicles with burning pain. Red, shining, as if glazed. Foul breath.

Pulse.—Slow, weak, intermitting; slow during day, rapid at night; intermits every third beat; small, frequent, feeble.

Analysis.—Typhoid or typhus; deep stupid sleep; unconscious while awake; loud moaning or muttering; tongue coated at edges, *shrunken, dry, leather-like, paralyzed;* involuntary fetid stools *while passing urine; sliding down in bed;* pulse intermits every third beat; hemorrhage of dark liquid blood; mouth full of bluish ulcers; great prostration.

NATRUM MURIATICUM.

Characteristic.—For the anemic and cachectic; whether *from loss of vital fluids*—profuse menses, seminal losses—or mental affections. **Great emaciation; losing flesh even while living well** (Abrot., Iod.); throat and neck of children emaciate rapidly during summer complaint (Sanic.).

Great liability to take cold (Cal., Kali c.).

Irritability: child cross when spoken to; crying from slightest cause; gets into a passion about trifles, especially when consoled with.

Awkward, hasty, drops things from nervous weakness (Apis, Bov.).

Marked disposition to weep; sad weeping mood, without cause (Puls.), but consolation from others < her troubles.

Headache: of school-girls (Cal. p.); *from sunrise to sunset;* beginning with blindness (Iris, Kali bi.); from eye strain; with left-sided clavus; as if bursting; with red face, nausea and vomiting before, during, and after catamenia; as if beaten with little hammers in the brain; during fever, better after sweat begins.

Hay fever: squirming sensation of the nostril, as of a small worm; brought on by exposure to hot sun or intense summer heat.

Sensation as of a hair on the tongue (Sil.).

Tongue: **mapped,** *with red insular patches;* like ringworm on sides (Ars., Lach., Mer., Nit. ac., Tarax.); heavy, difficult speech, children *slow in learning to walk.*

Fever blisters, *like pearls* about the lips, lips dry, sore and cracked, ulcerated (Nit. ac.).

Lachrymation; tears stream down the face whenever he coughs.

Constipation: sensation as of contraction of anus, torn, bleeding, smarting afterwards; stool hard, difficult, crumbling; stitches in rectum (see Nit. ac.); involuntary, knows not whether flatus or feces escape (Aloe, Mur. ac., Iod., Olean., Pod.).

Urine: involuntary, when walking, coughing, laughing; has to wait a long time *if others are present;* cutting *after* (Sars.).

Pressing, pushing toward genitals, every morning, must sit down to prevent prolapsus (Lil., Mur., Sep.).

The hair falls out when touched, in nursing women (Sep.—after fevers, Lyc.); face oily, shiny (Plb., Thuja).

For the bad effects: of anger (caused by offence); acid food; bread; Quinine; cauterizations of all kinds with silver nitrate; too much salt.

Hangnails: skin around the nails dry and cracked (Petr.); herpes about the anus, in border of hair (in bend of knees, Graph., Hep.).

Dreams *of robbers in the house,* and on waking will not believe to the contrary till search is made (of robbers, danger, Psor.); of burning thirst.

The heart's pulsations shake the body (Spig.).

Eczema: raw, red, inflamed, especially in edges of hair; < from eating too much salt, at seashore, from ocean voyage.

Warts on palms of hands (sore to touch, Nat. c.).

"Cannot often be repeated, in chronic cases, without an intercurrent."—DUNHAM.

Should not be given during paroxysm.

If vertigo and headache be very persistent or prostration prolonged, Nux vomica will relieve.

Relations.—Complementary to Apis: acts well both before and after it.

Natrum mur. is the chronic of Ignatia, which is its vegetable analogue. Is followed by Sepia and Thuja.

Aggravation.—At 10 or 11 A. M.; heat of sun or stove; in summer; at seashore or from sea air; mental exertion; talking, writing, reading; lying down.

Amelioration.—In open air (Puls.); cold washing; sitting up; fasting.

Type.—Every type of fever belongs to Natrum muriaticum: vernal, midsummer, autumnal, midwinter; quotidian; tertian; quartan. Simple type. Anticipating tertian. Malarial.

Time.—3, 4, 5, 6, 7, 8, 9 A. M.—10 to 11 A. M. Like Nux vom. the characteristic paroxysm is in the morning or forenoon; the lesser paroxysm occurs in afternoon or evening. 4 to 7 P. M.; 6 to 7 P. M.; 5.30 to 7.30 P. M. Chilly all day, with fever all night.

Fever without chill, 10 to 11 A. M.

Cause.—Exposure to emanations from salt or fresh water; living on, or in the vicinity of water, margins of streams, or ponds; in damp regions or near recently turned up soil, especially freshly plowed fields of virgin soil. When Quinine has perverted and temporarily suppressed the original or regular paroxysm.

Prodrome.—Patient dreads the chill. *Languor, headache, thirst;* knows the paroxysm is coming because of headache and thirst; nausea and vomiting sometimes present; if vomiting, it is water recently drunk; tearing pains in hands, feet, and kidneys.

Chill.—*With thirst.* Paroxysm at 8 A. M.; ***violent chill till noon; then heat till evening;*** without perspiration or thirst during the chill or heat; **unconscious, with violent headache;** sensation as if the head would fly into fragments, is stupefied, knows not where he is. Great chilliness every morning between 3 and 4 o'clock, with *languor, headache, great dyspnea,* followed by great heat and thirst, and terminated by profuse perspiration. **Long and severe chill from 10 to 11 A. M., beginning in the feet, fingers, and toes, or small of the back (Gels.), with blue lips and nails (Nux).** ***Thirst, drinking often and much at a time*** (drinking often and large quantities, but it produces vomiting, Eup.—drinks little and often, **Ars.**). **Bursting headache; nausea and vomiting; and sometimes complete unconsciousness.** Frequent creeping chills about

5.30 P. M., followed by heat and perspiration that lasted till 7.30. Violent chill, especially in a warm room, from 4.30 to 7 P. M.; relieved in the open air. Chilliness over the whole body between 6 and 7 P. M., with great sleepiness; was able to keep awake only by a great effort. Chill over the whole body in a warm room, between 4 and 7 P. M., with frequent yawning, though warm to the touch, except in the face.

Internal shivering from 4 to 7 P. M.; she is generally chilly; each night suffers excessively from rigors, followed by heat and profuse perspiration; as rigors come on, and during continuance, *excessive languor,* with *headache and dyspnea "almost indescribable." Chill predominates, mostly internal; hands and feet icy cold; could not be warmed.* **Chilliness, great thirst, tearing in the bones, blue nails, chattering of the teeth, at 10 A. M.** Chilliness, with *increasing headache in the forehead every day from 9 A. M. till noon;* afterwards *heat with thirst,* and *gradual appearance of sweat;* the headache *decreasing gradually as the sweat increases* until 5 o'clock in the evening. Chill of right side (**Bry.**—left, **Caust., Carbo v.**).

"Icy coldness about the heart (Arn., Camph., Helod., Kali c., Olean., Petr.), continuing after the paroxysm; blindness and unconsciousness during the chill, with great prostration, worse after chill; slight fever (Ars.)."—LIPPE.

"Chill predominates; chilliness internally, as from want of natural heat, with icy coldness of hands and feet. Continuous chilliness from morning till noon."—LIPPE.

Heat.—With *increased thirst; intolerable hammering headache (as if beaten with a thousand hammers),* with **stupefaction and unconsciousness** (**Bell., Cac., Op.**), or obscuration of sight and fainting.

Long severe heat, with *excessive weakness, which compels him to lie down* (weakness and prostration during chill, **Lyc.** —great prostration after paroxysm, **Ars.**). *Great thirst* for large quantities of water; drinks *much and often,* which refreshes (Bry.—drinks little and often, but it produces vomiting, **Ars.**). *Nausea and vomiting* (**Ipec.**).

"Fever blisters cover the lips like pearls."—RAUE.

Hydroa, especially on upper lip (Rhus—see Ign., Nux).

"Continuous heat in the afternoon, with violent headache and unconsciousness; they are gradually relieved during the perspiration which follows."—LIPPE.

Sweat.—With thirst; *profuse, gradually relieving all pains,* except headache, which may continue during and after sweating stage (Samb.—headache is increased, **Eup.**). *Profuse sweat breaks out easily during motion,* although he is very chilly (**Bry., Psor.**); over whole body at night and in the morning (over whole body, except legs, **Lyc.**); sour-smelling sweat.

Tongue.—Thin, yellowish-white coating on dry tongue; blisters on the mapped tongue or *looks like ringworm* (*herpes*) *on the sides* (**Lach., Tarax.**). Taste: water tastes putrid (water tastes bitter, **Ars.**); bitter, salt, sour; food has no taste at all. Longing for salt or bitter things. Aversion to bread.

Pulse.—*Irregular intermission when lying on left side;* at one time rapid and weak; at another full and slow; every third beat intermits (Mur. ac.). **The heart's pulsations shake the body.**

Apyrexia.—Never clear; *emaciation, languor, debility; livid, sallow complexion;* stitches about the liver and spleen; urine muddy, with *red, sandy sediment* (**Lyc.**); loss of appetite, loss of taste; *aversion to bread* (aversion to meat, **Arn.**); hiccup, after suppression by Quinine; *hydroa, like beads on the lips* (**Ign., Nux,** Rhus); *ulceration of labial commissures; sensation of fulness of the stomach after eating ever so little* (**Bry., Lyc.**); sexual desire diminished, or entirely lost, in men.

"Hard chill about 11 A. M., with great thirst, which continues through all stages; the heat is characterized by the most violent headache, relieved by perspiration."—RAUE.

Arsenicum.	Natrum mur.
Advancing type.	Receding type.
Worse afternoon and night.	Worse forenoon and daytime.
Headache beginning with fever, and continuing long after sweat.	Headache begins in chill, increased in fever, partially relieved by profuse sweat.
Vomiting of *bile* with the chill; of water after drinking, in every stage.	Vomiting of bile between chill and fever (Eup., Lyc.), or during heat.
Thirst, drinks little and often during chill and heat; large quantities during perspiration.	Thirst in all stages; drinks large quantities and often, which refresh him.
Hungry.	Loss of appetite.
Had been at seashore or summer watering-resorts during hot weather (Gels.).	Had been near freshly plowed or newly turned grounds, swamps, canals, or standing water.
Lips pale, dry and cracked.	*Lips covered with hydroa, like string of pearls.*

"It is taught by every writer, that the chill must come on about 11 A. M., for Natrum muriaticum to be curative. This is all bosh and nonsense. I have cured many, many cases of chronic and acute intermittents where the chill has come on late in the afternoon. If the rest of the symptoms indicate this remedy, it makes no difference when the chill commences. And let me say here, that Natrum will cure more cases of intermittent fever, both acute and chronic, especially the latter, than any known remedy. With the *thirtieth* potency, I have cured several hundred cases with this drug alone. It is the best friend a physician has in a malarious district."—BURT.

While it is true that time is but one element in a case, for one symptom, however prominent, never overides the totality, and that we must always obtain the totality or majority of symptoms, it is also true that the morning paroxysm predominates, especially at 11 A. M.

"During my travels in Hungary, in the malarious plains of the Theiss and Maros, as well as during a prolonged residence among the Guarosi Indians, of South America, I used a cheap remedy which radically cures every case of ague in twenty-four hours by taking one or, at the utmost, two doses of it. I order a good handful of fine, clean kitchen salt to be thoroughly roasted—if possible, in a new pan, or at least, in one thoroughly cleansed—over a slow fire, till it takes on a brown color, similar to that of lightly roasted coffee. From this roasted salt, a grown up man takes a full tablespoonful, rather more than less, dissolved in a glass of hot water, at once, on the morning following the paroxysm, on an empty stomach, and in quotidian fevers a few hours after the paroxysm is over. As the remedy is only sure of its action on an empty stomach, neither food nor drink must be taken. Though great thirst follow, the patient must only sip a little water through straws; and, when the patient becomes hungry, forty-eight hours after taking the salt, he might take a little chicken broth, or a little beef tea. Strict diet and great care not to catch cold are of the utmost importance. I have used this remedy for the last eighteen years, and it has never failed in a single case when rightly applied. Hundreds of cases in Hungary were cured by it; and, during my voyage to Buenos Ayres, the mate of the steamer Ibis was cured by a single dose in twenty-four hours from an ague which had troubled him periodically for years, and the cure remained permanent. In the tropics of America every European immigrant, as soon as he goes inland, is attacked by intermittent fever, which, if neglected, is too frequently fatal. Thus, four hundred English people succumbed to it in the most paludal forests of Stape, in spite of the immense doses of Quinine and brandy taken; whereas the equally suffering German colony in the adjacent department of Haqua and Paraguay took their roasted salt, and no death occurred among them."—Dr. Brooke, in *N. A. J.*, 1878.

There is, probably, no remedy in our Materia Medica (Arsenic alone excepted) so often indicated in severe cases—acute or chronic, even those maltreated by Arsenic and Quinine—as Natrum muriaticum. It will cure promptly when indicated;

and much quicker and more permanently in the attenuations *above* than *below* the thirtieth. Like Lyc., Cal., Sep., Sul., and some of the metals, it is comparatively inert in the crude form. Hydroa on the lips is a guiding symptom, although Ign., Nux and Rhus all have it. If hydroa be present in first onset of the fever, although after frequent suppression by Quinine it may not be present in old cases, Natrum muriaticum should be thought of. In nursing children, hydroa on the lips, and later the ulcers which succeed them with forenoon attack, are guiding.

Analysis.—The patient dreads the chill.

Chill; 10-11 A. M.; with thirst, long, severe; beginning in fingers, feet, toes, small of back, with blue lips and nails; headache, often unconscious; nausea and vomiting; bone pains.

Heat; more thirst; long, severe; headache, with stupefaction and unconsciousness.

Sweat; with thirst, profuse, sour, gradually > all pains except headache; thirst, drinking refreshes

Hydroa on the lips.

Pulsations shake the body.

NATRUM SULPHURICUM.

Characteristic.—Ailments which are < by, or which depend upon, *dampness of weather,* damp houses or cellars (Ant. t., Aran., Ter.).

Patient feels every change from dry to wet; cannot tolerate sea air, nor eat plants that thrive near water; a constitution in which the gonorrheal poison is most pernicious; recovers slowly from every sickness.

Every spring; skin affections reappear (Psor.).

Inability to think (Nat. c.).

Sad, gloomy, irritable; worse in morning; dislikes to speak or be spoken to (Iod., Sil.).

Depressed; *lively music makes her sad;* satiety of life; must use great self-control to prevent shooting himself.

Mental traumatism; mental effects from injuries to head; chronic effects of blows, falls.

Granular lids: *like small blisters* (Thuja); green pus and terrible photophobia; gonorrheal or sycotic.

Nosebleed during menses (instead of menses, Bry., Phos., Puls.).

Toothache > by cold water, cool air (Coff., Puls.).

Dirty, greenish-gray or brown coating on tongue.

Diarrhea: sudden, urging, gushing, much flatus; *on first rising and standing on the feet;* after a spell of wet weather; living or working in basements.

Gonorrhea; *greenish-yellow, painless,* thick discharge (Puls.); chronic or suppressed (thick, green, Kali iod.).

Dyspnea; desire to take a deep breath during damp, cloudy weather.

Humid asthma in children; *with every change to wet weather; with every fresh cold;* always worse in damp, rainy weather; sputa green, greenish, copious (greenish grey, Cop.).

Sycotic pneumonia; *lower lobe of left lung;* great soreness of chest, during cough, has to sit up in bed and hold the chest with both hands (Nic.—r. lung, Bry.).

Spinal meningitis: *violent crushing gnawing pains at base of brain;* head drawn back; spasms with mental irritability and delirium; violent congestion of blood to head; delirium; opisthotonos.

Aggravation.—Damp basements or dwellings; damp weather (Aran., Ars. i., Dul.); rest; lying.

Amelioration.—Dry weather; pressure; sitting up (cough); changing position (but > in wet weather, Caust.); open air.

Type.—Remittent, bilious, malarial, yellow; or yellow assumes a remittent or low continued form, instead of recovering.

Time.—4-8 P. M.

Cause.—Exposure; living in damp houses, basements, cellars; wet weather; sea air; living near water; every change from dry to wet (Aran., Dul., Rhus).

Chill.—Internal, with yawning and stretching. Chills; with icy coldness and goose-flesh, 4-8 P. M.; towards evening, without thirst; evening in bed, could not get warm all night; up the back, with shaking and chattering of the teeth, without internal coldness; waking at night with anguish and thirst.

Chilly in bed and shaking chills out of it, thirst, pulse very rapid. Chilly and feverish in evening.

Heat.—Day in afternoon; in sudden flashes towards evening; hot sensation on vertex; general heat and restlessness in evening.

Sweat.—Without thirst; on single parts, on face, on genitals; at night; in morning.

Tongue.—Dirty, greenish-grey, or greenish-brown coating on base of tongue; covered with mucus, slimy; taste bitter or lost.

Analysis.—Fevers, with icy coldness, no thirst in any stage; attacks come on suddenly; bilious vomiting; malarial, caused or < by wet weather or living near water or seashore, working in damp rooms or basements.

NITRIC ACID.

Characteristic.—Suitable especially to lean persons of rigid fibre, dark complexion, black hair and eyes—the brunette rather than blonde—nervous temperament.

Persons suffering with chronic disease who take cold easily; are disposed to diarrhea; rarely to those who suffer with constipation.

Old people, diarrhea and great weakness.

Excessive *physical* irritability.

Pains: **sticking, pricking, as from splinters**; suddenly appearing and disappearing; on change of temperature or weather; during sleep; gnawing here and there, as from ulcers forming.

Diseases: which depend on some virulent poison—mercury syphilis, scrofula—in broken-down, cachectic constitutions; hateful and vindictive.

Irritable, headstrong; hateful and vindictive; inveterate, ill-willed, unmoved by apologies.

After continued loss of sleep, long-lasting anxiety; over-exertion of mind and body from nursing the sick (Coc.); anguish from the loss of his dearest friend (Ign.).

Sensation: of a band around head, around the bones (Carb. ac., Sul.); *of a splinter* in affected parts, ulcer, piles, throat, ingrowing toe nail, < on slightest contact.

Often anxious about his own illness; constantly thinking about his past troubles; mind weakened and wanders; morbid fear of cholera.

Ozena: green casts from the nose every morning.

Diarrhea: great straining but little passes; as if stayed in rectum and could not be expelled (Alum.); pain as if rectum and anus were torn or fissured (Nat.); violent cutting pain *after stool,* lasting for hours (Rat., Sul.).

Very sensitive to rattle of wagons over paved streets.

Urine: *scanty, dark brown,* **strong-smelling,** like horse's urine; *cold when it passes;* turbid, looks like remains of a cider barrel.

Warts, condylomata: sycotic or syphilitic; large, jagged, pedunculated; bleeding readily on washing; moist, oozing; sticking pain (Staph., Thuja).

Ulcers: easily bleeding, *pricking pains* especially on contact (Hep.); zigzag, irregular edges; base looks like raw flesh; exuberant granulations; after mercury or syphilis or both, engrafted on a scrofulous base.

Hemorrhage: from bowels in typhoid or typhus (Crot., Mur. ac.); after miscarriage or post-partum; from over-exertion of body; profuse, bright or dark.

Affects especially the mucous outlets of the body where skin and mucous membrane join—mouth, nose, rectum, anus, urethra, vagina (Mur. ac.).

Relations.—Complementary: Arsenicum, Caladium.

Follows well: after Calcarea, Hepar, or Thuja, but is most effective after Kali carbonicum.

Should not be used before or after Lachesis.

Often difficult to distinguish from Mercury; but is adapted to black-haired people, while Mercury is more useful in light-haired persons.

Aggravation.—Evening and at night; contact; change of temperature or weather; on waking; while walking; rising from a seat.

Amelioration.—While riding in a carriage (the reverse of **Coc.**); from eructations.

Type.—Quotidian; tertian; typhoid; typhus; yellow fever.

Time.—Afternoon and evening.

Chill.—*Continuous chilliness in the evening; before going to bed and after lying down; in bed, worse from uncovering or moving* (**Nux**). Chill in the afternoon while in the open air, for an hour and a half; afterwards dry heat in bed, with delirium and a sort of half-waking, dreamy state; *sweat and sleep towards evening.* Chilliness in the afternoon, for an hour; then heat over the whole body, for a quarter of an hour; afterwards profuse perspiration over the whole body for two hours; there is no thirst in either cold or hot stages. Cold hands, with *extreme ill-humor. Constant coldness of the feet* as far up as the calves. *Icy coldness of soles of feet,* preventing sleep at night.

Heat.—Dry, internal at night; *desire to uncover* (**Acon.**); pricking all over, as from needles. Dry heat of hands and face in flushes, with sweat of hands. **Constant paroxysms of flushes of heat, of single parts or over entire body** (**Fer.**, **Sep.**). *The blood seemed hot at night, especially in the hands,* preventing sleep. Great heat in the face and hands; or heat in face, with icy cold hands. *Dryness of the throat.*

Sweat.—*All over the entire body after eating* (**Carbo a.**). **Sweat, with cold hands and blue nails. Sweat sour, offensive, like horse's urine.** Night-sweat, *on covering up in bed* (on being covered sweats profusely all over, **Cinch.**). *Night-sweat, only on the parts on which he is lying* (**Acon.**, **Bry.**—on the part not lain upon, **Benz.**). **Profuse night-sweat,** *every other night. Offensive axillary sweat* (**Bov.**). **Profuse sweat on the soles, causing soreness of the toes and balls of the feet, with sticking pain as if he were walking on pins. Perspiration in the morning.**

Tongue.—Coated white or lemon-color; dry in the morning; saliva profuse, fetid, acrid; corners of mouth sore and ulcerated; cadaverous odor. Taste, bitter after eating (**Puls.**); aversion to meat and bread; longing for fat (reverse of **Puls.**). Corners of mouth ulcerated. Cracking in the maxillary articulation when chewing or eating.

Pulse.—During fever full, hard and tense. In old cases irregular; fourth beat intermits; one normal beat is often followed by two rapid beats.

Analysis.—*Heat;* in flushes, in paroxysms, of single parts or over entire body.

Sweat; with cold hands, blue nails; sour, offensive, like horse's urine; profuse night sweat; profuse on soles causes soreness of toes and balls of feet; sticking pain as if walking on pins.

Chronic cases; a general anemic, cachectic condition.

NUX MOSCHATA.

Characteristic.—Adapted especially to women and children of a nervous, hysterical temperament; to people *with a dry skin who rarely perspire;* ailments of pregnancy.

All the ailments are accompanied by **drowsiness, sleepiness,** *or an inclination to faint;* **complaints cause sleepiness** (Ant. t., Op.).

Absence of mind, cannot think; great indifference to everything.

Changeable humor; one moment laughing, the next crying (Croc., Ign.).

"Sudden change from grave to gay, from lively to serene."

Great soreness of all the parts upon which one lies. Ten dency to bedsores (Bap., Bry., Pyr.).

Weakness of old age; dyspepsia of old people.

Oversensitive: to light; of hearing; of smell; to touch.

Weakness or loss of memory (Anac., Lac c., Lyc.).

Vanishing of thoughts while reading, talking or writing; uses wrong words; does not recognize well-known streets (Can. I., Lach.).

Great dryness of the mouth; dryness of eyes, too dry to close the lids; *tongue so dry it adheres to the mouth;* saliva seemed like cotton; throat dry, stiffened, no thirst.

Sensation of great dryness; without real thirst and without dryness of the tongue.

Eating a little too much causes headache; pain, fulness and distress in stomach *while eating* or immediately after (Kali bi.).

Diarrhea: in summer, from *cold drinks;* from boiled milk; during dentition; during pregnancy; with sleepiness and fainting; in autumn, epidemic, white, fetid (Colch.).

At every menstrual nisus, mouth, throat, and tongue become *intolerably dry,* especially when sleeping.

Leucorrhea, in place of menses (Coc); awakens with dry tongue (Lach.).

Pain, nausea and vomiting; caused by pessaries, during pregnancy, > by Nux moschata.

Sudden hoarseness from walking against the wind (Euph., Hep.).

Cough, caused by: getting warm in bed; overheated; during pregnancy (Con.); bathing; standing in water; living in cold, dark places (Aran., Ter.); loose after eating, dry after drinking.

Rheumatic affections; from getting feet wet; from exposure to drafts of air while heated (Acon., Bry.); < in cold, wet weather, or cold wet clothes (Rhus); of left shoulder (Fer.—right shoulder, Sang., Stron.).

Backache, while riding in a carriage.

Soreness of all parts on which one lies (Bapt.).

Fatigued, must lie down after least exertion.

Sleep: irresistibly drowsy; sleepy, muddled, as if intoxicated; coma, lies silent, immovable; eyes constantly closed (with stertorous breathing, Op.).

Aggravation.—Cold, wet, windy weather (Rhod.); weather changes; cold food, water and washing; riding in a carriage (**Coc.**); motion; lying on painful side.

Amelioration.—Rest; dry, warm weather; warm room; wrapping up warmly.

Type.—Tertian; double tertian; quartan; double quartan.

Time.—7 A. M., 1, 5, 6, 9 P. M.

Chill.—Without thirst. *Skin cold and blue over the whole body,* at 5.30 P. M. Became cold, chilly and pale on going into open, especially damp, cold air, disappeared at once in a warm room (worse in a warm room, **Apis**). Coldness *commencing in left arm and lower limbs* (in left hand and arm, **Carbo v.**), in frequent attacks, and clear intermissions, *with desire to sleep between attacks.* Chill from uncovering (**Nux**); hands and feet icy cold and as if numb from coldness (**Rhus**). As chill progressed became very drowsy, and at close of chill fell asleep (**Apis, Nux**); continued through heat, which was very light.

Heat.—With slight thirst, with redness of face and hot hands. Great heat, with prostration, hypochondriac mood; *mouth and throat dry; drowsiness and deep sleep* (**Apis, Op.**—falls asleep at climax of heat and breaks out with sweat. **Pod.**).

Sweat.—Drowsiness during sweat (**Pod.**); cannot bear to be uncovered (**Bar., Hep., Nux**). Sweat light, or wanting altogether; sweat red or bloody (**Lach.**).

"Double tertian intermittent fevers, with sleepiness, white tongue, rattling breathing, bloody expectoration, and very little thirst only during the hot stage."—LIPPE.

"Remittent fever with continuous drowsiness, sleepiness and frontal headache; wakes occasionally for a drink; face very red. Makes no complaint. Sleeps nearly all the time."—C. B. GILBERT.

"Fever, not paludal, purely nervous; its periodicity places it here. At seven o'clock every morning the chills set in and increase, but, in the midst of this progression of chills, the patient becomes drowsy, and, when the chills cease, is fast asleep. The hot stage is very slightly pronounced, the patient continues to sleep; on awakening great dryness of throat; fever, with colliquative diarrhea."—A. CHARGE.

Tongue.—Coated white, dotted with red papillæ. "Cotton" saliva, *sticky dry lips,* and *tongue adhering to roof of mouth,* without any actual dryness or real thirst. Can only digest highly seasoned food.

Analysis.—*Chill;* the whole body cold and blue. Sleepy, falls asleep at close of chill.

Heat; with very red face; sleepy or deep sleep.

Sweat; light or wanting; red or bloody; cannot bear to be uncovered. Sleeps during sweats. Sticky, dry lips, tongue and mouth; no thirst.

NUX VOMICA.

Characteristic.—Adapted to thin, irritable, choleric persons, with dark hair and bilious or sanguine temperament, disposed to be *quarrelsome, malicious; spiteful, melancholic.*

Debauchers of *a thin, irritable, nervous disposition* (debauchers with light hair, blue eyes, Lob.); prone to indigestion and hemorrhoids.

"Nux vomica is chiefly successful with persons of an ardent character; of an irritable, impatient temperament, disposed to anger, spite, or deception."—HAHNEMANN.

Anxiety with irritability and inclination to commit suicide, but is afraid to die.

Oversensitive: *to external impressions; noise; odors; light or music; trifling ailments are unbearable* (Cham.); *every harmless word offends* (Ign.).

Persons who are very particular, careful, zealous, inclined to become easily excited or angry; irascible and tenacious.

Bad effects: of coffee, tobacco, alcoholic stimulants; highly seasoned food; over-eating; long continued over-mental exertion (Arg. n.); sedentary habits; loss of sleep; aromatic or patent medicines; sitting on cold stones.

One of the best remedies with which to commence the treatment of cases that have been drugged by mixtures, bitters, vegetable pills, nostrums and quack remedies, especially aromatic or "hot medicines," *but only if symptoms are similar.*

Pains are tingling, sticking, hard, aching, worse from motion and contact.

Cannot keep from falling asleep in the evening, while sitting, hours before bedtime, and wakes at 3 or 4 A. M.; falls into a dreamy sleep at daybreak, from which he is hard to arouse, and then feels tired and weak (with many complaints)

Eructations: sour, bitter; nausea and vomiting every morning, with depression of spirits; after eating.

Nausea: constant; after eating; in morning; from smoking. "If I could only vomit I would be so much better."

Stomach: pressure an hour or two after eating as from a stone (immediately after, Kali bi., Nux m.); pyrosis, tightness, must loosen clothing; cannot use the mind for two or three hours after a meal; sleepy after dinner; from anxiety, worry, brandy, coffee, drugs, night watching, high living, etc.

Convulsions, *with consciousness* (Strych.); < anger, emotion, touch, moving.

Constipation: frequent unsuccessful desire, passing small quantities of feces, sensation as if not finished (no desire, Bry., Op., Sul.).

Alternate constipation and diarrhea (Sul., Ver.) in persons who have taken purgatives all their lives.

Menses: too early, profuse, last too long; or keeping on several days longer, with complaints at onset and remaining after; every two weeks; irregular, never at right time; stopping and starting again (San., Sul.); during and after < of old symptoms.

Labor pains *violent,* spasmodic; *cause urging to stool or to urinate;* < in back; prefers a warm room.

Strangulated hernia, especially umbilical.

Backache, must sit up to turn over in bed; lumbago; from sexual weakness, from masturbation.

Relations.—Complementary: Sulphur in nearly all cases.

Is often indicated after Ipecacuanha, which it follows well.

Nux should be given on retiring or, what is better, several hours before going to bed; it acts best during repose of mind and body.

Aggravation.—Morning; mental exertion; after eating or over-eating; spices; narcotics; contact, noise, anger; dry weather.

Amelioration.—Evening; rest; lying down, and in damp, wet weather (**Caust.**).

Type.—Fevers of every type. Simple; quotidian; tertian; quartan; but like Natr. mur. it is more frequently called for in the morning paroxysm and in the tertian type than perhaps in any other. Every spring (Lac c., Sul.). Anticipating; congestive; monthly; after the menses; apoplectic intermittents; malarial; continued; remittent; pernicious.

Irregular in paroxysm; may come on at any hour of the day, and return at the same hour, or earlier, or later.

Irregular in stage; may consist of heat, then chill, then sweat; or sweat, then chill, then sweat again; or external heat and internal chill or *vice versa.*

Time.—Night or **early morning, 6 to 7 A. M., 11 A. M.,** 12 M., 4, 5, 6 P. M.; 7 to 9 P. M. Evening paroxysm usually lasts all night (**Lyc., Polyp., Puls., Rhus**).

Fever without chill, at 6 or 7 P. M.

Cause.—Typical cases are apt to occur in men of active, "rushing," business habits; nervous, dyspeptic from worry, care, too much mental and too little physical exertion. Irregular, unseasonable, rapid eating; too much coffee, tobacco, stimulants; late suppers, late hours of debauches.

Prodrome.—Intolerable drawing pain through the thighs and legs, *that obliged him to draw them up and stretch them out.* Prostration. Sensation of paralytic weakness; especially in the limbs. *Often heat,* and sometimes *sweat* before the chill.

Chill.—Without thirst. Chilliness every morning after rising. *Violent, shaking chill, lasting three-quarters of an hour,* **with bluish cold face and hands,** followed by *violent heat* and moist skin.

Anticipating morning fever; chill with gaping, and *aching in the limbs* (sore, bruised pain in limbs, as if in periosteum, **Arn.**); **blue nails**; no thirst; then *long-lasting heat with thirst* (**Nat.**), and stitches in the temples; *sensation of chilliness on* *the back* and *limbs,* followed by light sweat *in the morning* with *painfulness of the skin, as if it had been frozen,* and *numbness of limbs, as if gone to sleep,* as they do in cold weather.

Afternoon paroxysm: chilliness and coldness with blue nails, for four hours, *followed by general heat and burning of the hands, with thirst at first for water, afterwards for beer,* without subsequent sweat. Shivering and chilliness *after drinking* (chill after every drink, **Caps., Eup.**). Drinking increases and hastens chill, and causes vomiting (**Ars., Eup.**—drinking relieves the chill, **Caust.**). *Coldness of the whole body,* with **blue hands** and **blueness of the skin. Great coldness, relieved neither by warmth of the stove, nor by covering in bed** (worse from uncovering, **Phos.**—worse in a warm room or near the stove, **Apis**—chill increased by external heat, **Ipec.**). Shivering and chilliness for an hour *from the slightest contact with the open air* (excessively sensitive to cold air, **Camph.**—coldness and chills as soon as she attempted to rise or put one limb out of bed, **Canth.**). Violent chill, and sleep for an hour in the evening after lying down, followed by heat, with headache and roaring in the ears. Chill evening and night in bed, *lasting till morning, worse when moving.* **Pain in sacrum** during chill (**pain in dorsal vertebræ, Chin. s.**). **Congestive chill,** with vertigo, headache, anguish, delirium, terrible coldness of body, with blue face, nails and hands, accompanied by vivid visions, distention of the stomach, stitches in the sides and abdomen; worse from the slightest attempt to uncover or move in bed. *Sleep after chill* (Nux m., Pod.—sleep during heat, **Apis**).

Heat.—*With thirst. Violent, long-lasting heat, with great thirst.* Flushing redness and heat of the cheeks on the slightest motion or exertion (heat relieved by moving about, **Caps.**); worse in the open air; averse to uncovering when in bed, day or night; desire to uncover, but chilled when uncovering (**Acon.**

—averse to uncovering, **Bell.**—cold and chilly on putting hands out from under bedclothes, **Bar. c.—cannot move or uncover in the least without feeling chilly, Arn.**); heat of hands and feet, which must be covered *because cold causes intolerable pain* (Stram.). *Great heat; whole body burning hot,* **yet patient must be covered up** (must be uncovered, **Sec.**). Heat and redness of face, cheeks, hands, with stitching headache, especially in the sinciput; anguish, vertigo, and delirium, with redness of the face (**Bell.**); roaring in the ears; pain in chest, sides, abdomen; feet cold and shivering.

"During the fever a round spot at the pit of the stomach of two inches in diameter, *feels hot to the patient,* but *is cold to the touch.* Cured by Nux vom."—C. LIPPE.

Sweat.—*Without thirst* (with great thirst, **Ars., Cinch.**). Usually, *sweating stage light,* **with chilliness from motion or allowing the air to strike him.** *Sweat relieves pains in limbs* (**Eup., Lyc., Nat.**). *Sweat alternating* with chill (**Ant. c.**—chill alternating with sweat, always either chilly or in a sweat, **Caust.**). Sweat *one-sided* (right), or only on upper part of the body (**Acon., Cinch., Nit. ac., Puls.**—sweat on trunk, but not on legs, **Lyc.**); cold on face; sour, clammy, offensive.

Profuse perspiration, *after the severest paroxysms,* or *attending the congestive chill* (**reverse of Eup., which has light chill and profuse sweat; or hard, shaking chill and** *light, scanty sweat*); *only on right side.*

Tongue.—Heavily coated, white or yellow. Taste so *bitter, sour, putrid,* **must rinse the mouth (Thuja).** Canine hunger; with *aversion to bread, water, coffee, tobacco.* Longing for brandy, beer, fat food (see **Puls.**).

Pulse.—Full, hard, quick; small, quick during fever heat; fourth or fifth beat intermitting.

Apyrexia.—Gastric and bilious symptoms are always present. Legs feel weak and paralytic; head heavy, dull, with vertigo and severe frontal headache, especially in morning; pains are pressive, pulsating, sticking, worse in temples and sinciput; face pale and waxy, as in chlorosis; debility; soreness of liver and spleen, which are sensitive to least pressure; loss of appetite and obstinate constipation, with frequent but ineffectual inclination (rarely canine hunger and diarrhea); great sensitiveness in and distention of the epigastrium. Vomiting of food or bitter fluids and sour mucus; emaciation; anxiety; and great weakness of the whole body. Chilly on the least movement, repugnance to cold, or cold air. Nightly paroxysm of dry cough. Many of the symptoms, after continuing with greater or less intensity, gradually pass into the succeeding prodrome.

Natrum mur.	**Nux vomica.**
Time.—5 to 8 A. M., 10 to 11 A. M., and 4 to 7 P. M. Fever without chill, 10 or 11 A. M.	**Time.**—6 to 7 A. M., 11 A. M., or 12 M.; and 5 to 9 P. M., lasting all night. Fever, without chill, 6 or 7 P. M.
Type.—Anticipating, every other day. Every day paroxysm, regular.	**Type.**—Anticipating. Paroxysm and stages usually irregular.
Prodrome.—*Dreads the chill.* Languor, headache, thirst, nausea and vomiting.	**Prodrome.**—Drawing pain in limbs; weak and paralyzed. Heat and sweat sometimes before the chill.
Chill.—With thirst, drinking often and much at a time, with blue lips and nails, and bursting headache; tearing in bones and chattering of teeth.	**Chill.**—Without thirst, shaking, with blue face and hands; pain and numbness of limbs, as if gone to sleep; relieved neither by warmth of stove nor covering in bed.
Heat.—With thirst; increased headache, unconsciousness and excessive weakness.	**Heat.**—With great thirst, violent and long-lasting. *Cannot move or uncover in the least without feeling chilly.*
Sweat.—With thirst, gradually relieving all pains except headache, which is not so severe. Profuse sweat breaks out easily on motion. Sour-smelling.	**Sweat.**—Without thirst; with chilliness from motion or allowing the air to touch him. Sweat on one side (right) or upper part of body. Relieves pains in limbs.
Tongue.—Mapped tongue, like herpes, on the side; yellow coat; salt taste.	**Tongue.**—Heavily coated white or yellow; putrid taste; must rinse the mouth.

"Children's intermittents; *shaking chill,* with *blue-mottled skin, especially on covered parts.* Morning chill, very severe, with *skin blue-mottled;* thirst very great during chill and fever; great tendency to spasms (and even convulsions), as *the chill went off* and *sweat came on.* Bowels constipated, with ineffectual urging to stool, especially in nursing children; appetite poor, urine red and fetid, and generally a dry, hacking cough (Crotalus, if right side was *most mottled*)."—DR. HIGGINS, *N. A. J.*, p. 182.

The anticipating chill always denotes increasing severity of the fever, and the remedies which correspond to it are among the most prominent and frequently called for, viz., Arsenic, Bryonia, Cinchona, Chininum s., Natrum mur., and Nux vomica. Ipecacuanha may anticipate. Ignatia anticipates and postpones.

By many professing homeopaths Nux vomica is used in alternation with Ipecacuanha, and they boast of their success in the treatment of ague. However successful such treatment may be, it is routine practice, and, like the empiricism which leads the other school to the indiscriminate use of Quinine, must often fail. Nux vomica deserves, and will repay, a careful individualization.

OPIUM.

Characteristic.—Especially adapted to children and old people; diseases of first and second childhood (Bar. c., Mill.); persons with light hair, lax muscles, and want of bodily irritability.

Ailments: with insensibility and partial or complete paralysis that originate *from fright;* bad effects of fright, the fear still remaining (Acon., Hyos.); from charcoal vapors; from inhaling gas; of drunkards.

All complaints: with great sopor; painless, complains of nothing, wants nothing.

Spasms: of children, from approach of strangers; from nursing after fright of mother (Hyos.—after anger of mother, Cham., Nux); from crying; eyes half opened and upturned.

Screaming before or during a spasm (Apis, Hell.).

Deep stertorous respiration on inhalation and exhalation.

Sleep: heavy, stupid; **with stertorous breathing,** *red face, eyes half-closed,* blood-shot; *skin covered with hot sweat;* after convulsions.

Sleepy, but cannot sleep (Bell., Cham., Stram.); sleeplessness with acuteness of hearing, clock striking and cock crowing at a great distance keep her awake.

Loss of breath on falling asleep (Grind., Lach.).

Bed feels so hot she cannot lie on it (bed hard, Arn., Bellis, Bry., Pyr.); moves often in search of a cool place; must be uncovered.

Want of susceptibility to remedies; lack of vital reaction, the well chosen remedy makes no impression (Carbo v., Laur., Val.).

Digestive organs inactive: peristaltic motion reversed or paralyzed; bowels seem closed.

Constipation: of children; of corpulent, good-natured women (Graph.); from inaction or paresis, no desire; from lead poisoning; stool hard, round, black balls (Chel. Plumb., Thuja); protrude and recede (Sil., Thuja).

Stool: involuntary, especially after fright (Gels.); *black and offensive;* from paralysis of sphincter.

Urine: retained with bladder full; retention, post-partum or excessive use of tobacco; in nursing children, after passion of nurse; in fever or acute illness; paralysis of bladder or sphincter. (In Stramonium we have suppression; while in Opium the secretion is not diminished, the bladder is full but fullness is unrecognized.)

"Opium renders the intestines so sluggish that the most active purgatives lose their power."—HERING.

"Persistent diarrhea in those treated with large doses of the drug."—LIPPE.

Delirium: constantly talking; eyes wide open, face red, puffed; or unconscious, eyes glassy, half-closed, face pale, deep coma; preceded by stupor.

Thinks she is not at home; this is continually in her mind.

Picking of bed clothes during sleep (while awake, Bell., Hyos.).

Sudden retrocession of acute exanthema results in paralysis of brain or convulsions (Zinc.).

Marasmus; child with wrinkled skin, looks like a little dried up old man (Abrot.).

Aggravation.—Warmth; while perspiring; from stimulants; night and morning; during and after sleep (Apis).

Amelioration.—From cold; motion, during day and evening.

Type.—Congestive. Epileptiform. Regular paroxysms; irregular stages. Sleepy. Typhoid, typhus.

Time.—11 A. M. Afternoon; night; after midnight.

Chill.—Without thirst. *Shaking chill at 11 A. M.; body cold,* or *coldness only of the limbs, abdomen, back, hands, and feet.* Shaking chill, followed by heat, *with deep soporous sleep,* during which she *sweats profusely.* Chill with pains in limbs, **hot head and deep sleep.** Chilliness on going to bed; **sleep, with profuse sweat about the head.**

Heat.—Over *whole body, burning even when bathed in sweat,* with *red face.* **Soporous, snoring sleep,** with *open mouth,* twitching of the limbs. Spasmodic contraction of the muscles of the face; sardonic smile; unconsciousness, and *desire to uncover* (must be uncovered, **Apis, Puls.**). Headache, great prostration and often fainting when waking from sleep.

Sweat.—Over entire body, which is burning hot; *deep sleep,* *with stertorous breathing and open mouth. Hot, profuse morning sweat, wants to be uncovered.* Sweat on the upper part of the body, lower part hot and dry; heat and sweat intermingled. Cold sweat on forehead. Profuse sweat about the head. *Worse during sweat* (**Ipec.**—better after sweat, **Bell.**).

Tongue.—Coated dirty yellow, *quivering.* Loss of appetite; aversion to food. Longing for spirituous liquors.

Pulse.—Full and hard; or weak, slow, scarcely perceptible.

Apyrexia.—Symptoms of *cerebral congestion,* with profound stupor; complete indifference; the patient makes no audible complaint. Intermittents of old persons and children.

Analysis.—*Chill;* with hot head and deep sleep; profuse sweat about the head; coldness of single parts.

Heat; deep, soporous sleep; desire to uncover.

Sweat: hot, profuse; < during; profuse about head.

PARIS QUAD.

Characteristic.—Head feels too large; as if distended; as if the walls were thin (as if elongated, Hyp.).

Headache of spinal origin, arises from nape and produces a sensation as if head were immensely large.

Eyes feel as if too large, they seem to have no room in sockets; as if lids could not close.

Aggravation.—Thinking; mental exertion, excitement; using the eyes; motion; smoking tobacco.

Eyes feel as if projecting, with a sensation as if a thread was tightly drawn through the eyeball and backward into the middle of the brain; sight weak.

Dull pain in nape of neck; feels stiff and swollen on turning it; weary, as from a great weight lying upon it; worse from exertion, better from rest and in open air.

Chill.—Mostly towards evening; in the chest, abdomen and lower limbs, with gooseflesh, yawning and icy cold feet; with internal trembling. Coldness of the whole right half of the body, from the head to the feet, while the other half was of natural warmth (see Rhus). Small icy cold spots here and there in the skin. The coldness produces a drawing, contracting sensation in skin and all parts of the body as if drawn together by the cold.

Heat.—Starts from nape of neck and descends the back; in the face; with sweat of upper part of the body. The fingers are alternately hot and cold as if dead and of a dead color (Ced., Sep., Stann.).

Sweat.—In the morning; when waking, with biting-itching that compels scratching; profuse; on waking, about 3 A. M.

PETROLEUM.

Characteristic.—Adapted to persons of light hair and skin; irritable, quarrelsome disposition (Nux v.); offended at trifles; vexed at everything.

Symptoms appear and disappear rapidly (Bell., Mag. p.).

During sleep or delirium: imagines that one leg is double; that *another person lies alongside of him in the same bed; that there are two babies in the bed* (Bry., Val.).

Vertigo: on rising; *in occiput;* as if intoxicated; *like seasickness.*

Headache: *in occiput, which is as heavy as lead;* pressing, pulsating pain; as if everything in the head were alive; numb, bruised; as if made of wood.

Gastralgia: of pregnancy; with pressing, drawing pains; *whenever the stomach is empty; > by constant eating* (Chel., Sep.).

Diarrhea: yellow, watery, *gushing;* after cabbage, sour

krout: during pregnancy, stormy weather; *always in the day-time.*

Complaints: from riding in a carriage, railroad car, or in a ship (Coc., San.); < before and during a thunderstorm.

Sweat and moisture of external genitals, of both sexes; fetid, of axillæ (Graph., San.).

Tips of fingers rough, cracked; fissured, *every winter;* skin of hands rough and cracked; of whole body, sore and painful.

Painful, itching chilblains and chapped hands < in cold weather; decubitus.

Sensation of coldness about the heart (Ars., Carbo an., Helod., Kali m., Nat. m.).

Relations.—The skin symptoms are worse in winter, better in summer (Alum., Psor.); if suppressed, cause diarrhea.

Aggravation.—Carriage riding; during a thunderstorm; in winter (skin symptoms).

Amelioration.—Warmth; warm air.

Type.—Quotidian. Cold stage predominates.

Time.—*10 A. M.,* 3, 4, 6, 7 and 10 P. M. *Evening paroxysm predominant.*

Fever without chill, 5 to 6 P. M.

Chill.—Without thirst at 10 A. M. for half an hour, with coldness of the hands and face. Chilliness lasting two hours, every afternoon, at 3 or 4 o'clock, with cold hands and *dryness of the mouth.* Shaking chill at 7 P. M., with sweat over whole body, except lower extremities, which were quite cold. Violent internal shaking chill at 10 P. M. *Shaking chill every evening. Chilliness with trembling, face cold, cheeks, fingers and nails blue. Chilliness at 6 P. M., with blue nails. Chilliness in the open air.* Chilliness in evening, with flushes of heat in the face. *Frequent chilliness through the whole body,* **followed by violent itching of the skin** (pricking of the skin, **Nit. ac.**).

Heat.—And chill at same time, at 10 P. M. Heat at night, *bedclothes were intolerable, and was obliged to uncover* (external warmth is intolerable, **Puls.**). *Flushes of heat over whole body. Heat of head; redness of face; burning pain in the mouth, and dryness of the trachea.* Heat in the evening after the chill.

Sweat.—*Of single parts at different times, as hands, palms, head, back, chest, axilla, arms, legs, feet* (Thuja). *Profuse perspiration of the forearms, lower legs, feet;* on the soles. Sweat; with partial chills; or immediately after the chill. Offensive, of axilla and soles. No heat intervening.

Tongue.—Coated white in the centre, with a dark streak along the sides (white, with red edges, or red and white in alternate streaks, **Ant. t.**); offensive saliva. Taste, slimy, pappy, putrid; *aversion to fat meat, and all warm cooked food.* Ravenous hunger, or loss of appetite.

Pulse.—Full, rapid; accelerated by every motion; becomes slow again during rest. Cold feeling about the heart (Nat. m.).

Analysis.—*Chill;* of single parts, $<$ in open air; followed by violent itching of the skin.

Heat; of head, red face; flushes over whole body.

Sweat; of single parts at different times; after chill, no intervening heat. Chronic cases maltreated by drugging and Quinine.

PETROSELINUM.

Characteristic.—In the herbarium of Horstius, as early as 1630, this remedy is mentioned as having cured catarrhal, quotidian and tertian fevers. But like all similar cures, they were purely empirical and practically worthless.

Sudden urging to urinate.

Child suddenly seized with desire to urinate; if he cannot be gratified immediately he jumps up and down with pain.

When chronic urethritis or stricture, gonnorrheal or traumatic, cause or complicate the case (Clem.).

Vesical or urinary symptoms are usually present as valuable concomitants.

There is frequent desire to urinate, recurring nearly every half hour, caused by a crawling, stitching, titillating in the fossa navicularis.

Drawing, burning, sticking in fossa navicularis, **that after urinating changed to a cutting-biting** (Canth., Med., Sars.).

Type.—Quotidian by preference; tertian. Periodicity strongly marked; the stages are regular both in their evolution and succession (Quinine). Adapted to acute, non-miasmatic fevers, which appear to depend upon defective assimilation or perverted innervation.

Apyrexia.—There are twitching, jerking pains in the epigastrium, flatulent eructations, colic, nausea and vomiting; stools white, clay-colored (Pod.).

PHELLANDRIUM.

Adapted to persons of a feeble, irritable, lymphatic constitution, with weak and defective reaction.

Time.—From 4 to 10 P. M.—4, 6, 7, 8, 9, 10 P. M.

Chill.—Coldness and chilliness, with frequent shaking, about 8 P. M., continuing even after lying down; internal, could scarcely get warm in bed until midnight, though the skin was not cold to the touch. Shivering; as if dashed with cold water (Rhus, Sabad.); not > by warmth of stove. Chilliness and shivering over whole body, with gooseflesh on the arms and cutting pains in epigastric region. Chill every third day at 4 P. M., continuing one hour and preceded by severe rheumatic pains in arms.

Heat.—Of the head and face, with burning and redness of the face. Heat and sweat lasted two hours, followed by violent headache, nausea and stitching pains in feet.

Sweat.—Slight; intermingled with heat; often wanting altogether.

There may be present as concomitants catarrhal and pulmonary affections, loss of appetite, emaciation, sleeplessness, diarrhea and night-sweats.

Generally on the day after the attack there would be entire inability to urinate, or it would pass off in small quantities with urging and burning pains.

"Jn. Frank reports (*Path. Med. Trans.,* Paris, 1835) that he cured, without a failure, the intermittent fevers which prevailed during the spring and summer of 1801 with Phellandrium. But, he adds, immediately after that, in the following years, the same employed in the same disease failed. What more evident proof of the necessity of absolutely and always individualizing in pathology and therapeutics? The law of cure is immutable; there is no caprice about it; caprice is the appanage of physicians! Phellandrium cured the fever of 1801; with the testimony of Jn. Frank no one has a right to doubt it; and if it failed in the following epidemics it was because the medical constitution was no longer the same; and, not knowing how to individualize, Jn. Frank has left us a memento, but a sterile one. If, however, he had left us the minutely exact portraiture of the fever of 1801, he would have left us the characteristics of Phellandrium, and the success which he obtained, instead of being lost to us, might have been repeated."—A. Charge, M. D.

PHOSPHORIC ACID.

Characteristic.—Adapted to persons of originally strong constitutions, who have become debilitated by **loss of vital fluids**; sexual excesses (Cinch.); violent, acute diseases; chagrin or a long succession of moral emotions, as grief, care, disappointed affection.

Mild, yielding disposition (Puls.).

Pale, sickly complexion, eyes sunken and surrounded by blue margins.

Is listless, pathetic; *indifferent to the affairs of life;* to those things that used to be of most interest; *prostrated with grief.*

In children and young people who grow too rapidly (Cal., Cal. p.); pains in back and limbs as if beaten.

Delirium: muttering, unintelligible; lies in a stupor or a stupid sleep, unconscious of all that is going on around him; when aroused is fully conscious, answers slowly and correctly and relapses into stupor.

Patient trembles, legs weak, stumbles easily, or makes missteps.

Interstitial inflammation of bones; scrofulous, syphilitic, mercurial; periosteum inflamed, pains burning, tearing, as if scraped with a knife (Rhus); caries, rachitis, but not necrosis; growing pains.

Vertigo: head sinks forward and backward; on closing the eyes; in typhus, they fall when sitting up; when lying in bed, as if feet were going up with head remaining still.

Headache: *crushing weight on vertex,* from long lasting grief or exhausted nerves; in occiput and nape; usually from behind forward, < by motion, noise, especially music, > lying (Bry., Gels., Sil.).

Headache of school girls from eye strain or over use of eyes (Cal. p., Nat.); of students, who are growing too fast.

Diarrhea: *painless; not debilitating; white* or yellow; involuntary with flatus (Aloe, Nat.); from acids, choleraic, from fear.

Urine; looks like milk mixed with jelly-like, bloody pieces; decomposes rapidly; profuse urination at night, of clear watery urine which forms a white cloud at once (excess of phosphates, nerve waste).

Onanism; when patient is greatly distressed by the culpability of the act (Dios., Staph.).

Boring, drawing, digging pains in nerves of extremities; neurosis in stump after amputations (Cepa).

Emissions: *frequent, profuse, debilitating;* after coitus; most desire, after; several in one night; *abashed, sad, despairs of cure* (with irresistible tendency to masturbate, Ust.).

Chest: weak from talking or coughing (Stan.); in phthisis; nervous, from loss of vital fluids, too rapid growth, depressing mental emotions.

Aggravation.—From mental affections; loss of vital fluids, especially seminal; self abuse; sexual excesses; talking causes weakness in chest (Stan.).

Amelioration.—Motion; warmth; wet weather; (Caust., Nux).

Type.—Periodicity not marked. Apt to become remittent or typhoid, with cerebral symptoms predominant; typhus.

Time.—9 to 10 A. M.; 4, 6, 7, 8, 9, 10; afternoon till 10 P. M.

Chill.—Without thirst. Shaking chill, with blue nails, coldness in tips of fingers, in abdomen, tearing in wrists, and paralytic weakness of the arms. Chilliness and palpitation (palpitation during sweat, **Mer.**—see **Bar.**). Violent shaking chill from afternoon till 10 P. M., *followed by such great heat that he almost lost consciousness.* Chilliness for an hour towards evening, without subsequent heat (**Sul.**). Chill 9 P. M. with great prostration which continues all through the paroxysms. Chill and heat, alternate frequently. Shaking chill over whole body, with ice cold fingers (**Ced., Sep.**). *The evening chill predominates.*

Heat.—Without thirst; *excessive, depriving one almost of consciousness;* internal without being hot to the touch. Fever all night with frequent passing of large quantities of clear, watery urine; not much thirst; side on which she lies painful.

Hot face, on the side on which he is not lying. Heat, yet cannot be uncovered (**Bell.**—must be uncovered, **Ign., Puls.**). Hot head; cold feet.

Sweat.—*Thirst only during sweat* (**Cinch.**—drinks often and in large quantities, **Ars.**—thirst after sweating stage, **Lyc.**). Perspiration, with heavy dreams of dead people and of being pursued. *Profuse morning sweat; clammy; exhausting;* most on occiput and neck.

Tongue.—Red streak in the middle of the tongue. *Craves refreshing, juicy food.*

Pulse.—Weak, small, frequent; irregular; intermitting one or two beats.

Analysis.—Cerebral typhoid or typhus; **complete apathy and stupor**; takes no notice, "lies like a log," utterly regardless of surroundings; intestinal hemorrhage, blood dark; night sweats.

Chill.—Shaking over whole body; fingers icy cold.

Heat; excessive, depriving of consciousness.

Sweat; profuse, exhausting. Thirst only in sweat.

PHOSPHORUS.

Characteristic.—Adapted to *tall, slender persons* of sanguine temperament, *fair skin, delicate eye lashes, fine, blonde or red hair,* quick, lively perceptions and sensitive nature.

Young people, who grow too rapidly, are inclined to stoop (walk stooping, Sul.); chlorosis; anemia; old people, with morning diarrhea.

Oversensitiveness of all the senses to external impressions, light, noise, odors, touch (Ign., Nux, Tar.).

Restless, fidgety; moves continually, cannot sit or stand still a moment (fidgety feet, Zinc.).

Burning: *in spots* along the spine; *between the scapulæ* (as of a piece of ice, Lachn.); or intense heat running up the back; of palms of hands (Lach.); in chest and lungs; of every organ or tissue of the body (Ars., Sulph.); generally in diseases of nervous system.

Pain: acute, especially in the chest, < from pressure, even slight, *in intercostal spaces, and lying on left side;* excited by slightest chill; open air intolerable.

A weak, empty, all-gone sensation in head, chest, stomach and entire abdomen.

Apathetic; unwilling to talk; answers slowly; moves sluggishly.

Weary of life; full of gloomy forebodings.

Nervous debility; trembling; desires to be magnetized.

Weakness and prostration; of whole body; weariness, from loss of vital fluids.

A weak, empty, all-gone sensation in head, chest, stomach and *entire abdomen.*

Longs for: cold food and drink; juicy, refreshing things; ice cream > gastric pains.

As soon as water becomes warm in stomach it is thrown up.

Constipation; feces slender, long, dry, tough and hard like a dog's; voided with difficulty (Caust., Prunus, Staph.).

Diarrhea: as soon as anything *enters the rectum;* profuse, pouring away as from a hydrant; watery with sago-like particles; **sensation of the anus remaining open** (Apis, Sec.); involuntary; during cholera time.

During pregnancy: unable to drink water; sight of it causes vomiting; must close her eyes while bathing (Lys.).

Hemorrhagic diathesis; slight wounds bleed profusely (Kreos., Lach.).

Hemorrhage: frequent and profuse, pouring out freely and then ceasing for a time; hemoptysis; metrorrhagia, cancer, vicarious, from nose, stomach, anus, urethra in amenorrhea.

Cannot talk, the larynx is so painful; cough, going from

warm to cold air (rev. of Bry.), laughing, talking, reading, eating, *lying on left side* (Dros., Stan.).

Acts more beneficially when patients suffer from chronic diarrhea.

Relations.—Complementary: Arsenic, with which it is also in isomorphic relation.

Incompatible: with Causticum, must not be used before or after.

Follows well: after Cinchona or Calcarea.

Hahnemann says: "Acts more beneficial when patient suffers from chronic loose stool or diarrhea."

Aggravation.—Evening before midnight (Puls., Rhus); when alone; lying on left or painful side; from light; during a thunderstorm; change of weather, either hot or cold; eating something warm.

Amelioration.—In the dark; lying on right side; after sleep; eating something cold; rubbing, or being mesmerized.

Cold air relieves the head and face symptoms, but aggravates those of the chest, throat and neck.

Type.—Quotidian. Typhoid, typhus, yellow.

Time.—1, 6, 5 to 6, 7 P. M. Afternoon and evening. *Same hour every day.*

Chill.—Without thirst. Towards evening, *not > by heat of stove* (**Meny., Nux**). Chill at 1, lasting till 5 P. M. Chilliness over whole trunk, as if in cold water, *not relieved by external covering* (**Nux**). Chilliness in the evening on falling asleep; from 6 P. M. till midnight, falling asleep from weakness. **Chilliness every evening, with shivering,** *with aversion to uncovering.* Violent shaking chill at night, with diarrhea, followed by heat and perspiration. *Chill alternating with heat* (**Ars.**); *veins of hands swollen;* yawning; goose-flesh. *Chill descends; heat ascends,* the back (**Ver.**). **Coldness in the knees at night in bed** (**Carbo v.**). *Coldness of limbs;* **icy coldness of the hands and feet, even in bed.**

Heat.—With thirst. Violent chill; he could not get warm at 5 to 6 P. M., followed by heat and internal chilliness; then heat and perspiration all night. Heat at night, beginning in stomach; faint and hungry; then chill followed by internal heat, especially in the hands, the cold continuing externally. **Heat and sweat at night, with ravenous hunger,** *that could not be appeased* (hunger in every stage, **Cina**—hunger after paroxysm, **Eup.**—hunger before chill, **Cinch.**). Hot flushes over whole body, beginning in the hands, both afternoon and evening; cold externally. Urine turbid, whitish, brick dust sediment.

Sweat.—Profuse over whole body and on slight exertion. *Morning sweat, most profuse during sleep* (**Cinch.**). *Profuse exhausting morning sweat,* sometimes clammy. Sweat on head, hands, feet, fore part of body, alternating with chilliness; urine turbid and milky. Perspiration has the odor of sulphur.

Tongue.—Coated with a thick fur, white or brown, dark centre and red edges; or coated only in the middle.

Hunger, must eat during chill and heat, before he can get up; feels faint; wants cold food, ice water, ice cream. Regurgitation of food, in mouthfuls, with nausea. Food scarcely swallowed, comes up again.

"Intermittent fever; heat and perspiration at night, with faintness and ravenous hunger, which could not be satisfied by eating; afterwards chilliness, with chattering of teeth and external coldness; chilliness succeeded by internal heat, especially in hands, the external coldness continues."—LIPPE.

Apt to become remittent or typhoid; or a remittent fever takes on after a time—or after a partial or complete suppression—an intermittent type, usually the quotidian.

Analysis.—*Chill;* chilliness every evening, with icy coldness of extremities.

Heat; and sweat at night, with ravenous hunger.

Sweat; profuse, over whole body and on slight exertion.

PLANTAGO.

Characteristic.—Suitable to chronic cases with regular type, which Quinine will neither change nor suppress.

Persons of irritable, morose disposition; impatient, restless mood, with dull stupid feeling in the brain.

Great mental prostration, increased by mental exertion, which also causes rapid respiration and a feeling of great anxiety.

Teeth (left side) elongated, sore; pain unbearably severe, boring, digging in sound teeth; worse from contact and extremes of heat and cold.

Bad effects of excessive use of tobacco, especially the mental anxiety; digging toothache and frequent attacks of sudden sneezing with profuse, watery, bland coryza.

Nocturnal enuresis; profuse colorless urine, depositing a white sediment; occurs from midnight to morning.

Type.—Every type. Quotidian, tertian, quartan. Every two, three, four, seven, or fourteen days. Remittent; continued.

Time.—2 P. M. Any time during the day.

Cause.—Abuse of Quinine.

Prodrome.—Erratic pains in chest, dullness in head and stretching of limbs.

Chill.—Without thirst. Cold chills with goose-flesh at 2 P. M., running over the body, worse when moving about; fingers cold. Coldness of body with shivering; head feels irritable; feet and legs cold; hands cold even in a warm room.

Heat.—With thirst; great excitability, anxiety, mental agony, restlessness; room seems hot and close; oppression of chest, rapid respiration; breathing difficult, as if there was no air in the room (anxious, oppressed breathing, **Ipec.**—air of room intolerable, **Apis**). Burning heat of head, face, hands and feet; head feels hot, painful, dull and stupid. Hands hot and clammy.

Sweat.—Cold over lumbar and sacral region Heat of room was unbearable, producing perspiration.

Tongue.—White coated; breath putrid, offensive. Taste dirty, putrid. Food tasteless. Eructations tasting of sulphur, last all day.

PODOPHYLLUM.

Characteristic.—Adapted to persons of bilious temperament, who suffer from gastro-intestinal derangement, especially after abuse of Mercury; "bilious attacks."

Pains: sudden attacks of jerking pain.

Depression of spirits; imagines he is going to die or be very ill (Ars.); disgust for life.

Headache; alternating with diarrhea (Aloe); headache in winter, diarrhea in summer.

Painless cholera morbus; violent cramps in feet, calves, thighs; watery, painless stools; cholera infantum (Phyt.).

Difficult dentition: moaning, grinding the teeth at night; *head hot and rolling from side to side;* intense desire to press the gums together (Phyt.).

Patient is *constantly rubbing and shaking the region of liver with his hands.*

Diarrhea: of children; during teething; after eating; *while being washed; of dirty water, soaking napkin through* (Benz. ac.); *early in morning,* continues through forenoon, followed by natural stool in the evening (Aloe), and accompanied by sinking or weakness in abdomen and rectum; of long standing.

Stool: green, *watery, fetid, profuse* (Cal.); gushing out (Jatro., Phos.); chalk-like, jelly-like (Aloe); undigested (Cinch., Fer.); yellow, meal-like sediment; prolapse of rectum, before or with stool.

Prolapsus uteri: *from overlifting or straining;* after parturition. In early months of pregnancy, can lie comfortably only on stomach.

Affects right throat, right ovary, right hypochondrium.

Pain and numbness in right ovary, running down thigh of that side (Lil.).

Suppressed menses in young girls (Puls., Tub.).

Aggravation.—In early morning (**Aloe, Nux, Sul.**); in hot weather (diarrhea); during dentition.

Amelioration.—Evening; external warmth; pressure.

Type.—Quotidian; tertian; quartan. Periodicity marked. Morning paroxysm predominates. Bilious; malarial. Intermittent may become bilious, remittent or continued.

Time.—7 A. M., characteristic. Light paroxysms may occur in the evening.

Prodrome.—Backache; *severe* in lumbar region. *Gastric and bilious symptoms are marked, sometimes for days before the paroxysm.*

Chill.—Without thirst, *with pressing pains in both hypochondria* and dull aching in *knees, ankles, elbows* and *wrists.* Feverish during the afternoon, with occasional chilliness, which *was not > by the heat of the stove,* but *was > by covering up warmly in bed.* **Great loquacity;** consciousness, but cannot talk, because he forgets the words; or tries to talk continually, but forgets the words he wishes to employ (**Marum v.**). Chilly on first lying down in the evening, with incoherent talking during the imperfect semi-sleep.

Heat.—*With thirst.* The heat begins *during the chill,* or *while he is yet chilly.* The shaking and sensation of coldness continue for some time *after the heat commences.* **Violent headache with excessive thirst.** Chilliness while moving about and in the act of lying down; with sweat at once. **Great loquacity,** *constantly talking* (**Carbo v., Lach.**), *which continues with delirium until fever* reaches its climax, when **he**

falls asleep *and transpires profusely,* with forgetfulness of all he had said (falls asleep during evening fever, and wakes when it stops, **Calad.**—see **Apis, Nux m.**).

Sweat.—Profuse sweating, so that it dropped off the finger-ends. Warm on head and legs. **Sleep during perspiration;** > headache. Bathed in cold perspiration.

Tongue.—Coated white, moist, dirty, pappy, pasty, shows imprint of teeth (**Mer.**); dry, yellow. Offensive odor of breath, *which disgusts him* (offensive odor from mouth; *not perceptible to himself,* **Puls.**). Taste foul; total loss of taste, or everything tastes sour. **Gastric symptoms predominate.**

Apyrexia.—Total loss of appetite; even the smell of food produces loathing (**Colch.**); offensive breath; foul taste; profuse salivation; eructations smelling like rotten eggs. Constipation or diarrhea.

Analysis.—*Chill;* with aching in hypochondria, knees, ankles, elbows, wrists; *great loquacity* during semi-sleep.

Heat; thirst, headache, *great loquacity,* delirium: falls asleep at climax of fever and sweats profusely.

Sweat; profuse, sleeps during perspiration. Gastric symptoms predominate.

The loquacity *during chill* and *far into heat,* with complete forgetfulness afterwards of all that had passed, is characteristic. *Falls asleep at climax of heat, and sleeps during perspiration* resembles Apis, but the urticaria is wanting, and the perspiration is more profuse.

POLYPORUS OFFICINALIS.

Type.—Quotidian; tertian. Sporadic or endemic, of spring, summer, winter. Rarely called for in autumn.

Time.—5, 10 and 11 A. M.—1, 3, 4, 3 to 4 and 9 P. M.

Prodrome.—Great languor and aching in the large joints.

Chill.—Chills, with slight thirst, alternate with heat several times a day. Chilliness with disposition to yawn and stretch. *Frequent creeping chills along the spine between the shoulder-blades, up the back to nape of neck,* intermingled with hot flushes (chills along the spine, running up the back in successive waves, **Gels.**). **Chills commencing in the back between the shoulder-blades** (**Caps.**). *Coldness of nose, hands and feet. Great languor, with severe aching pains in back, large joints, and bones of legs* (**Eup., Pod.**); *yawns and stretches.* Severe chills, lasting two hours, followed by heat and perspiration. *Unusual chilliness when the open air is encountered, with icy coldness of the nose.*

Heat.—With thirst; constant, lasting all night (after evening chill, **Lyc., Puls., Rhus**). Skin extremely hot and dry. *Face hot and flushed,* with prickly sensation (**Nit. ac.**); *hands, palms, feet hot and dry.* Thirst not excessive, nausea and vomiting often occur during heat.

Sweat.—*Profuse after midnight;* sweat all night; mild in recent, profuse in old chronic cases.

Tongue.—Coated white: or yellow thick coat, with red tip. Taste, bitter, coppery. Loss of appetite. Desire for sour things, which always relieved symptom.

Apyrexia.—Pain in liver, with jaundice of the skin and great lassitude. Pain in abdomen between stomach and navel; loud rumbling in the bowels. Constipation, dull headache and great languor; or congestion of blood to the head with vertigo. Intermission very short; fever almost continuous in severe cases, and apt to become remittent.

Best adapted to old, long standing cases that have been saturated with Quinine, and remained proof against all febrifuges.

PSORINUM.

Characteristic.—Especially adapted to psoric constitutions; lack of reaction after severe acute diseases, appetite will not return.

Extremely scrofulous patients; nervous, restless, easily startled, sleepless from intolerable itching and frightful dreams of robbers, danger, etc.

In chronic cases, when **well-selected remedies fail to relieve or permanently improve** (in acute diseases, Sul.); **when Sulphur is indicated but fails to act**; in fevers with *a personal or family history of eczema, quinsy or hay fever.*

Children are pale, delicate, sickly; sick babies will not sleep day or night, but worry, fret, cry (Jalapa); child good, plays all day; restless, troublesome, screaming all night (rev. of Lyc.).

Great weakness and debility; from loss of fluids; *remaining after acute diseases;* without any organic lesion, or apparent cause.

Despairs of recovery; *hopeless, thinks he will die,* especially *after fevers;* during climaxis.

Religious melancholy; despairs of salvation (Melil.).

Body has a filthy smell, even after bathing.

Headache: chronic, at every change of weather; awakened from sleep with pain; *hungry during headache; > while eating,* by washing, by nosebleed; preceded by dim vision or blindness, black spots or rings.

Great sensitiveness to cold air or change of weather; wears a fur cap, overcoat or shawl, even in the hottest summer weather.

Stormy weather affects him severely; feels restless for days before, and during a thunder-storm (Phos.).

Cough and dry scaly eruptions return every winter.

All excretions—diarrhea, leucorrhea, menstrual flow, perspiration—**have a carrion-like odor.**

Ailments: from suppressed skin diseases, when Sulphur fails to >; severe, from even slight emotions; from some eruptive disease of childhood.

Feels unusually well, day before an attack.

Quinsy: to > acute attack and eradicate the constitutional tendency.

Hay fever; annually, same day of month and often same hour of day; should be treated in winter to eradicate the diathesis and prevent return.

Hungry in the middle of the night; must have something to eat.

Eructations tasting of rotten eggs (in A. M., Arn.—at night, Ant. t.—in A. M. only, disappearing after rinsing the mouth, Graph.).

Diarrhea; stool watery, dark brown, fetid, *carrion-like odor.*

Leucorrhea; clotted, *large lumps,* of an *unbearable odor.*

Vomiting of pregnancy, obstinate cases when the best selected remedy fails; fetus moves too violently.

Asthma: < sitting up, in open air; > lying down and keeping arms spread wide apart; thinks he will die.

Skin: abnormally susceptible to skin diseases; dry, inactive, rarely sweats; looks dirty, as if never washed; coarse, greasy as if oiled; bad effects of ointments.

Aggravation.—Evening, before midnight; in open air; stormy weather, thunder-storm; sitting.

Amelioration.—Lying down; in the room; moving; **sweating.** Always feels better before the paroxysm.

Type.—Periodicity of fever paroxysms not marked. Attacks (of other diseases) at same hour every day. Every alternate day; headache, thirst, cold. Typhoid, typhus, continued, yellow, the bubonic plague.

Time.—Evening.

Chill.—With thirst, especially in the evening, *on the upper arms and thighs,* with horripilations, hot flashes, creeping chills, great weakness, debility, sleepiness. *Internal shivering, creeping chills,* and *icy cold feet.* **Drinking causes cough** (causes cough and gagging, **Cimex**).

Heat.—And sweat on the face in the evening; *when riding in a carriage* (better when riding in a carriage, **Nit. ac.**). *Evening heat with delirium, great thirst,* followed by *profuse sweat.* Heat, sweat, thirst, during both chill and heat (**Cal., Sul.**).

Sweat.—Profusely and freely when walking, with consequent debility (Bry., Cinch., Carbo a.). Takes cold easily (Cal., Bar.). *Copious perspiration on face, palms of hands* and *perineum,* **when moving about** (profuse from *walking, reading, riding, talking,* **Sep., Sul.**). Profuse at 3 A. M.

After the sweat all the complaints cease (Bry., Calad., *Nat.*).

Sweat at night > the headache.

Sweat profuse, stinking, at night.

Sour smelling, viscous sweat.

Tongue.—Coated white or yellowish-white; tip dry and feels burnt as far as the middle (red, triangular tip, **Rhus**). Taste bitter, goes off after eating or drinking (reverse of **Nit. ac., Puls.**); foul taste. Great hunger without appetite.

Analysis.—The constitutional symptoms are guiding.

Sweats profusely; takes cold easily.

In all fevers, but, especially typhoid, Psorinum will prevent a protracted case, if there be a history of eczema, suppressed eruption or quinsy. In such cases the symptoms are never clear.

Patient has never been well since typhoid fever.

Psorinum will often clear up a case where there is lack of vital reaction after severe attacks, when other remedies, although well chosen, fail to relieve or permanently improve.

The constitutional symptoms are reliable; the chief symptoms do not come to the surface during the paroxysm. It has cleared up many a case for me in psoric constitutions after Sulphur failed. More frequently indicated than used (reverse of Quinine).

See "True Cause of Typhoid," introduction, page 36.

PULSATILLA.

Characteristic.—Adapted to persons of indecisive, slow, phlegmatic temperament; sandy hair, blue eyes, pale face, easily moved to laughter or tears; affectionate, mild, gentle, timid, yielding disposition—the woman's remedy.

Weeps easily; almost impossible to detail her ailments without weeping (weeps when thanked, Lyc.).

Women inclined to be fleshy, with scanty and protracted menstruation (Graph.).

The first serious impairment of health is referred to puberic age, have "never been well since"—anemia, chlorosis, bronchitis, phthisis.

Secretions from all mucous membranes are thick, bland and yellowish-green (Kali s., Nat. s.).

Pains: drawing, tearing, **erratic, rapidly shifting** *from one part to another* (Kali b., Lac c.); are accompanied with constant chilliness, and the more severe the pain the harder the chill; appear suddenly, leave gradually, or tension, which increases until very acute, and then "lets up with a snap" (toothache, neuralgia); on first moving (Rhus).

Symptoms ever changing; no two chills, no two stools, no two attacks alike; very well one hour, miserable the next.

Thirstlessness *with nearly all complaints.*

Gastric difficulties from eating rich food, cake, pastry, especially fat pork or sausage; the sight or even thought of pork causes disgust; "bad taste" in the morning.

"All-gone" sensation in stomach, in tea drinkers especially.

Diarrhea: only, or usually, at night; watery; greenish-yellow, very changeable; soon as they eat; from fruit, cold drinks, ice-cream (Ars., Bry.—eating pears, Ver., China; onions, Thuja; oysters, Brom., Lyc.; milk, Cal., Nat. c., Nic., Sul.; drinking impure water, Camp., Zing).

Derangements at puberty; catamenia, suppressed from getting the feet wet; *too late, scanty,* slimy, *intermitting flow,* with evening chilliness; *flows more during the day* (Lil.—on lying down, Kreos.; only at night or when lying, Mag. c.).

Sleep: wide awake in the evening, does not want to go to bed, first sleep restless, sound asleep when it is time to get up; wakes languid and unrefreshed (rev. of Nux).

Styes, especially on upper lid, *from eating fat, greasy, rich food or pork* (compare, Lyc., Staph.).

Threatened abortion: flow ceases and then returns with increased force; pains spasmodic, excite suffocation and faintness; must have fresh air; during chill.

Relations.—Complementary: Kali m., Lyc., Sil., Sulph. ac.

Follows well: after Kali bi., Lyc., Sep., Sil., Sul.

Ailments: from Cham., Quinine, Mer., Sul., tea-drinking.

Silicea is the chronic of Pulsatilla in nearly all ailments.

One of the best remedies with which to begin the treatment of a chronic case (Cal., Sulph.).

Patients, anemic or chlorotic, who have taken much iron, Quinine and tonics, even years before.

Aggravation.—In a warm, close room; evening, at twilight; lying on the left or painless side; indigestible food, fats, pork, ice cream, etc.; on beginning to move; heat, warm applications (Kali m.).

Amelioration.—In open air; lying on painful side (Bry.); cold room; eating or drinking cold things; cold applications.

Type.—Every type; simple and compound. Quotidian; tertian; quartan. Monthly (Nux, Sep.); every fourteen days (Ars., Cinch., Plan.). Irregular type; irregular stages; *long chill, little heat, no thirst* (short chill, long heat, no thirst, Ipec.); stages not marked and apt to run into each other (Ars., Nux, Pod.). Bilious, remittent, continued.

Time.—1, 8 and 11 A. M. 1 and **4 P. M.** Afternoon and evening. The 4 o'clock paroxysm predominates. Evening paroxysm lasts all night (Lyc., Nux, Rhus).

Cause.—Dietetic irregularities. Eating rich, fat food, pastries, pork, often originates an attack, or during convalescence produces a relapse (Ant. c., Ipec.).

Prodrome.—Thirst; drowsy and sleepy all day, with mucous diarrhea; nausea or vomiting of mucus. If morning chill *diarrhea previous night without thirst.*

Chill.—*Cold chills all over; chilliness all the time; feels cold even in a warm room, in the evening. Chilliness the whole evening before bedtime,* even while walking. *Chilliness; on going from a warm room into the cold air; with pains in the evening.* **Chill at 4 P. M.,** *no thirst;* vomiting of mucus when the chill comes on; anxiety; dyspnea; flitting chilliness; in spots, now here, now there; worse in the evening. *One-sided coldness,* with numbness (**Bry., Nat.** right side;—**Caust., Carbo v., Lyc., Thuja**—the left). *Chilliness over the abdomen extending around the sacrum and back.* Shivering on the back extending into the hypochondria, especially into the anterior portion of the *arms* and *thighs,* with a coldness of the limbs, and a feeling as if they would fall asleep, about 4 P. M. Shivering running up the back all day; creeping-shivering over the arms, with heat of the cheeks; *the air of the room seems hot. Cold hands and feet, they seem dead* (**Lyc., Sep.**—whole body numb, **Ced.**). Hand and foot of one side cold and red; the other side hot, in the evening. The morning paroxysm at 8 A. M. has nausea, vomiting, headache and vertigo; chilliness, heat and sweat intermingled, or simultaneous (Ars.), and usually much thirst during entire attack. Evening paroxysm; violent chill, with external coldness, without shivering or thirst; in the morning sensation of heat, as if sweat would break out, without thirst or external heat, though with hot hands and aversion to uncovering.

Heat.—With thirst; with *red face,* or *one cheek red* and *one pale* (**Acon., Cham.**). *Heat of right side* (left side and left arm, Rhus), *or on upper part of body,* lessened by motion or washing (**Caps.**—increased by motion, **Nux**); heat of face, or of one hand, with coldness of the other; body hot, limbs cold (**Bell., Carbo v.**). **Anxious heat,** *as if dashed with hot water* (**Rhus**). **Intolerable burning heat at night in bed with uneasiness. Dry heat of the body in the evening, with distended veins and burning hands, that seek out cool places** (**Opium**). **He is hot, wishes to be uncovered** (**Apis, Camph., Sec.**). **Moans and groans, licks the lips, but does not drink.** Heat of the whole body, except the hands, which are cool, with pressive headache above the orbits. Internal dry heat with thirst; flushes of heat; with clothes on was too warm, on taking them off was chilly. **External warmth is intolerable** (heat of room is intolerable, **Apis**); **the veins are enlarged** (**Bell., Cinch.**). **Fever; thirst at 2 P. M., followed by chill at 4 P. M., without thirst, with coldness of the face and hands; anxiety and oppression of the chest; afterward, when lying down, drawing pains in the back, extending to the occiput, and thence into the temples and vertex; after three hours, heat of the body, without thirst; the skin was burning hot, but there was sweat only on the face, trickling down in large drops like pearls, sleepiness without sleep, and restlessness; next morning sweat over whole body.**

"The intermittent fever that Pulsatilla is able to excite has thirst only during heat (not during chill), seldom after the heat or before the chill. When there is only a sensation of heat, without externally perceptible heat, the thirst is wanting."—HAHNEMANN.

"When heat follows the chilliness, if it be only a sensation of heat with no objective warmth, there is no thirst; but if the heat be, as it sometimes is, both objective and subjective, it is then attended by thirst. Remember this, because absence of thirst is said to be a characteristic of Pulsatilla, and presence of thirst, therefore, to contra-indicate. This is true with the limitation stated."—DUNHAM.

Sweat.—One-sided; only on the left, or *only on the right side* of the body; sweat on the *right side of the face* (sweat on the side on which he lies, **Acon., Chin. s.**—on the side not lain upon, **Benz., Sanicula**—on single parts only, **Bry.**); sweat worse at night or in the morning, *ceases when waking* (see **Samb.**). Perspiration on the head, face, and scalp. Sweat all night, with **loquacity during stupefied slumber** (loquacity during chill, **Pod.**—during heat, **Lach.** and **Pod.**). Pains continue during sweat (**Eup., Lach., Nat., Nux**—worse during sweat, Ipec.).

Tongue.—Coated *white* or *yellow,* and covered with *a tenacious mucus;* too large, too broad. *Taste foul, of putrid meat; disgusting; bitter, slimy,* bilious taste after eating, drinking and smoking. Desire for beer, alcohol, stimulants, sour, refreshing things. *Aversion to fat pork,* milk, bread.

Pulse.—Weak, small, but accelerated. Pulsations through the whole body; in violent paroxysms; from chagrin, fright, joy; with anemia, chlorosis; great anxiety, was obliged to throw off his clothes.

Apyrexia.—Spleen enlarged and sensitive. *Constant chilliness during apyrexia.* Headache, moist cough, painful oppression of the chest, somnolence, loss of appetite, bitterness of the mouth, sour eructations, nausea and vomiting of mucus, diarrhea of glairy, watery stools, with prevalence of gastric and bilious symptoms

After abuse of Quinine, with bitter taste of food and clean tongue. Suppression of menses, or irregular menses (**Sep.**). Slightest derangement of the stomach will cause a relapse (**Ipec.**). *Mild, tearful disposition* of women and children often becomes converted into a peevish, irritable, fretful mood; symptoms of threatened abortion during paroxysm in early months of pregnancy. **Paroxysm of increasing severity and ever changing symptoms; no two attacks alike.**

Analysis.—*Chill;* evening, 4 P. M.; cold all over; one-sided.

Heat; of single parts, or heat of one hand, coldness of the other, or body hot, limbs cold; thirst and < from external warmth.

Sweat; one sided; of single parts; with loquacity during stupefied sleep.

No two paroxysms alike, ever changing symptoms; increasing severity.

Abuse of Quinine; relapse from slight errors in diet.

PYROGEN.

A Product of Sepsis. *A Nosode.*

For saprenia or septicemia: puerperal or surgical; from ptomaine or sewer gas infection; during course of diphtheria, typhoid or typhus; **when the best selected remedy fails to > or permanently improve.**

The bed feels hard (Arn.); *parts lain on feel sore and bruised* (Bapt., Nux m.); rapid decubitus (Carb. ac.).

Great restlessness; must move constantly to > the soreness of parts (Arn., Bellis, Eup.).

Taste: *sweetish; terribly fetid;* **pus-like**; as from an abscess.

Vomiting: persistent; brownish, coffee-ground; offensive, stercoraceous; with impacted or obstructed bowels (Op., Plb.).

Diarrhea: horribly offensive (Psor.); brown or black (Lep.); painless, involuntary; uncertain, when passing flatus (Aloe, Nat., Olean.).

Constipation: with complete inertia (Op., Sanic.); *obstinate from impaction, in fevers;* **stool, large, black, carrion-like**; *small, black balls,* like olives (Op., Plb.).

Menses: horribly offensive, carrion-like; a rotten odor; last but a day, then a bloody leucorrhea of the same horrible odor.

Fetus: or secundines retained, decomposed; dead for days, black; horribly offensive discharge, "never well since" septic fever, following abortion or confinement.

Lochia; thin, acrid, brown, very fetid (Nit. ac.); suppressed, followed by chills, fever and profuse fetid perspiration.

Distinct consciousness of a heart; it feels tired; as if enlarged; purring, throbbing, pulsating, constant in ears, preventing sleep; cardiac asthenia from septic conditions.

Pulse abnormally rapid, out of all proportion to temperature.

Skin; pale, cold, of an ashy hue (Sec.); obstinate, varicose, offensive ulcers of old persons (Psor.).

Relations.—Compare: Arn., Ars., Bap., Carbo v., Op., Rhus, Sec., Ver.

Latent pyogenic process, patient continually relapsing after apparent simillimum.

Type.—Septic and zymotic; tends rapidly to malignancy. Puerperal and surgical fevers, with a rapid tendency to septic typhus.

Time.—Forenoon; 10 or 11 A. M. most marked. When distinctly remittent, evening fever lasts all night. Every alternate day.

Cause.—Sepsis intestinalis from eating ice cream, cheese, sausage, or canned meats undergoing the putrefactive process; sepsis following abortion, labor or surgical operations; septicemia. Sewer gas poisoning.

Prodrome.—Bone pains: *aching in the limbs,* or over the entire body as from a severe cold; with great *muscular soreness;* **the bed feels hard.** Coldness and numbness of hands and feet, of arms and legs.

Chill.—Begins in the back between scapulæ (Caps., Eup., Polyp.).

Chilliness. Chilly all night; *the bed feels hard.*

Chilly when getting into bed, teeth chattered.

Chilly as soon as he touches the cold sheets (Aran.).

Coldness and chilliness all day that no fire would warm; sits by the fire and breathes the heat from the stove; chilly when leaving the fire; at night when fever came on had a sensation as if lungs were on fire, must have fresh air, which relieved.

Chilly, with increased action of the heart.

Intense restlessness, must move constantly to > the aching bones and sore muscles.

Heat.—Feels hot, as if he had a fever, as if temperature was 105, but actually was only 99.

Frequent urging to urinate as soon as fever came on; urine profuse and clear as spring water; could tell when fever was coming on from frequent calls to urinate.

Great throbbing of temporal arteries, every pulsation felt through the head.

Circumscribed redness of the cheeks.

Sweat.—Cold sweat over the entire body.

Perspiration horribly offensive; carrion-like (Psor.).

Profuse, offensive, exhausting perspiration.

Sweat: of single parts; of chest and neck; of genital organs; of affected parts; during sleep, stops when he wakes; fetid, cold, viscid, musty.

Tongue.—Large, flabby, leaves imprint of teeth; white, or yellowish-white, brown on base; heavy, yellowish-gray fur; tip and edges red; clean and smooth as if varnished; fiery red, then dark red and very dry; yellow-brown streak down centre;

dry in central third from base to apex; dry, cracked, articulation difficult (compare, Arn., Ars., Crot., Ter.).

Taste: bitter; fetid in mouth and throat as if full of pus; breath horribly offensive.

Analysis.—For the first use of Pyrogen in typhoid and septic conditions we are indebted to our English homeopathic brethren. It is adapted to the most malignant type, cases in which we formerly zig-zagged a cure with Arsenic, Carbo veg., Rhus or Terebinth are met directly by this powerful nosode. But it is in puerperalism that it bids fair to occupy a unique place in our therapeutics; here it is almost without a rival, in prompt and effective action, when the best selected remedy fails to > or improve.

Prodrome; aching and soreness of the limbs.

Chill; begins between scapulæ, as soon as he touches the cold sheets; **the bed feels hard.**

Heat; frequent urging to urinate as soon as the chill comes on; circumscribed redness of the cheeks.

Sweat: profuse, exhausting, carrion-like; cold, musty, viscid; of single parts.

Chill: *begins in the back,* between scapulæ; **severe,** *general of bones and extremities;* marking onset of septic fever; temperature 103 to 106; heat sudden, skin dry and burning; pulse rapid, small, wiry, 140 to 170; cold clammy sweat follows.

In septic fevers, especially puerperal, Pyrogen has demonstrated its great value as a homeopathic dynamic antiseptic.

RHUS TOXICODENDRON.

Characteristics.—Adapted to persons of a rheumatic diathesis.

Bad effects of getting wet, especially after being overheated.

Ailments: from spraining or straining *a single part,* muscle or tendon (Bellis, Cal., Nux); overlifting, particularly from stretching arms high up to reach things; lying on damp ground; summer bathing in lake or river.

Affects the fibrous tissue especially (Rhod.—the serous, Bry.); right side more than left.

Pains: as if sprained; as if a muscle or tendon was torn from its attachment; as if bones were scraped with a knife; < after midnight; in wet weather; affected parts sore to touch.

Great restlessness, anxiety, apprehension; cannot remain in bed; must change position often to obtain relief from pain (restlessness from mental anxiety, Acon., Ars.).

Muscular rheumatism, sciatica, left side (Col.); aching in left arm, with heart disease.

Great sensitiveness *to open air;* putting the hand from under the bed-cover brings on the cough (Bar., Hep.).

Great apprehension at night; fears he will die of being poisoned; cannot remain in bed.

Headache: brain feels loose when stepping or shaking the head; sensation of swashing in brain; stupefying; as if torn; *from beer;* returns from least chagrin; < from sitting, lying, in cold; > by warmth and motion.

Vertigo when standing or walking, is worse when lying down (better when lying down, Apis); < rising from lying (Bry.).

Dreams of great exertion; rowing, swimming, working hard at his daily occupation (Bry.).

Corners of mouth ulcerated, fever-blisters around mouth; exanthema on chin (Hep., Nat.).

Back: pain between the shoulders on swallowing; pain and stiffness in small of back < sitting or lying; > by motion or lying on something hard.

Relations.—Complementary: to Bryonia.

Inimical: to Apis, must not be used before or after.

Aggravation.—Before a storm; *cold, wet, weather;* at night, especially at midnight; anything cold. **Rest.**

Amelioration.—Warmth; warm, dry weather, wrapping up, warm or hot things; *motion; change of position; moving the affected parts.*

"The great characteristic of Rhus is that, with few exceptions, *the pains occur and are aggravated during repose and are ameliorated by motion.* This statement, however, requires some explanation. In addition to the symptoms of Rhus, which resemble paralysis, there are also groups of symptoms resembling muscular and articular rheumatism. These rheumatic symptoms come on with severity during repose and increase as long as the patient keeps quiet, until they compel him to move. Now, on first attempting to move, he finds himself very stiff, and the first movement is exceedingly painful. By continuing to move for a little while, however, the stiffness is relieved and the pains decidedly decrease, the patient feeling much better. But this improvement does not go on indefinitely. After moving continuously for a longer or shorter period, and finding comfort therein, the paralytic symptoms interpose their exhausting protest, and the patient is compelled, from a sensation of lassitude and powerlessness, to suspend his movements and to come to repose. At first this repose, after long-continued motion, is grateful, since it relieves, not the aching and severe pains, but only the sense of prostration. Before long the pains come on again during this repose and the patient is forced to move again as before."—DUNHAM.

The *pains* of Rhus are aggravated by rest, while the pains of Bryonia are relieved by rest. It is the languor and paralysis of Rhus that are relieved by rest, not the pains.

Type.—Every type. Quotidian; tertian, double tertian; quartan, double quartan. First two stages often irregular. Remittent; continued; endemic and epidemic typhoid and typhus; dengue; mountain; yellow fever.

Time.—5, 6, 7, 8 and 9 P. M. All periods except forenoon. Morning fever without chill 6 to 10 A. M. Evening paroxysm predominant; that at 7 P. M. lasts all night (Nux, Lyc., Puls.); every seventh day.

Cause.—Rheumatic exposure, especially getting wet when overheated; after a drenching from rain and neglecting the precaution of changing the wet clothes; too frequent cold bathing in ponds or streams; "going in swimming" too often in midsummer. Living in damp rooms; sleeping in damp beds; fevers occurring in damp, wet weather.

Prodrome.—Yawning; stretching and aching of the limbs; increase of saliva in mouth; burning in the eyes and painful weariness of the limbs. **"A dry, teasing, fatiguing cough, coming on first sometimes hours before, and continuing during the chill (Samb.).** I have often cured intermittents with Rhus, guided by this symptom alone."—DUNHAM.

Chill.—Begins in one thigh, only on one side, the right by preference (Bry., Thuja); sometimes, though rarely, between the scapulæ; or with severe rheumatic pains over whole body. The arm and leg of this side first feel the cold. Shaking chill about 5 P. M., even in a warm room or by a hot stove, with thirst and salivation, relieved by covering up in bed (not relieved by covering, **Nux**); salivation and all symptoms disappeared during sleep or on rising. *Stretching and pain of the limbs, shivering over the whole body, with much thirst, cold hands, heat and redness of the face;* in the evening in bed shivering; in the morning perspiration over the whole body. Chill, with intense muscular pains, must walk about for relief. *Chilliness and heat in the evening; the face very hot, though the cheeks were cold to touch and pale; with very hot breath.* Shaking chill on going from the open air into a warm room without thirst (reverse of **Puls.**). *Shivering heat* and *perspiration* over body at the same time (chill and heat alternating or simultaneously, **Ant. t., Ars., Cal.**), without thirst. Shaking chill in open air, not relieved by covering. *Internal coldness of limbs* (like falling asleep) *but no trace of external coldness.* Extremely cold hands and feet. Chill in all the limbs for an hour at 6 P. M., with diarrhea (without thirst), then violent heat and profuse perspiration lasting three hours, with thirst. **Severe chill at 7 P. M., as though dashed with ice cold water (Ant. t.), or as if the blood were running cold through the vessels; cold when he moves; increased by eating and drinking;** *became hot by lying down and covering, pain between the shoulders and stretching of the limbs during fever at night, sweat in morning.* Chill at 8 P. M., without thirst, with diarrhea and cutting pains in abdomen with the heat, for several hours, with thirst; followed by light sweat, sleep and morning diarrhea. **Cough during chill; dry, teasing, fatiguing** (dry, racking with pain and pleuritic stitches in chest, **Bry.**). **Great restlessness in chill** (in all stages, **Ars.**). The restlessness is because he finds that tossing about relieves, not from mental anguish, as in Arsenicum.

Heat.—*With thirst. General heat at 10 a. m.,* with *yawning, drowsy, tired feeling as if dashed with hot water,* **excessive heat, as from hot water running through the blood-vessels,** *without thirst,* but with *throbbing, dull headache,* pressure and swelling at pit of stomach, and *diarrhea with cutting pain in abdomen,* may last all night. **No cough in heat, but urticaria breaks out over entire body with violent itching, increased by rubbing,** *with great heat and thirst, drinks little and often;* lips dry. (Urticaria as chill passes off, Apis—before and during chill, Hep.—during heat and sweat, Rhus—during heat only, Ign.) She was too hot internally and chilly externally. Head and hand hot, rest of body chilly, or *vice versa.* Heat on the left side and *coldness of right side of body.* Hot, flushed face and burning heat of skin, yet not warm to the touch. Heat, after the chill, with *sweat, which relieves,* or chill in some parts and heat in others, both at the same time. **Restless, constantly changing position (Ars.).** *Shuddering on moving or uncovering.*

"The urticaria is intolerable; appears in spots or weals over the whole body; even the palms of the hands and soles of the feet, driving the patient frantic."—CLEMENT PEARSON.

Sweat.—*Profuse sweat, odorless and not exhausting* (**Samb.**). *Morning sweats, not debilitating.* **Urticaria, with violent itching, which passes off with the sweat.** Sweat, with violent trembling. Night-sweat; sometimes sour; musty; putrid (rare). Sweat over whole body, except face (reverse of **Sil.**), or *vice versa.* **Sleep during sweat (Pod.).** Sweat does not relieve all pains (like **Nat.**). Sweat may be profuse and debilitating in old cases, after frequent suppression by Quinine and "ague cures."

Tongue.—Coated white, often on one side only; takes imprint of teeth (**Mer., Pod.**); **with red, triangular tip**; sore, cracked. Bread tastes bitter, after eating. Hunger, without appetite; **craving for milk**; *cold water;* beer, to relieve the dry mouth. Aversion to alcoholic liquors and meat (reverse of **Puls.**).

Apyrexia.—Not characteristic. Symptoms of the paroxysms continue in a modified form, particularly of the skin. *Continual motion only relieves. Constant restlessness, cannot sit quiet, turns in bed frequently without finding an easy place* (because bed is so hard, **Arn., Pyr.**). Hydroa on upper lip, not as pearly, but as characteristic as **Natrum.**

In July, 1881, I cured three cases of ague in one family, where hydroa on upper lip was characteristic. Nat. m. had been given in each case without success, and one prescription of Rhus cured. Since verified by W. A. Allen and A. McNeil.

Natrum mur.	**Rhus tox.**
Time.—4 to 9; 10 to 11 A. M.; 4 to 7 P. M. Fever without chill at 10 to 11 A. M.	**Time.—10 A. M.; *7 P. M.* and evening, lasting all night.**

Natrum mur.	Rhus tox.
Cause.—Exposure to emanations from salt or fresh water streams, ponds; near recently turned-up (especially virgin) soil.	**Cause.**—Rheumatic exposure, especially by cold bathing. Swimming in ponds, rivers and small lakes.
Prodrome.—*Dreads the chill.* Languor, headache, thirst, nausea and vomiting.	**Prodrome.**—Burning in eyes, stretching and severe pain in limbs; dry, teasing, fatiguing cough.
Chill.—With thirst; blue lips and nails; bursting headache; severe shaking; chattering of teeth and tearing in bones; nausea and vomiting, and sometimes unconsciousness. *Begins in fingers and toes.*	**Chill.**—Mixed and irregular; severe chill, as if ice water were dashed over him, or blood running cold through the vessels. Coldness of *left tibia, arm* and *left side of body.* Shaking chill on going from open air into warm room. Dry, teasing, fatiguing cough.
Heat.—With thirst; increased headache, unconsciousness and excessive weakness. Long and severe. Nausea and vomiting.	**Heat.**—Excessive heat, as if dashed with hot water, or as if hot water were running through the vessels. Urticaria over entire body, itching violently. Restless, constantly changing position, without finding an easy place.
Sweat.—With thirst; profuse, gradually relieving all pains. Chilly.	**Sweat.**—Over whole body, except face, or *vice versa.* Profuse, but not debilitating. Violent trembling during sweat.
Tongue.—Mapped; herpes like ringworm on the tongue; yellow coating; salt taste. Aversion to bread. Longing for salt. Hydroa around the mouth, like strings of pearls.	**Tongue.**—Coated white, or on one side white; red, dry, triangular tip. Aversion to alcoholic liquors, putrid taste after eating or drinking. Hydroa on upper lip.

Analysis.—From rheumatic exposure, summer bathing.

Chill; severe, as if dashed with ice water; as if blood was running cold through vessels; intense rheumatic pains; cough dry, teasing, fatiguing; restlessness, must move or walk about.

Heat; intense, as if blood were molten lead; restless; urticaria over whole body, with violent itching < by rubbing.

Sweat; sleeps during sweat; profuse, urticaria passes off.

Hydroa on the lips.

Diarrhea with profuse, watery or bloody stools, with marked prostration are premonitory symptoms of typhoid or typhus.

ROBINIA.

Characteristic.—Excessive acidity of stomach; the child smells sour; sour vomiting and sour stool (Hep., Rheum).

Eructations and vomiting of intensively sour fluid, setting the teeth on edge (Lyc., Sulph. ac.).

Sick headache, with irritability, despondency, very acid eructations and acid vomiting (with sweet saliva, sweet vomiting, Iris).

Time.—Paroxysm, from 3-4 P. M. to 3-4 A. M.

Chill.—Especially in afternoon and evening; feels frozen, as if blood did not circulate (Lyc.). Hands cold. Unconscious.

Heat.—With intense thirst; frothy saliva; pasty, nauseous taste; delirium, cerebral congestion; soporous sleep; flatulence and eructations; violent cramps of extremities and great prostration. Heat and sensation of drowsiness over the whole body; face pale with circumscribed redness of cheeks, headache, nausea, colic and thirst (Lach.).

Sweat.—Copious, oily, fetid, especially on the scalp and face.

SABADILLA.

Characteristic.—Suited to persons of light hair, fair complexion, with a weakened, relaxed muscular system.

Worm affections of children (Cina, Sil., Spig.).

Nervous diseases: twitching, convulsive tremblings, catalepsy; from worms (Cina, Psor.).

Nymphomania from ascarides.

Many symptoms go from right to left (Lyc., Pod.); chilliness from feet to head.

Illusions: that he is sick; parts shrunken; that she is pregnant, when only distended with flatus; that she has some horrible throat disease that will be fatal.

Delirium during intermittents (Pod.).

Headache: from too much thinking, too close application or attention (Arg. n.); from tenia.

Sneezing: in spasmodic paroxysms; followed by lachrymation; copious watery coryza; face hot and eyelids red and burning.

Diphtheria, tonsillitis; *can swallow warm food more easily;* stitches and most symptoms, especially of throat, go from left to right (Lach., Lac c.).

Sensation of a skin hanging loosely in throat, must swallow over it (of a lump, Lach.).

Dryness of fauces and throat.

Parchment-like dryness of skin.

Relations.—Compare: Col., Colch., Lyc. where < is from 4 to 8 P. M.; Puls. > in open air.

Follows Bryonia and Ranunculus well in pleurisy, and has cured after Aconite and Bryonia failed.

Aggravation.—Cold; sensitive to cold air; during rest; forenoon.

Type.—Quotidian; tertian; quartan. Periodicity well marked; paroxysms return at same hour with great regularity (**Aran., Ced., Gels.**). Stages irregular, incomplete.

Time.—3, 4, 5 P. M.; 9 and 10 P. M. Afternoon and evening.

Chill.—Without thirst, and **often without subsequent heat.** *Violent chilliness,* at 5 P. M., over the back as if *dashed with cold water* (**Ant. t., Rhus**); *relieved by warm stove* (**Ign.** —*not relieved by heat of stove,* **Ver.**). Chilliness at 9.30 P. M., has to go to bed, followed by shaking chill; after half an hour, alternately hot and cold for half an hour; afterwards profuse perspiration. Recurring fits of shuddering coming and going quickly (Nux m.). *Chill always runs from below upward* (reverse of **Ver.**). **Dry spasmodic cough, with pain in the ribs and tearing in all the limbs and bones** (dry teasing cough *before* and *during chill,* **Rhus**—*during chill and heat,* racking cough with pleuritic stitches, **Bry.**). Chill beginning in hands and feet. *Thirst begins* as chill leaves. **Chill predominates.**

Heat.—With slight thirst *for warm drinks* (**Casc., Ced.**), *before heat begins* (between cold and hot stages), little after. Mostly on head and face; flushes of heat with redness of face, alternating with shivering; yawning; stretching; delirium. Sweat, often *during* or *with the heat* (**Pod.**). Redness and burning of face; hands and feet cold.

Sweat.—Profuse sweat about head and face, which were hot to touch, rest of body cold. Sweat after midnight, towards morning; *sweat of soles of feet.* Sleep only during sweat (Pod., Rhus—after chill, **Nux m.**). Sweat in axillæ.

Tongue.—Coated white in centre, tip bluish and sore, as if full of blisters; as if scalded.

Apyrexia.—Constantly chilly; loss of appetite; eructations sour, rancid; vomiting of bile and bitter mucus; oppressive bloatedness of stomach; pain in chest; *debility.* Sour eructations (**Lyc.**).

The gastric symptoms predominate as in Nux and Pulsatilla.

Analysis.—*Chill;* often without subsequent heat. Severe, from below upwards; with dry spasmodic cough and bone pains; predominates.

Heat; with thirst for warm drinks (Casc., Ced., Eup. p.).

Sweat: profuse, hot, of head and face, rest of body cold; of soles of feet.

Apyrexia; sour eructations (Lyc.).

SAMBUCUS.

Characteristic.—Adapted to diseases of scrofulous children: of the air passages especially.

Persons formerly robust and fleshy suddenly become emaciated (Iod., Tub.)

Bad effects of violent mental emotions; anxiety, grief, or excessive sexual indulgence (Phos. ac., Kali p.).

Edematous swellings in various parts of the body, especially in legs, instep and feet.

Dry coryza of infants; nose dry and completely obstructed preventing breathing and nursing; snuffles (Am. c., Nux).

Dyspnea; child awakens suddenly, nearly suffocated, face livid, blue, sits up in bed; turns blue, gasps for breath, which it finally gets; attack passes off, but is again repeated; **child inspires, but cannot expire** (Chlor., Meph.); sleeps into the attack (Lach.—compare, Arum drac.).

Attacks of suffocation as in last stage of croup.

Cough: suffocative, with crying children; worse about midnight; hollow, deep, whooping, with spasm of chest; with regular inhalations, but sighing exhalations.

Aggravation.—During rest; midnight; after eating fruit.

Amelioration.—Sitting up in bed. Motion: most of the pains occur during rest and disappear during motion (Rhus).

Follows well: after Opium in fright. Antidotes abuse of Arsenic.

Type.—Irregular.

Time.—3, 4, 5 and 6 P. M. Afternoon and evening.

Prodrome.—Cough, *deep and dry, for half an hour,* with nausea and thirst (dry, teasing, fatiguing cough, **Rhus**). *Sweat* (**Carbo v., Nux**).

Chill.—Without thirst. Coldness creeps over the whole body, especially hands and feet, which are cold to touch. Shaking chill creeping over whole body, though face was warm. *Hands and feet icy cold;* the rest of body warm as usual. *Chill lasts half an hour. Spasmodic, deep, dry cough* from lower part of chest, without expectoration; *may occur during chill if absent in prodrome.* Rarely occurs both before and during chill (see **Rhus**).

Heat.—Without thirst; dread of uncovering. *Sensation of burning heat in the face, with warmth of body and icy coldness of the feet, without thirst. Dry heat on falling asleep.* Intolerable dry heat all over the body, with dread of uncovering; thinks he would take cold or have an attack of colic *if uncovered* (Hep.). **Dry heat while he sleeps.**

Sweat.—Profuse sweat breaks out on the face, without thirst, while awake, from 7 P. M. to 1 A. M.; stood in drops upon the face, and extends over the entire body during waking hours; on going to sleep again the dry heat returns (sweat when he sleeps, stops when he wakes, **Thuja**). *Profuse non-debilitating sweat, day and night,* with relief of all symptoms (**Nat.**).

Apyrexia.—*Profuse sweat continues during this stage;* may become weakening from its profuseness alone, which is out of all proportion to the chill and heat.

Analysis.—Cough deep, dry, precedes the fever paroxysm. Fever: *dry heat while he sleeps; on falling asleep;* after lying down; without thirst; *dreads uncovering* (must be covered in every stage, Nux).

Profuse sweat over entire body **during waking hours;** on going to sleep, dry heat returns (sweats as soon as he closes his eyes to sleep, Cinch., Con.).

Sambucus is almost the only remedy which has *dry heat while asleep,* **profuse sweat while awake,** then *dry heat again when he sleeps.* (Sweat on waking from a sound sleep, Rum.)

The profuse sweat is *rarely debilitating,* and *never in proportion to its profuseness;* always without thirst. Cinch. has *profuse debilitating* sweat with *great thirst;* the reverse of Sambucus. *Deep, dry, racking cough before the chill, for half an hour,* with nausea and thirst, *is characteristic* (Rhus has dry, teasing cough, like Rumex crispus, before and during chill).

CLINICAL.

CASE I.—Irregular paroxysm occurring every other day. Quinine had no effect. *Cough deep and dry for half an hour,* with nausea and thirst. *Chill* for half an hour, without cough, nausea or thirst; slight fever with moist skin; profuse sweat at night not debilitating. Apyrexia complete. Prescribed for the profuse sweat at night, not debilitating, Sambucus, a drop dose of the tincture, which resulted in a perfect cure, no other attack occurring.—DUNHAM.

CASE II.—Mrs. H——. Chills and fever; type quotidian. Paroxysm commenced at 3 P. M., with hard dry cough, from lower part of the chest, racking and shaking the whole body, and producing a pain over the whole head which is relieved by pressure or having the head tightly bound up. No expectoration with the cough. Great thirst for large quantities of water very often. Longing for acids.

Chill.—Severe and shaking, continuing for *half an hour.* Lips and nails blue. Nausea and vomiting, aggravated by drinking, the substance vomited having a bitter, sour taste. Bitter, sour taste in the mouth during the paroxysm. Tongue coated white, chills running down the back. Back and limbs ache, particularly during the chill, and worse when they come in contact with the bed. Cough, headache and thirst continued.

Heat.—Great, with stupor and prostration. Thirst and cough continue, but no headache. Pains in the back and limbs. Great difficulty in speaking. With the heat a profuse perspiration.

Delirium.—Is distressed because she imagines some one in bed with her. This oppresses her respiration, as she has to breathe for two. Continual talking. Sense of suffocation, with a fluttering at the heart. Great distress in the region of the heart, whence the cough seems to proceed. Moaning and weeping during sleep.

Sweat.—At night a drenching sweat, smelling sour-fetid, staining yellow, not debilitating. Ineffectual desire to urinate, passing water once in twenty-four hours, a small quantity of turbid, loam-colored urine.

Attempts to cover the totality of the symptoms with any one remedy, resulted in the conviction that it was impossible. Eup., Bry., Ipec., Ars., Cal., and Sabad., were successively given without benefit. Dr. Dunham now suggests that the "hard, dry cough before the chill," "the half-hour chill," and the "profuse, non-debilitating sweat at night," reminded him of a case he had cured with Sambucus. The cough and sweat, however, seemed the characteristics in this case, and Sambucus 1000 was given. To my surprise and gratification I found the entire train of symptoms removed, till the seventh day, the cough returning, was removed by a repetition of the remedy.—SWAN.

SABINA.

Characteristic.—Chronic ailments of women; arthritic pains; tendency to miscarriages, especially at third month.

Music is intolerable; produces nervousness, goes through bone and marrow (causes weeping, Thuja).

Drawing pains in small of back, **from sacrum to pubes,** in nearly all diseases (from back, going round the body to pubes, Vib. op.).

Ailments: following abortion or premature labor; hemorrhage from uterus; flow partly pale red, partly clotted; *worse from* **least motion** (Sec.); often relieved by walking; *pain extending from sacrum to pubes.*

Menses: too early, too profuse, too protracted; partly fluid, partly clotted (Fer.); in persons who menstruated very early in life; flow in paroxysms; with colic and labor-like pains; *pains from sacrum to pubes.*

Discharge of blood between periods, with sexual excitement (Amb.).

Retained placenta from atony of uterus; intense afterpains (Caul., Sec.).

Menorrhagia: during climacteric, in women who formerly aborted; with early first menses.

Inflammation of ovaries or uterus after abortion or premature labor.

Promotes expulsion of moles or foreign bodies from uterus (Canth.).

Fig warts with intolerable itching and burning; exuberant granulations (Thuja, Nit. ac.).

Aggravation.—From least motion; warm air or warm room (Apis, Puls.).

Amelioration.—In cool, open, fresh air.

Chill.—In evening, with attacks of shivering chilliness all day; one chill after another. Shivering with obscuration of sight, followed by sleepiness.

Shuddering, with gooseflesh.

Cold sensation in r. limb, as if standing in ice water (Sep.).

Heat.—Burning of whole body, with great restlessness.

Flushes of heat in face, rest of body chilly; with icy cold hands and feet.

Sweat.—Night sweats. Sweats easily; every night; profuse on feet.

SARRACENIA.

Type.—Quotidian; tertian.

Time.—5 P. M.; afternoon and evening.

Chill.—General chills between the shoulder-blades (Caps., Led., Polyp., Eup. purp.). Horripilations between shoulder-blades in afternoon or evening. Coldness of extremities, as from deficient circulation. Chills, heat and sweat at 5. P. M., of a tertian or quotidian type. Chills, with cold perspiration and a desire to lie down after meals.

Heat.—Beginning in the afternoon and *lasting all night* (Lyc., Puls., Rhus). Fever, with heat and redness of the face, burning in the stomach, great prostration, delirium and loss of consciousness. Burning heat of the skin, with *excoriation and fissures,* as if it had been *excessively stretched.* Heat and continual burning in the legs; heat in the whole right lumbar region. *General heat,* with dryness of the skin, excessive thirst, and as *if hot vapors rise up to the brain.* Heat in the feet, as if *he had been cut.*

Sweat.—Copious night-sweat. Great sweat on the limbs, especially in the evening and during rest.

Tongue.—Coated brownish-white. Bad taste in the mouth, with loss of appetite.

SECALE.

Characteristic.—Adapted to women of *thin, scrawny, feeble, cachectic appearance;* irritable, nervous temperament; face ashy, pale, sunken.

Very old, decrepit, feeble persons.

Women of very lax muscular fibre; *everything seems loose and open; no action, vessels flabby;* passive hemorrhages, copious flow of thin, black, watery blood; the corpuscles are destroyed.

Hemorrhagic diathesis: the slightest wound causes bleeding for weeks (Lach., Phos.); discharge of sanious liquid blood, with a strong tendency to putrescence; tingling in the limbs and great debility, particularly when the weakness is not caused by previous loss of vital fluids.

Leucorrhea; green, brown, offensive.

Boils: *small, painful, with green contents;* mature very slowly and heal in the same manner; very debilitating (Tub).

Unnatural, ravenous appetite; even with exhausting diarrhea he is hungry; craves lemonade, acids.

Diarrhea: involuntary, profuse, watery, putrid, brown; discharged with great force (Gamb., Crot. t.); very exhausting; urine suppressed; anus wide open (Apis, Phos.).

Enuresis; of old people, pale, watery, bloody urine.

Burning; in all parts of the body, as if sparks of fire were falling on the patient (Ars.).

Cholera collapse: face pale, sunken, distorted, particularly around the mouth; skin cold, yet cannot bear to be covered.

Senile, dry gangrene; < by external heat.

The skin feels cold to the touch, yet the patient cannot tolerate covering; icy coldness of extremities.

Menses: irregular; copious, dark, fluid; with pressing, labor-like pains in abdomen; continuous discharge of watery blood until next period.

Threatened abortion, especially at third month (Sab.); prolonged, bearing down, forcing pains.

During labor: pains irregular; too weak; feeble or ceasing; everything seems *loose and open, but no expulsive action;* fainting.

After-pains: too long; too painful; hour-glass contraction.

Suppression of milk; in thin, scrawny, exhausted women; the breasts do not properly fill.

Pulse small, rapid, contracted and often intermittent.

Relations.—Similar: to Arsenicum, but cold and heat are opposite.

Resembles Colchicum in cholera morbus.

Aggravation.—*Heat: warmth from covering;* of all affected parts; in all diseases *worse from heat.*

Amelioration.—In cold air; getting cold; uncovering affected parts; rubbing.

Type.—No periodicity. All types of fever; tendency to typhoid, and typhus, yellow fever, hemorrhagic stage.

Time.—At all periods.

Prodrome.—Vomiting.

Chill.—*With thirst. Violent, shaking,* followed by violent heat with anxiety, delirium and almost *unquenchable thirst. Shaking chill,* with creeping coldness in different parts of body, as from snow (**Petr.**). **Intense icy coldness of the skin,** *particularly of face and extremities* (**Camph., Meny., Nux, Ver.**). **Cold limbs, cold skin,** *with shivering; pale, sunken* *face,* with coldness of the back and abdomen. Temperature of body diminished (**Camph., Ver.**). *Lips bluish* (**Nux**).

Heat.—*With thirst* and hot skin. *Burning heat, interrupted by shaking chills, then internal burning heat* with *great thirst.* During heat great pain in stomach, abdomen, limbs (cramps and pain in stomach and abdomen, with vomiting and purging, **Elat., Ver.**) *Severe, long-lasting, dry heat, with great restlessness and violent thirst* (**Ars., Nat., Rhus**).

Sweat.—*All over the body, except the face* (**Rhus**—reverse of, **Sil.**). General sweat, relieving all the symptoms (**Nat., Samb.**). *Profuse cold sweat on limbs. Cold, clammy sweat over whole body. Sweat from head to pit of stomach.*

Pulse.—Accelerated during heat; generally slow, contracted, at times intermittent; often unchanged even with the most violent attacks.

Tongue.—Sticky, yellow coating; tongue *deathly pale* (mucous membrane of mouth and tongue pale, **Fer.**); or clean, with dry, red tip; or red tip and edges, centre coated. Desire for sour things; lemonade (**Eup. purp.**). Disgust for food, meat and fats.

Apyrexia.—Aversion to heat or to being covered. *May feel cold, but does not wish to be covered* (**Camph.**). **Face pale, drawn, collapsed, hippocratic.** Great tendency to typhoid.

Analysis.—*Chill;* intense icy coldness; lips and fingers blue; face and extremities cold; great thirst.

Heat; severe, long, great thirst and very restless.

Sweat; profuse, cold clammy; all over body, except the face (Rhus).

Aversion to heat and cannot be covered; pernicious and sinking fevers.

SEPIA.

Characteristic.—Adapted to persons of dark hair, rigid fibre, but mild and easy disposition.

Diseases of women; particularly those occurring during pregnancy, child-bed, and lactation; or diseases attended with sudden prostration and sinking faintness (Murex, Nux m.).

"The washerwoman's remedy;" complaints that are brought on or are aggravated after laundry work.

Pains extend from other parts *to the back* (rev. of Sab.), are attended with shuddering (with chilliness, Puls.).

Particularly sensitive to cold air, "chills so easily;" lack of vital heat, especially in chronic disease (in acute disease, Ledum).

Faints easily: after getting wet; from extremes of heat or cold; riding in a carriage; while kneeling in church.

Sensation of a ball in inner parts; during menses, pregnancy, lactation; with constipation, diarrhea, hemorrhoids, leucorrhea and uterine affections.

Coldness on the vertex with headache (Ver.—heat of vertex, Cal., Graph., Sul.).

Anxiety: with fear, flushes of heat over face and head; about real or imaginary evils; toward evening.

Great sadness and weeping. Dread of being alone; of men; of meeting friends; with uterine troubles.

Indifferent: even to one's family; to one's occupation (Fl. ac., Phos. ac.); *to those whom she loves best.*

Indolent; does not want to do anything, either work or play, even an exertion to think.

Headache: in terrific shocks; at menstrual nisus, with scanty flow; in delicate, sensitive, hysterical women; pressing, bursting < motion, stooping, mental labor, > by external pressure, continued hard motion.

Great falling of the hair, after chronic headaches or at the climacteric.

Yellowness of the face; conjunctivæ; yellow spots on the chest; *a yellow saddle across upper part of cheeks and nose.*

Herpes circinnatus *in isolated spots* on upper part of body (in intersecting rings over whole body, Tell.).

Painful sensation of *emptiness,* "all-gone feeling," in the epigastrium, not > by eating (Chel., Murex, Phos.).

Pot-belliedness of mothers (of children, Sulph.).

Tongue foul, but becomes clear at each menstrual nisus, returns when flow ceases; swelling and cracking of lower lip.

Constipation: during pregnancy (Alum.); stool hard, knotty, in balls, insufficient, difficult; pain in rectum during and long after stool (Nitr. ac., Rat., Sul.); sense of weight or ball in anus, not > by stool.

Urine: deposits a reddish, clay-colored sediment, which adheres to the vessel as if it had been burnt on; fetid, so offensive must be removed from the room (fetid after standing, Indium).

Enuresis: the bed is wet almost as soon as the child goes to sleep (Kreos.); always during *the first sleep.*

Gleet: painless, yellowish, staining linen; meatus glued together in morning; obstinate, of long standing (Kali iod.); sexual organs, weak and exhausted.

Violent stitches upward in the vagina; lancinating pains from the uterus to the umbilicus.

Prolapse of uterus and vagina; **pressure and bearing down as if everything would protrude from pelvis;** must cross her limbs to prevent it; with oppression of breathing (Agar., Lil., Murex).

Irregular menses of nearly every form—early, late, scanty, profuse, amenorrhea or menorrhagia—when associated with above-named symptoms.

Morning sickness of pregnancy; the sight or thought of food

sickens (Nux); the smell of cooking food nauseates (Ars., Colch.).

Dyspnea: < sitting, after sleep, in room, > dancing or walking rapidly.

Erythism: flushes of heat from least motion; with anxiety and faintness; followed by perspiration over whole body; *climacteric* (Lach., Sang., Sulph., Tub.); *ascend* from pelvic organs.

Itching of skin; of various parts; of external genitalia; is not > by scratching, and is apt to change to burning (Sulph.).

Relations.—Complementary: Natrum mur.

Inimical: to, Lach., should not be used before or after; to, Puls., with which it should never be alternated.

Often indicated after: Silicea, Sulphur.

A single dose often acts curatively for many weeks.

Aggravation.—In afternoon or evening; from cold air or dry east wind; sexual excesses; at rest, sultry, moist weather; *before a thunderstorm.*

Amelioration.—Warmth of bed, hot applications; violent exercise.

Many symptoms, especially those of head, heart and pelvis, are both < and > by rest and exercise.

Type.—Many types; quotidian most common. **Monthly** (**Nux, Puls.**—every six or twelve months, **Lach.**). Quotidian; tertian; quartan. Bilious, remittent, malarial, typhoid.

Time.—9 or 10 A. M.—4 to 6 P. M. Indefinite periods; time not marked.

Cause.—In women, uterine diseases, menstrual delays, suppression or irregularities are often present. Constitutional chronic disease usually found.

Chill.—*With thirst. Shaking chill for an hour in the evening,* with brown, acrid-smelling urine; *he must lie down.* **Chilliness from every motion,** *though in a warm room* (**Nux**). Chill commencing in *fingers* and *toes* (**Nat.**) in *chest*

(**Apis**) and *between shoulder-blades in back* (**Caps.**). Violent headache *during chill,* **external warmth is unbearable** (**Puls.**). *Icy coldness of the whole body,* she could not get warm in warm room. *At 11 A. M. a shaking chill, beginning with very cold feet, thence over whole body; she had to lie down,* became hot at 4 A. M., and slight sweat during night over whole body. Chill, with icy cold hands and warm feet, or *vice versa.* **Very cold feet, with headache, evening and in the morning. Icy cold and damp feet all day, like standing in cold water up to ankles,** (**Lyc., Puls.**—icy coldness of right limb, as in cold water, **Sab.**). *Coldness, with* **deadness of the limbs and fingers.**

Heat.—With less thirst than in chill. *Attacks of flushes of heat,* **as if hot water were poured over one** (**Rhus**), **with redness of face,** *sweat of the whole body,* **with anxiety, without thirst or dryness of throat.** *Flushes of heat from the least exercise.* Violent rising of heat to the head, alternating with chilliness in lower limbs. **Heat ascends** (**Nat., Ver.**). Face hot from talking. Feet hot at night. **Vertigo,** *unable to collect one's senses.*

Sweat.—*Profuse in the morning* **after awaking** (see **Samb.**). *Sweat worse from least exertion, mental* or *physical, walking, writing, eating* (**Bry., Psor., Sul.**); smelling like elder blossoms. Cold night sweat on *breast, back, thighs* and *male genitals.* Sour night sweat. Sweat from above downwards to calves of legs, *every third night.*

Pulse.—Pulsations in all the blood vessels (Nat.); violent beating after waking, *from anger or mental emotions;* pulse full, quick, intermitting, with an occasional hard "thump" of the heart.

Tongue.—Coated white, with vesicles in old cases. Food tastes too salt (Carbo v., Cinch.). Aversion to meat (**Arn.**).

Apyrexia.—Canine hunger, or complete loss of appetite.

Analysis.—*Chill; monthly,* with thirst, < by every motion,

< by external warmth; icy cold feet up to ankles; deadness of limbs and fingers.

Heat; without thirst, red face, in flushes, as if hot water were poured over body; heat ascends; sweat with heat.

Sweat: profuse after waking (Rum., Samb.); from least exertion, mental or physical; of single parts; odor of elder blossoms.

A good picture of a spoiled case—of Cinchonism—of suppression of paroxysm, of menses, of rheumatism, of eruptions. The face is yellow, sallow, dirty, doughy, yellow patches here and there; the so-called "old malarial," often found in the tropics.

SILICEA.

Characteristic.—Adapted to the nervous, irritable, sanguine temperament; persons of a scrofulous diathesis.

Constitutions which suffer from deficient nutrition, not because food is lacking in quality and quantity, but from imperfect assimilation (Bar. c., Calc.); oversensitive, mentally and physically.

Scrofulous, rachitic children *with large heads;* **open fontanelles and sutures**; much sweating about the head (lower than Cal.), which must be kept warm by external covering (Psor., Sanic.); *large bellies;* weak ankles, slow in learning to walk.

Persons of light complexion; fine, dry skin; pale face; weakly, with lax muscles.

Diseases: caused by suppressed foot-sweat; exposing the head or back to any slight draft of air; from vaccination (Thuja); chest complaints of stone cutters, with total loss of strength.

Want of vital heat, always chilly, even when taking exercise (Led., Sep.).

Nervous debility; exhaustion with erythism; from hard work and close confinement; weariness, wants to lie down; may be overcome by force of will.

Has a wonderful control over the suppurative process—soft tissue, periosteum or bone—maturing abscesses when desired or reducing excessive suppuration (chiefly affecting soft tissues, Calend., Hep.).

Children are obstinate; headstrong, cry when kindly spoken to (Ant. t., Sanic., Iod.).

Restless, fidgety, starts at least noise.

Anxious, yielding, faint hearted.

Mental labor very difficult; reading and writing fatigue, cannot bear to think.

Vertigo: spinal, ascending from back of neck to head; as if one would fall forward; from looking up (Puls.—looking down, Kal., Spig., Psor.).

Chronic sick headaches, since some severe disease of youth (Psor.); *ascending from nape of neck to the vertex,* as if coming from the spine and locating in one eye, especially the right (left, Spig.); < draught of air or uncovering the head; > pressure and wrapping up warmly (Mag. m., Stron.); > profuse urination.

Constipation: *always before and during menses* (diarrhea before and during menses, Am. c., Bor.); difficulty, *as from* **inactivity of rectum**; with great straining, as if rectum was paralyzed; **stool when partly expelled, recedes again** (Thuja); remains a long time in rectum.

Discharge of blood from vagina every time *the child takes the breast* (compare Crot. t.).

Nipple is drawn in like a funnel (Sars.).

Night walking; gets up while asleep, walks about and lies down again (Kali br.).

Unhealthy skin; every little injury suppurates (Graph., Hep., Merc.).

Crippled nails on fingers and toes (Ant. c.).

Takes cold from exposure of feet (Con., Cup.).

Sweat of hands, toes, feet and axillæ; **offensive.**

Intolerable, sour, carrion-like odor of the feet, without perspiration, every evening.

Desire to be magnetized, which > (Phos.).

Promotes expulsion of foreign bodies from the tissues; fish bones, needles, bone splinters.

Relations.—Complementary: Thuja, Sanicula.

Graphites, Fluoric acid and Hepar follow well.

Silicea is the chronic of Pulsatilla.

Aggravation.—Cold; during menses; *during new moon;* uncovering, especially the head; *lying down.*

Amelioration.—Warmth, especially from wrapping up the head; all the symptoms except gastric, which are < by cold food (Lyc.).

Type.—Periodicity not characteristic. Stages ill defined. All kinds of fever.

Time.—Midnight to 8 A. M.; 10 A. M. to 8 P. M.

Evening chill from 5 to 6 P. M. **Chilly all day.**

Fever without chill 12 to 1 P. M.

Cause.—If the fever can be traced to a suppressed foot-sweat, Silicea is the first remedy to be thought of.

Chill.—Without thirst, **on every movement** (**Arn., Nux**); **very chilly all day**; *in the morning fell asleep from excessive weariness. Very chilly even in a warm room. Cramp-like chill in the evening in bed,* with shivering. *She did not dare to put her foot out of bed on account of consequent chilliness* (**Bar., Canth.**). **Shaking chill at 6 P. M.**; *was obliged to lie down and could not get warm in bed for a long time.* **Icy cold shivering frequently creeps over the body,** ***not relieved by heat of fire*** (**Phos.**). **Affected parts feel cold. Coldness with ravenous hunger** (**Cina**). *Coldness of knees and arms;* finger-nails *white* (coldness of knees, **Apis, Carbo v., Phos.**). *Nose cold as ice.* **Icy coldness of the feet and legs as far as knees.**

Heat.—*With thirst* and chilliness, at 11 A. M. **Violent heat in the head, and dark redness of the face** (face of a mahogany red, **Eup.**). **Fever in evening, worse at night** (**Cina**). *Afternoon paroxysm, consisting of heat with intense thirst and very short breath.* **Great heat all night, with catching respiration.** *Heat returning periodically during day,* followed by slight sweat.

Sweat.—**Profuse and general at night** (**Cinch.**). **Sweat only on the head or head and face** (reverse of, **Rhus, Sec.**). *Sweats periodically; 6 A. M., 3 to 5 P. M., 11 P. M. Sweat only on the head, running down the face. Profuse night-sweat, offensive, sour, debilitating; worse after midnight; from least exertion* (**Sep., Sul.**). **Offensive sweat of feet, they become sore while walking** (**Graph.**).

Tongue.—Clean or coated with brown mucus. Loss of taste and appetite; or taste of blood; of soap-suds; rotten eggs; oil. *Sensation as if a hair were lying on the forepart of the tongue.* Disgust for meat. *Averse to warm food; desire only for cold things* (Lyc.).

Apyrexia.—The constitutional symptoms developed during this stage are numerous and always reliable.

SPIGELIA.

Characteristic.—Adapted to anemic, debilitated subjects, of rheumatic diathesis; to scrofulous children afflicted with ascarides and lumbrici (Cina, Stan.).

Persons with light hair; pale, thin, bloated, weak; wrinkled, yellow, earthy skin.

Body painfully *sensitive to touch; part touched feels chilly;* touch sends shudder through the whole frame (Kali c.).

Afraid of sharp, pointed things, pins, needles, etc.

Rheumatic affections of heart (Kal., Led., Naja); systolic blowing at apex. Aneurism.

Nervous headache; periodical, beginning in morning at base of brain, spreading over the head and locating in eye, orbit and temple of left side (right side, Sang., Sil.); pain, pulsating, violent, throbbing.

Headache; at sunrise, at its height at noon, declines till sunset (Nat., Tab.).

Intolerable, pressive pain in eyeballs; could not turn the eyes without turning the whole body; worse, especially on making a false step.

Sensation: as if eyes were too large for the orbits (Act., Com.); *sensitive to touch;* as if a band around head (Cac., Carb. ac., Sulph.).

Copious offensive mucus from posterior nares, drops into throat, causing choking at night (Hydr.).

Sharp, stabbing, sticking pains through eyeballs back into the head; *from cold, damp, rainy weather.*

Prosopalgia: periodical, left-sided orbit, eye, malar bone, teeth; *from morning until sunset;* pain tearing, burning, cheek dark red; *cold, rainy weather;* from tea.

Toothache from *tobacco smoking;* > only on lying down and *while eating* (Plan.); worse from cold air and water; returns from thinking about it.

Scirrhus of sigmoid or rectum, atrocious unbearable pain (Alumen).

Dyspnea: must lie on right side or with head high (Cac., Spong.); pains in chest are stitching, needle-like.

Chest affections with stitching pains synchronous with pulse < from motion, < cold, wet weather.

Palpitation: *violent, visible and audible;* from least motion; when bending forward; systolic blowing at apex.

Stammering, repeats first syllable three or four times, with abdominal ailments; helminthiasis.

Aggravation.—From motion, noise, touch, turning the eyes; *from every shaking, commotion, or concussion.*

Amelioration.—Lying on right side with the head high (Ars., Cac., Spong.).

Type.—Quotidian; periodicity marked.

Time.—Morning; at same hour. Evening paroxysm is rare.

Cause.—Rheumatic exposure; or occurring in connection with periodic neuralgia of head, face or chest.

Chill.—*Every morning, at same hour;* alternates with heat or perspiration, especially on the back.

Sudden creeping chills, at one time only in the feet, at another only in the head and hands, at another on the back of chest and abdomen, at another over whole body, without thirst. Chill spreads from the chest (Apis, Carbo a., Sep.); least movement of the body causes chilliness.

Heat.—Especially in the back; in flushes at night; on the face and hands with chill in the back. Heat in back, hands, abdomen, gradually increasing until he becomes hot all over. Thirst for beer, not water (**Nux**).

Sweat.—Putrid smelling night-sweat. Sweat of hands clammy; cold all over body; on slightest covering (**Cinch.**).

Pulse.—Irregular, generally strong but slow; trembling.

Tongue.—Coated yellow or white; cracked. Taste like putrid water. Ravenous hunger with nausea and thirst. Desire for alcoholic drinks.

STANNUM.

Characteristic.—Extreme exhaustion of mind and body.

Sinking, empty, all-gone sensation in stomach (Chel., Phos., Sep.).

Sad, despondent, feels like crying all the time, but crying makes her worse (Nat., Puls., Sep.); faint and weak, especially when *going down stairs;* can go up well enough (Bor.—rev. of Cal.).

Headache or neuralgia; pains begin lightly and *increase gradually* to the highest point and then *gradually decline* (Plat.).

Colic: > by hard pressure, or by laying abdomen across knee or on shoulder (Col.); lumbrici; passes worms.

Menses; too early, too profuse; sadness before; pain in malar bones, during.

Leucorrhea; great debility; weakness seems to proceed from chest (from abdomen and pelvis, Phos., Sep.).

Prolapsus, worse during stool (worse with diarrhea, Pod.); *so weak she drops into a chair* instead of sitting down.

While dressing in the morning has to sit down several times to rest.

Nausea and vomiting; in the morning; from the odor of cooking food (Ars., Colch., Sep.).

When singing or using the voice, aching and weakness in deltoid and arms.

Great weakness in chest; < from talking, laughing, reading aloud, singing; **so weak, unable to talk.**

Cough: deep, hollow, shattering, strangling; concussive, in paroxysms of three coughs (of two, Mer.); dry, while in bed, in evening; *empty sensation in chest.*

Expectoration: profuse, like the white of an egg; *sweetish, salty* (Kali i., Sep.); sour, putrid, **musty**; yellow-green pus (heavy, green, salty, Kali i.); during day.

Hoarseness: deep, husky, hollow voice; relieved for the time by coughing or expectorating mucus.

Sweat: mouldy, musty odor; after 4 A. M. every morning; on neck and forehead; very debilitating.

Relations.—Complementary: Pulsatilla.

Aggravation.—Laughing and singing, talking, *using the voice;* lying on right side; *drinking anything warm* (from cold drinks, Spong.).

Amelioration.—Coughing or expectoration relieves hoarseness; hard pressure (Col.).

Type.—Suppressed by Quinine or some anti-periodic; low fever, with bronchial or pulmonary complications.

Time.—10 A. M.; 4-5 P. M.

Chill.—Over whole body at 10 A. M.; with coldness of the hands, deadness of the fingers, and numbness of the finger tips (Paris, Sep.); in the evening over the back; slight, but with chattering of the teeth, as from convulsion of the masseter muscles; only in left arm, or left leg (Carbo v.—right arm, Mercurialis); knees and feet very cold (Carbo v.).

Heat.—From 4-5 P. M., with sweat; of single parts, of back, chest, abdomen, limbs.

Anxious heat, as if sweat would break out.

Burning heat in limbs. Hectic fever.

Sweat.—Profuse after 4 A. M. every morning.

Morning sweat, chiefly on the neck, nape of the neck and forehead; mouldy, musty odor; debilitating from the least movement.

Tongue.—Red; yellow; coated with yellow mucus.

Taste: sour; sweetish; offensive; everything bitter but water. Fetid odor from mouth.

STAPHISAGRIA.

Characteristic.—For the mental effects of onanism and sexual excesses.

Very sensitive to slightest mental impressions; least action or harmless word offends.

Great indignation about things done by others or by himself: grieves about consequences.

Apathetic, indifferent, low-spirited, weak memory from sexual abuses (Anac., Aur., Nat., Phos. ac.).

Ailments from pride, envy or chagrin.

Ill-humored children cry for things which, after receiving, they petulantly push or throw away (Kreos.).

Was insulted; being too dignified to fight subdued his wrath and went home sick, trembling and exhausted (the rev. of, Nux).

Mechanical injuries from sharp-cutting instruments; *post-surgical operations;* stinging, smarting pains, like the cutting of a knife.

For the bad effects of: onanism, sexual excesses, loss of vital fluids; chagrin, mortification, unmerited insults; indignation, with vexation or reserved displeasure (Aur.).

Styes, chalazæ on eyelids or upper lids, one after another *leaving hard nodosities in their wake* (Con., Thuja).

Toothache: *during menses;* sound as well as decayed teeth; painful *to touch of food or drink,* but not from biting or chewing; < drawing cold air into mouth (Ant. c., Mer.); < from cold drinks and after eating.

Extreme hunger even when stomach is full of food.

Teeth are black, show dark streaks through them; cannot be kept clean; crumble; *decay on edges* (at the roots, Mez., Thuja); scorbutic cachexia.

Sensation as if stomach and abdomen were hanging down, relaxed (Agar., Ipec., Tab.). *Craving for tobacco.*

Colic: after lithotomy or ovariotomy; attending abdominal section (Bis., Hep.).

Urging to urinate, has to sit at urinal for hours; in young married women; after coition; after difficult labor (Op.); burning in urethra when *not urinating;* urging and pain *after* urinating in prostatic troubles of old men; prolapse of bladder.

Painful sensitiveness of sexual organs, vulva so sensitive can scarcely wear a napkin (Plat.).

Onanism: persistently dwelling on sexual subjects; constantly thinking of sexual pleasures.

Spermatorrhea: with sunken features; *guilty, abashed look;* emissions followed by backache, weakness; prostration and relaxation or atrophy of sexual organs.

Cough: only in the daytime, or only after dinner, worse after eating meat; after vexation or indignation; excited by cleaning the teeth.

Croupy cough in winter alternating with sciatica in summer; *cough excited by tobacco smoke* (Spong.).

Bachache, < at night in bed, and in the morning before rising.

Arthritic nodosities of joints, especially of the fingers (Caul., Colch., Lyc.); inflammation of phalanges with sweating and suppuration.

Sleepy all day, awake all night; body aches all over.

Fig-warts; dry, pediculated, cauliflower-like; after abuse of mercury (Nit. ac., Sab., Thuja).

Aggravation.—*Mental affections;* from anger, indignation, grief, mortification; loss of fluids; tobacco; onanism; sexual excesses; from the least touch on the affected parts.

Type.—Intermittent, quotidian, tertian; typhoid, typhus, zymotic, yellow.

Time.—9 A. M.; daily, same time; 3 P. M.

Prodrome.—Ravenous hunger for days (see **Cina, Sil.**).

Chill.—Without thirst. **Chill predominates.** *Shaking chill of whole body,* with hot cheeks, cold hands, warm forehead, **without subsequent heat or thirst (Sep., Sul.).** Shivering over whole body, *without thirst* or **subsequent heat.** Chill with goose-flesh about 3 P. M., which was relieved by exercise in open air. Chill ascends from the neck over the head and face, or transient shivering running down the back (transient chills run up the back, **Sul.**). Chill worse in a warm room (**Apis**).

Heat.—With thirst; at night; could not sleep after 3 A. M., with shaking chill at 9 A. M. Great heat at night, especially of the hands and feet, must be uncovered (**Sul.**—external heat is unbearable, **Puls.**). Heat without subsequent sweat. Burning heat at night (**Ars., Sep.**).

Sweat.—Profuse in afternoon, without thirst, but with heat over the whole body (**Nux**). Warm night-sweat on abdomen, feet, genitals. Night-sweat of bad odor, like rotten eggs; with desire to uncover. Sweats when sitting quiet (**Psor.**). *Cold sweat on forehead and feet.*

Pulse.—Very fast, but small and trembling.

Tongue.—White coating; food tastes bitter. Gums white, spongy, ulcerated, bleed when touched.

Apyrexia.—Extreme hunger, even when stomach is filled with food; putrid taste in mouth, gums bleed easily; constipation. Longing for fluid food, soup, bread and milk (longing for eggs, **Cal.**).

STRAMONIUM.

Characteristic.—Adapted to diseases of young plethoric persons (Acon., Bell., Ver. v.); especially children, in chorea; mania, fever, delirium.

Delirium: loquacious, talks all the time, sings, makes verses, raves; simulates Belladonna and Hyoscyamus, yet differs in degree. The delirium is more furious, the mania more acute, while the congestion though greater than Hyoscyamus is much less than Belladonna, never approaching a true inflammatory condition.

Loquacious: disposed to talk continually (Cic., Lach.); incessant and incoherent talking and laughing; **praying, beseeching, entreating**; with suppressed menses.

Convulsions with consciousness (Nux—without, Bell., Cic., Hyos., Op.); renewed by sight of a light, a mirror, or water (Canth., Bell., Lys.).

Desires light and company; *cannot bear to be alone* (Bis.); *worse in the dark and solitude;* cannot walk in a dark room.

Awakens with a shrinking look, as if afraid of the first object seen.

Hallucinations which terrify the patient.

Desire to escape, in delirium (Bell., Bry., Op., Rhus).

Imagines all sorts of things; that she is double, lying crosswise, etc. (Petr.).

Head feels as if scattered about (Bap.).

Eyes wide open, prominent, brilliant; pupils widely dilated, insensible; contortion of eyes and eyelids.

Pupils dilate when child is reprimanded.

Face hot and red with cold hands and feet; circumscribed redness of cheeks, blood rushes to face; risus sardonicus.

Painlessness with most complaints (Op.).

Hydrophobia: fear of water, with excessive aversion to liquids (Bell., Lys.); spasmodic constriction of throat.

Stammering; has to exert himself a long time before he can utter a word; makes great effort to speak; distorts the face (Bov., Ign., Spig.).

Vomiting as soon as *he raises his head from pillow;* from a bright light.

Twitching of single muscles or groups of muscles, especially of upper part of body.

Aggravation.—In the dark; when alone; looking at bright or glistening objects; touch; after sleep (Apis, Lach., Op.); swallowing.

Amelioration.—From company; bright light; warmth.

Type.—Quotidian; double quotidian; typhoid; typhus; yellow.

Time.—6 to 7 A. M. All periods, day or night.

Fever without chill, *noon* and *midnight* (11 A. M. and 11 P. M., **Cac.**).

Chill.—Without thirst. Shaking chill through whole body, with single jerks, partly of whole body or only of single limbs, elbows and knee-joints. Chilliness runs *down* along the back as from cold water (as if dashed with cold water, **Rhus, Sabad.**). *General coldness of the whole body,* with red face (Arn.), hot head, and twitchings of the limbs. *Chills,* with **great sensitiveness to uncovering** (excessively sensitive to cold air, **Camph.**—chill through and through from the slightest uncovering in warm air, **Thuja**). *Skin icy cold, and covered with cold sweat, hands and feet livid* (Ver.). *Face, hands* and *feet* **blue and cold (Camph., Ver.). Coldness of the limbs.** *Hands and feet extremely cold, bluish* and *almost immovable; coldness and paralysis of limbs* (**Nux**—numbness of limbs, **Ced.**).

Heat.—With thirst. Violent fever at noon, returning at midnight (11 A. M., returning at 11 P. M., **Cac.**). Heat of head and face, then coldness of the whole body, then general heat, with anguish; sleeps during heat (**Apis, Ign.**—falls asleep during heat and sweats profusely, **Pod.**). Nausea and vomiting in evening followed by violent, anxious heat. Heat over whole body from least motion (least motion relieves the heat, **Caps.**). Dry, glowing heat over whole body, with redness of head and face, and coldness and paleness of rest of the body (**Bell., Op.**). Skin hot and burning, with sweat at same time (**Sep.**). During heat, pains became violent if he put out a finger from under the cover (chilly, if she puts a limb from under the cover, **Bar., Canth.**). **Covers up closely.** During chill, *heat in head and face;* during the hot stage, *cold feet and legs;* during sweat, *cannot bear to be uncovered. Vertigo; delirium; epileptiform convulsions* (**Hyos.**).

Sweat.—*With thirst* (Ars., Cinch.). Profuse sweat, with burning in the eyes and dim vision. During sweat, good appetite, diarrhea, distention of abdomen, and colic. *Cold sweat over whole body.* Perspiration of forehead and face, *rest of* *body red, dry and hot.* **Oily sweat** (**Phos.**—as if mixed with oil, **Cinch.**).

Tongue.—Clean or whitish coated, with red papillæ; or swollen, dry and difficult to protrude. Juicy fruit tastes dry; *food tastes like straw.*

During fever, in children, they cry out in sleep; start suddenly, twitch and jerk; eyes half open; pupils dilated; urine suppressed.

Stramonium, like Nux, cannot bear to be uncovered in any stage; but not for the same reason. The Nux patient is cold and chilly, if uncovered in the slightest, even cold on moving in bed; while the Stramonium patient is cold, and with the coldness comes immediately violent pain.

SULPHUR.

Characteristic.—Adapted to persons of a scrofulous diathesis, subject to venous congestions, especially of portal system.

Persons of nervous temperament, move quickly, quick tempered, plethoric, skin excessively sensitive to atmospheric changes (Hep., Kali c., Psor.).

For lean, stoop-shouldered persons who walk and sit stooped; walk stooping like old men.

Standing is the worst position for Sulphur patients; they cannot stand; every standing position is uncomfortable.

Dirty, filthy people, prone to skin affections (Psor.).

Aversion to being washed; *always worse after a bath.*

Children: *cannot bear to be washed or bathed* (in cold water, Ant. c.); emaciated, big-bellied; restless, hot, kick off the clothes at night (Hep., Sanic.); have worms, but the best selected remedy fails.

When carefully selected remedies fail to produce a favorable effect, especially in acute diseases, it frequently serves to rouse the reactive powers of the system; clears up the case (in chronic diseases, Psor.).

Scrofulous chronic diseases that arise from suppressed eruptions (Caust., Psor.).

Complaints that are continually relapsing (menses, leucorrhea, etc.); patient seems to get almost well when the disease returns again and again.

Congestions to single parts—eyes, nose, chest, abdomen, ovaries, arms, legs—or any organ of the body marking the onset of tumors or malignant growths, especially at climacteric.

Sensation of burning: on vertex; and smarting in eyes; in face, without redness; of vesicles in mouth; and dryness of throat, first r. then l.; in stomach; in rectum; in anus, and itching piles, and scalding urine; like fire in ripples (Ars.); in chest, rising to face; of skin of whole body, with hot flushes; in spots, between scapulæ (Phos.).

Sick headache every week or every two weeks; prostrating, weakening (Sang.); with hot vertex and cold feet.

Constant heat on vertex; cold feet in daytime, *with burning soles at night,* wants to find a cool place for them (Sang., Sanic.); puts them out of bed to cool them off (Med.); cramps in calves and soles at night.

Hot flushes during the day, with weak, faint spells, passing off with a little moisture.

Bright redness of lips as if the blood would burst through.

Weak, empty, gone or faint feeling in the stomach about 11 A. M. (10 or 11 A. M. > by eating, Nat. c.); cannot wait for lunch; frequent weak, faint spells during the day.

Diarrhea: after midnight; painless; **driving out of bed early in the morning** (Aloe, Psor.); as if the bowels were too weak to retain their contents.

Constipation: stools hard, knotty, dry as if burnt (Bry.); **large, painful,** *child is afraid to have the stool on account of* *pain,* or pain compels child to desist on first effort; alternating with diarrhea.

The discharge, both of urine and feces, is *painful to parts over which it passes;* passes large quantities of colorless urine; **parts around anus red, excoriated**; *all the orifices* of the body are *very red;* all discharges acrid, excoriating wherever they touch.

Menses: too early, profuse, protracted.

Menorrhagia, has not been well since her last miscarriage. "A single dose at new moon."—LIPPE.

Boils: coming in crops in various parts of the body; or a single boil is succeeded by another as soon as first is healed (Tub.).

Skin: itching, voluptuous; scratching >; "feels good to scratch;" scratching causes burning; < from heat of bed (Mer.); soreness in folds (Lyc., San.).

Skin affections that have been treated by medicated soaps and washes; hemorrhoids, that have been treated with ointments.

To facilitate absorption of serous or inflammatory exudates in brain, pleura, lungs, joints, when Bryonia, Kali mur. or the best selected remedy fails.

Chronic alcoholism; dropsy and other ailments of drunkards; "they reform," but are continually relapsing (Psor., Tub.).

Nightly suffocative attacks, wants the doors and windows open; becomes suddenly wide awake at night; drowsy in afternoon after sunset, wakefulness the whole night.

Happy dreams, wakes up singing.

Everything looks pretty which the patient takes a fancy to.

Movements in abdomen as of a child (Croc., Thuja).

Relations.—Complementary: Aloe, Psor.

Ailments from the abuse of metals generally.

Sulph., Calc., Lyc.; or Sulph., Sars. and Sep. frequently follow in given order.

Calcarea must not be used before Sulphur.

Sulphur is the chronic of Aconite and follows it well in pneumonia and other acute diseases.

Aggravation.—At rest; *when standing; warmth in bed;* washing, bathing; changeable weather.

Amelioration.—Dry, warm weather; lying on the right side (Stan.).

Type.—Quotidian; double quotidian; tertian. In regular paroxysms. Yearly (Ars., Carbo v., Lach., Nat., Psor., Thuja). Typhoid, typhus, bilious, yellow; fever of every kind and every type.

Time.—Not characteristic; at all periods. Morning; afternoon; evening; night. Evening predominant; 8, 9, 10 A. M., 12 M.; 1, 2, 5, 6, 7, 8, 9, 11 and 12 P. M.

Prodrome.—Evening fever without chill. *Thirst* (**Caps., Eup., Puls.**—but *can only drink* in prodrome and apyrexia, **Cimex**).

Chill.—Without thirst. **Frequent internal chilliness.** *Chilliness, with headache in the evening* (**Sep.**), disappearing after lying down. Aching in forehead with restlessness, relieved when sweat comes on. *Chilliness and shivering over whole body,* **without subsequent heat or thirst (Bov.).** **Chilliness and rigor, with blue nails, pale face, heavy, giddy head, not relieved by heat of stove, but by lying down.** **Chilly in open air, as if naked.** Shivering on slightest movement in bed (**Nux, Stram.**). Coldness transient, of the *nose, hands, feet, chest, arms, back, abdomen.* **Chilliness in the back,** *in the evening for an hour, without subsequent heat.* **Chilliness constantly creeps from the sacrum up the back, without subsequent heat or thirst,** sometimes relieved by warmth of stove. **Icy coldness of the genitals.** Coldness through all the limbs. Hands and feet very cold, with livid, pale face. **Shaking chill for an hour in the P. M., with blue face and cold hands and feet; subsequent heat and perspiration (Ars., Bell.,**

Rhus). Headache, vertigo, delirium. Chill begins in hands, fingers, feet and toes (**Carbo v., Nat., Sep.**).

Heat.—With thirst. *Frequent flushes of heat in the face, with shivering sensation over the body* (**Sep.**). **Burning heat of the palms of the hands and soles of the feet**; or *cold feet, with hot, burning soles; was obliged to put them out of bed to find a cool place.* Heat and redness of face, with burning in single parts, as on malar bones, around the eyes, ears, nose, mouth. **Orgasm of the blood, and violent burning of the hands.** Alternate heat (of body and face) with chilliness (**Ars., Cal.**). *Frequent flushes of heat, ending in moisture and faintness.* **Intense, persistent, long-continued fever; skin dry, hot, burning; temperature 103-105, little or no remission, day or night, patient literally being consumed with fever.**

Sweat.—*Copious morning-sweat, setting in after waking* (sweat while awake, dry heat when sleeping, **Samb.**). **At night profuse sweat all over the body and restless sleep** (sweat all night without relief, **Kali c.**). Profuse sweat on occiput. *Perspiration on slightest motion* or *manual labor* (**Bry.**—sweat on least exertion or every mental effort, **Sep.**). *Profuse sweat* when **walking,** *reading, riding, writing, talking. Profuse sour night-sweat,* of a sour, burnt odor (**Lyc.**); vomiting; morning diarrhea; tenesmus.

Tongue.—Coated white or yellow, which wears off during the day, and becomes red and clean in evening. Bitter taste in mouth in morning; food tastes natural. Longing for sweets, beer, brandy. Aversion to meat. Milk disagrees, causes sour taste, sour eructations.

Apyrexia.—Great prostration after every paroxysm (**Ars.**), with thirst for beer. Burning heat on vertex. Early morning diarrhea. Feels as if he was just convalescing from a severe illness.

Sulphur bears the same relation to chronic cases that Ipecacuanha does to acute, viz.: if the indications for the remedy be not clear and well defined, *Sulphur may clear up the case, or completely cure it alone.* Intermittent fever is a terrible searcher after weak organs; and Sulphur is frequently required in all forms of the disease—acute and early, or chronic and later—to combat some latent malady aroused during the course of the fever. If we would use Sulphur more and Quinine less, our success would be much more satisfactory, both to our patients and ourselves.

"The antiperiodic virtue of Sulphur does not apply simply to pyrexial intermittents, but it also comprehends intermittent neuralgias, which consist of attacks of pain on the right side of the face and head, which begins at the maxillaries and finally extends along the orbital nerves, and thence involves the whole side of the head, there being no dental caries. The pains begin toward evening, last three to four hours, then cease, reappear later, and again cease up to the hour of attack in the evening. Psoric subjects; after the suppression of an exanthem: after the abuse of Quinine."—A. CHARGE, M. D.

Sulphur worn next the skin, in the form of flowers of Sulphur, is an effective antidote to the malarial poison which is supposed to produce intermittent fever, typhus and diphtheria, as well as cholera.*

---

*"Just as the milk of Sulphur applied to the skin (worn in the stockings) is the best preventive of cholera, so Carbo v. is the best preventive of yellow fever."—HERING.

"In Memphis, in 1873, charcoal came much into favor as a prophylactic; out of more than fifty persons who took it and were constantly exposed to the fever not one was attacked; the usual dose was half a teaspoonful of the crude powder, two or three times a day."—DR. MORSE.

SULPHURIC ACID.

Characteristic.—Adapted to the light-haired; old people, especially women; flushes of heat in climacteric years.

Unwilling to answer questions not from obstinacy, but inaptness.

Feels in a great hurry; everything must be done quickly (Arg. n.).

Pain of gradual and slowly-increasing intensity which ceases suddenly when at its height, often repeated (Puls.).

The pain is pressure as of a blunt instrument. Tendency to gangrene following mechanical injuries, especially of old people.

Child has a sour odor despite careful washing (Hep., Mag. c., Rheum).

Sensation as if the brain was loose in forehead and falling from side to side (Bell., Bry., Rhus, Spig.).

Aphthæ; of mouth, gums, or entire buccal cavity; gums bleed readily; ulcers painful; offensive breath (Bor.).

Chronic heartburn, *sour eructations, sets teeth on edge* (Rob.).

Water drunk causes coldness of the stomach unless mixed with alcoholic liquor.

Sensation as if trembling all over, without real trembling; internal trembling of drunkards.

Bad effects from mechanical injuries, with bruises, chafing and livid skin; prostration (Acet. ac.).

Ecchymosis; cicatrices turn blood-red or blue, are painful (turn green, Led.).

Petechia: purpura hemorrhagica; blue spots; livid, red itching blotches.

Hemorrhage of black blood from all the outlets of the body (Crot., Mur. ac., Nit. ac.).

Concussion of brain from fall or blow where skin is cold and body bathed in cold sweat.

Weak and exhausted from some deep-seated dyscrasia; no other symptoms (Psor., Sulph.).

Relations.—Complementary: Puls.

In contusion and laceration of soft parts it vies with Calendula.

Follows well: after, Arn. with bruised pain, livid skin and profuse sweat; after, Led. in ecchymosis.

Ailments, from brandy drinking.

Type.—Pernicious, malarial, putrid, typhoid, typhus, septic, yellow, zymotic; regular periods.

Time.—Not characteristic; evening most marked.

Chill.—With thirst; frequent during the day; running downward; < in the room, > in open air when exercising. Shivering, in paroxysms; shaking chill over whole body; pains in back and loins. Attacks begin with coldness and trembling, then general vigor.

Heat.—With thirst; in evening and in bed; after cold shivers gets warm and perspires.

Fever with great disposition to hemorrhage from capillaries and rapid sinking of the vital forces; oozing of dark, liquid blood; face deathly pale; tendency to collapse and gangrene. Black vomit of yellow fever. Flushes of heat (Lach., Sulph.). Urine involuntary.

Sweat.—With thirst; profuse mostly on upper part of the body; sour; cold, soon after eating warm food; mornings; at night, > by drinking wine; with great debility. Nose-bleed.

TARAXACUM.

Characteristic.—For gastric and bilious attacks, especially gastric headaches.

Mapped tongue (Lach., Mer., Nat.); covered with a white film with sensation of rawness. This film comes off *in patches,* leaving dark red, tender, *very sensitive spots* (Ran. s.).

Jaundice with enlargement and induration of liver (mapped tongue).

Debility, loss of appetite, *profuse night sweats,* especially when convalescing from bilious or typhoid fever.

Restlessness of and pain in thighs and limbs in typhoid and typho-malarial fevers (Rhus, Zinc.).

Relations.—Compare: Bry., Chel., Hydr., Nux, in gastric and bilious affections.

Aggravation.—Almost all symptoms appear when sitting; lying down; resting.

Type.—Malarial, typho-malarial and typhoid; when attack develops into a slow fever, in dry, nervous, bilious subjects. Periodicity not marked.

Time.—8 P. M.; at night, with gastric ailments.

Chill.—Great chilliness after eating, and especially after drinking (Bell., Caps., Kali c., Lob., Marum). Long-lasting chill; when he falls asleep, sweat breaks out, mostly on the head. Nose, hands and tips of fingers are icy cold (Sabad., Stan.).

Heat.—Sensation of heat, and heat in face, with redness (Lach.).

Sweat.—With thirst; *copious;* at night; with pain in spleen; all over body on falling asleep in the evening (Cinch.); *debilitating night-sweats,* causing biting of the skin.

Analysis.—The *abundant, debilitating, night-sweat* is the guiding symptom of Taraxacum. It occurs invariably at night, and differs from Cinchona, that while the latter, though profuse and debilitating, occurs during sleep or when covered. The tongue and gastric symptoms also serve to differentiate.

TARENTULA.

Characteristic.—Adapted to highly nervous organisms, especially choreic affections where whole body, or right arm and left leg are affected (of l. arm and r. leg, Agar.).

Constant movement of the legs, arms, trunk, with inability to do anything; twitching and jerking of muscles.

Restlessness, *could not keep quiet in any position;* must keep in motion, *though walking < all symptoms* (rev. of Rhus, Ruta).

Hyperesthesia: least excitement irritates, followed by languid sadness; **extreme, of tips of fingers.**

Slight touch along the spine provokes spasmodic pain in chest and cardiac region.

Headache; intense, as if thousands of needles were pricking in the brain.

Abscesses, boils, felons, affected parts of *a bluish color* (Lach.), and *atrocious burning pain* (Anth., Ars., Euphor.); the *agony of a felon,* compelling patient to walk the floor for nights.

Malignant ulcers; carbuncle, anthrax; gangrene.

Symptoms appear periodically.

Headache, neuralgic < by *noise, touch, stronger light,* > by pressure and rubbing head against the pillow.

At every menstrual nisus, throat, mouth and tongue intolerably dry, especially when sleeping (Nux m.).

Sexual excitement extreme even to mania; spasms of uterus; pruritus vulva becomes intolerable.

Relations.—Similar: to, Apis, Crot., Lach., Plat., Mygale, Naja, Ther.

Aggravation.—Motion; *contact;* **touch of affected parts;** noise; change of weather.

Amelioration.—In open air; music; *rubbing affected parts.*

Termini of nerves became so irritated and sensitive that some kind of friction was necessary to obtain relief.

Type.—Intermittent, remittent, nervous typhoid, toxemic, septic; fevers of tropics.

Prodrome.—Constant pain in hepatic region, with nausea and vomiting.

Chill.—Predominant cold stage. Constant coldness for days. Intense coldness, with shaking; blueness of nails and fingers (Nux); lasting two or three hours.

Chills and fever with choreic convulsions; shakes almost constantly with involuntary movements of limbs, abdomen, chest, face < l. side; could not speak, tongue and pharynx involved; after a severe scolding or punishment (Ign.).

Heat.—*Without thirst.* Scorching intense heat of whole body alternating with icy coldness; skin of a scarlet color; during heat continued *coldness of feet;* great dryness of mouth, no thirst (Nux m., Puls.); lasted five or six hours, lies in a comatose condition with eyes closed.

Sweat.—Profuse for three or four hours, followed by debility and prostration.

Tongue.—Coated yellowish; loss of appetite; dry mouth.

Apyrexia.—General emaciation, especially of face; skin yellow, jaundiced; marked hepatic derangement for months preceding attack.

Analysis.—*Choreic, hysterical, nervous subjects.* Predominant coldness; scorching heat, with dry mouth, without thirst; comatose condition or convulsions. Hepatic pain, nausea and vomiting generally precede attack in chronic cases.

TEREBINTH.

Characteristic.—For the hemorrhagic diathesis; "bleeders." Complaints of old people; sedentary habit; from living in basements and damp dwellings.

Abdomen: extremely sensitive to touch; distention, flatulence, *excessive tympanitis;* meteorism (Colch.).

Diarrhea: stool, watery, greenish, mucous; *frequent, profuse, fetid, bloody; burning* in anus and rectum, *fainting* and *exhaustion,* after (Ars.).

Worms: with foul breath, choking (Cina, Spig.); dry hacking cough; tickling at anus; ascarides, lumbrici, tapeworm segments passed.

Hematuria: blood, *thoroughly mixed with urine;* sediment, like coffee-grounds; *cloudy, smoky, albuminous; profuse, dark or black, painless.*

Congestion and inflammation of viscera; kidneys, bladder, lungs, intestines, uterus; with hemorrhage, and malignant tendency.

Purpura hemorrhagica; fresh ecchymoses in great numbers from day to day (Sulph. ac.).

Hemorrhages: *from bowels,* with ulceration; passive, dark with epithelial degeneration.

Ascites anascarca, in organic lesions of kidneys; dropsy after scarlatina (Apis, Hell., Lach.).

The urine has the odor of violets.

Violent burning and drawing pains in kidney, bladder and urethra (Berb., Can., Canth.).

Violent burning and cutting in bladder; tenesmus; sensitive hypogastrium; cystitis and retention from atony of fundus.

Albuminuria: acute, in early stages, when blood and albumin abound more than casts and epithelium; after diphtheria, scarlatina, typhoid.

Urine rich in albumin and blood, but few if any casts; < from living in damp dwellings.

Strangury; spasmodic retention of urine.

Relations.—Compare: Alumen, Arn., Ars., Canth., Lach., Nit. ac.

Is recommended as a prophylactic in malarial and African fevers.

Type.—Malarial; *tropical;* **African fevers**; toxemic; septic; typhoid; typhus; yellow; tend to a low malignant type, with hemorrhage.

Chill.—Violent, cold limbs, body hot; great coldness with restless tossing about; rigors, followed by heat through whole body.

Coldness and chill in abdomen.

Irregular chills and flushes of heat.

Heat.—With great thirst; red face; skin and mucous membranes hot and dry; pulse hard and frequent.

Stupor, muttering delirium; subsultus tendinum; pupils contracted; meteorisms and excessive tympanitis; copious hemorrhage, black, fluid, from nose, stomach, kidneys, lungs, bowels, with ulceration of Peyer's patches; great prostration and emaciation.

Sweat.—Profuse, with great prostration; cold, clammy, over whole body.

Tongue.—Smooth, glossy, red, as if deprived of papillæ, or as if glazed (Pyr.); elevated papillæ; coating peels off in patches, leaving bright red spots, or entire coating cleans off suddenly (in exanthemata); dry and red; burning in tip (compare, Mur. ac.).

Pulse.—Irregular, intermitting, with great weakness; small, wiry, thready, scarcely perceptible; feeble and slow in diarrhea.

THUJA OCCIDENTALIS.

Characteristic.—Adapted to the hydrogenoid constitution of Grauvogl, related to sycosis as effect is to cause. It possesses a capacity to contain water; hence rain, cold, damp weather, baths, and food that increases the amount of water in the system < the symptoms of the hydrogenoid constitution.

Thuja bears the same relation to the sycosis of Hahnemann —figwarts, condylomata and wart-like excrescences upon mucous and cutaneous surfaces—that Sulphur does to psora or Mercury to syphilis.

Acts well in lymphatic temperament, in very fleshy persons, dark complexion, black hair, unhealthy skin.

Ailments: from bad effects of vaccination (Ant. t., Sil.); from suppressed or maltreated gonorrhea (Med.).

Fixed ideas: as if a strange person were at his side; as if soul and body were separated; as if a living animal were in abdomen; of being under the influence of superior power.

Insane women will not be touched or approached.

Vertigo, when *closing the eyes* (Lach., Ther.).

Headache: as if a nail had been driven into parietal bone (Coff., Ign.); or as if a convex button were pressed on the part; < from sexual excesses; overheating; from tea (Sel.); chronic, of sycotic or syphilitic origin.

White scaly dandruff; hair dry and falling out.

Eyes: ophthalmia neonatorum, sycotic or syphilitic; *large granulations, like warts or blisters;* > by warmth and covering; if uncovered, feels as if a cold stream of air were blowing out through them.

Eyelids: agglutinated at night; dry, scaly on edges; styes and tarsal tumors; chalazæ, thick, hard knots, like small condylomata; after Staphisagria partially > but does not cure.

Ears: chronic otitis; discharge purulent, like putrid meat; granulations, condylomata; **polypi,** *pale red, cellular, bleeding easily.*

Teeth decay at the roots, crowns remain sound (Mez.—on edges, Staph.); crumble, turn yellow (Syph.).

Toothache from tea drinking.

Abdomen: as if an animal were crying; motion as of something alive; protrudes here and there like the arm of a fetus (Croc., Nux m.).

Distressing, burning pain in left ovarian region when walking or riding, must sit or lie down (Croc., Ust.); worse at each menstrual nisus.

Constipation: violent pains in rectum compel cessation of effort; stool *recedes, after being partly expelled* (Sanic., Sil.).

Piles swollen, pain *most severe when sitting.*

Diarrhea: early morning; expelled forcibly with much flatus (Aloe); *gurgling, as water from a bunghole;* < after breakfast, coffee, fat food, onions, vaccination.

Anus fissured, painful to touch, surrounded with flat warts, or moist mucous condylomata.

Coition prevented by extreme sensitiveness of the vagina (by dryness, Lyc., Lys., Natr.).

Skin: looks dirty; brown or brownish, white spots here and there; *warts, large, seedy, pedunculated* (Staph.); eruptions only on covered parts, burn after scratching.

Flesh feels as if beaten from the bones (Phyt.—as if bones were scraped, Rhus).

Sensation after urinating, as of urine trickling in urethra; severe cutting *at close of urination* (Sars.).

When walking the limbs feel as if made of wood.

Sensation as if the body, especially the limbs, **were made of glass and would break easily.**

Suppressed gonorrhea: causing articular rheumatism; prostatitis; sycosis; impotence; condylomata, and many constitutional troubles.

Nails: deformed, brittle (Ant. c., Med., Sil.).

Relations.—Complementary: Med., Sab., Sil.

Cinnab. is preferable for warts on the prepuce.

Follows well: after, Med., Mer., Nit. ac.

Aggravation.—At night; from heat of bed; at 3 A. M. and 3 P. M.; from cold, damp air; narcotics.

Type.—Quotidian, same time every day. Yearly; remittent (Carbo v., Lach., Psor., Tub., Sul.).

Time.—3 A. M., characteristic; 10 *A. M.*, 3 *P. M.*, 5, 6, 7, 7.30 *P. M.* After midnight.

Fever without chill 10 to 11 A. M., or 10 to 11 P. M. (Cac.—12 M. and 12 P. M., Sul.).

Cause.—The indication is more certain if the system be contaminated with sycotic or gonorrheal poison. Always chilly from least change of weather.

Prodrome.—Chilly and weak some time before the paroxysm.

Chill.—With thirst. **Chill beginning in the thighs.** *Violent shaking chill, for a quarter of an hour, about 3 A. M.*, followed by thirst, then profuse perspiration all over except on the head. *Shaking chill, with much yawning; warm air seems cold* and the *hot sun does not warm him.* **Shivering through and through, from the slightest uncovering of the body in warm air** (shivering from the slightest contact with the open air, **Nux**—great aversion to cold air, **Camph.**—chill as soon as he gets out of bed, **Canth.**). Chilliness every evening from 6 to 7.30, with excessive heat of the body, dryness of the mouth, and thirst. Chill of *left side of the body,* which felt cold to the touch (**Carbo v., Caust., Lyc.**). About 7 P. M., *shaking chill, beginning in thighs,* with *blueness of nails, chattering of teeth, rapid* and *difficult respiration,* for half an hour; then *thighs hot, like a glowing coal,* with *cold hands and feet;* gradually became warm, though had a shaking chill *every time he moved* (**Nux**); fell asleep after two hours, and awoke in a profuse perspiration—had to change his shirt eight times up to 3 A. M.—with headache, mild delirium and some thirst. Morning headache, chill at 10 A. M., lasting till noon, followed by heat, nausea, *constant one-sided headache,* and repeated bilious vomiting and diarrhea in the evening. Chill internal, with external heat and violent thirst (chill, then sweat, **Ant. t.**).

Heat.—*With thirst, neither preceded nor followed by chilliness. Sensation of burning heat in the face,* which causes neither *real heat, redness* nor *perspiration, with icy cold hands. Burning heat only in the face and cheeks, lasting the whole day* (**Bell., Cal.**). Dry heat of covered parts. Heat mornings, chill afternoons. *Deadness of fingers* (**Ced., Sep.**).

Sweat.—Only on uncovered parts; or **all over, except the head** (reverse of Sil.). Sweat, *when he sleeps, stops when he awakens* (reverse of **Samb.**). *Chill, then sweat* (**Ant. t., Ipec.**). *Profuse night-sweat, staining the clothes yellow,* as if **saturated with oil** (**Bell.**—as if mixed with oil, **Cinch.**). *Sour-smelling or fetid sweat almost every night* (**Arn., Lyc., Nat.**). *Scrotum, perineum* and *inner surface of the thighs* dripping with sweat (**Hep., Petr.**). Profuse night-sweat, so that he changes his shirt several times at night. Sweat on side not lain on (Benz., San.). *Congestion of blood to the head.*

Pulse.—Full and accelerated in the evening; slow and weak in the morning; throbbing in blood vessels; swelling of the veins.

Tongue.—*Swollen, clean or red, the tip is painfully sore to the touch.* Vesicles or blisters on the margin. Bitter, sour, taste; had to get up at night and rinse out the mouth (**Nux**). Ranula; bluish, or varicose veins on tongue or in mouth (Amb.).

Thuja helped in some cases, where the fever consisted in mere chills, with external and internal coldness (with thirst in same), followed by general sweat, without any previous heat.

CLINICAL.

Andrew Mc———, æt. 26, a resident of East Saginaw, Michigan. Eight years ago had intermittent fever, which was "broke up" with massive doses of *Quinine,* only to return from time to time, especially every Spring and Autumn, to be again suppressed in a similar manner with *Quinine.* When fever first appeared, paroxysm came every alternate day, at 10 to 11

A. M., attended with bone pains, violent headache, and at times nausea and vomiting.

February, 1882.—Has now had chills and fever every day for seven weeks. Chill from 5 to 7 P. M.; severe, shaking; must sit close to stove, although external heat does not relieve. Chill begins in *knees and thighs,* and gradually extends to hips, thence over body, lasting one to two hours. Some thirst in chill, but drinking aggravates. Heat, with thirst; drinking refreshes; continues until 1 or 2 A. M.; very restless, severe headache. Sweats: profusely on his legs, where chill began; less on his body; never on his head; when he sleeps, ceases when he wakes. Tongue clean; appetite and digestion good, and feels perfectly well as soon as paroxysm is over. The chill beginning in *knees* and *thighs,* the *time* of its appearance, the *character of the sweating stage,* and the entire freedom from ill-feeling during apyrexia, determined the selection of Thuja[30], four doses during intermission. Cured.—H. C. ALLEN, *Medical Advance,* XII., p. 296.

TUBERCULINUM.

Characteristic.—Adapted to persons of light complexion; blue eyes, blonde in preference to brunette; tall, slim; flat, narrow chest; active and precocious mentally, weak physically; the tubercular diathesis.

When with a family history of tubercular affections *the best selected remedy fails to relieve or permanently improve,* without reference to name of disease.

Symptoms ever changing; ailments affecting one organ, then another—the lungs, brain, kidneys, liver, stomach, nervous system—beginning suddenly, ceasing suddenly.

Takes cold easily without knowing how or where; seems to take cold "every time he takes a breath of fresh air" (Hep.).

Emaciation rapid and pronounced; losing flesh while eating well (Abrot., Cal., Con., Iod., Nat.).

Melancholy, despondent; morose, irritable, fretful, peevish; taciturn, sulky; naturally of a sweet disposition, now on the borderland of insanity.

Everything in the room seemed strange as though in a strange place.

Headache: chronic, tubercular; pain intense, sharp, cutting, from above right eye to occiput; as of an iron hoop around the head (Anac., Cac.); when the best selected remedy only palliates.

School-girl's headache; < by study or even slight mental exertion; when using eyes in close work and glasses fail to >; with a tubercular history.

Acute cerebral or basilar meningitis, with threatened effusion; nocturnal hallucinations; wakes from sleep frightened, screams; when Apis, Hell., or Sulph., though well selected, fail to improve.

Crops of small boils, intensely painful, successively appear in the nose; *green, fetid pus* (Sec.).

Plica polonica; several bad cases permanently cured after Bor. and Psor. failed.

Diarrhea: early morning, sudden, imperative (Sulph.); emaciating though eating well (Iod., Nat.); stool dark brown, watery, offensive; discharged with great force; great weakness and profuse night sweats.

Menses: too early; too profuse; too long lasting; tardy in starting; with frightful dysmenorrhea; in patients with a tuberculous history.

Eczema: tubercular, over entire body; itching intense < at night when undressing, or from bathing; immense quantities of white bran-like scales; oozing behind the ears, in the hair, in the folds of the skin with a rawness and soreness; fiery red skin. Ringworms.

Tubercular deposit begins in apex of lungs, usually the left (Phos., Sulph., Ther.).

Relations.—Complementary: Psor., Sulph.

When Psor., Sulph., or the best selected remedy fails to relieve or permanently improve.

Belladonna, for acute attacks, congestive or inflammatory, occurring in tubercular diseases.

Hydrastis to fatten patients cured with Tuberculinum.

VALERIANA.

Characteristic.—For nervous, irritable, hysterical subjects, in whom the intellectual faculties predominate and who suffer from hysterical neuralgia of the limbs; changeable disposition.

Mental confusion; replies incoherently (Arn., Bap.).

Delirium: hallucinations; sees figures, animals, men; delusions, thinks she is someone else, moves to edge of bed to make room; imagines animals lying near her which she fears she may hurt.

Great nervous excitement and trembling.

Red parts become white (Fer.).

Feels light as if floating in the air (Asar., Lac c.—as if legs were floating, Stic.).

Oversensitiveness of all the senses (Cham., Cof., Nux).

Sensation: of coldness in head (on vertex, Sep., Ver.); as if a thread were hanging down throat (on tongue, Nat., Sil.).

Child vomits: *curdled milk in large lumps;* same in stools (Eth.); *as soon as it has nursed, after anger of mother.*

Sciatica: pain < **when standing** and letting foot rest on floor (Bell.); in straightening out limb, during rest from previous exertion; > when walking.

Type.—Continued; typhoid, especially nervous typhoid.

Chill.—Short; *with thirst;* begins in neck and runs down back (heat begins in neck and runs down the back, Paris); with fainting during chill (during heat, Acon.).

Heat.—Long-lasting, severe, *with thirst* and dull headache; with restlessness and neuralgia of the limbs; indigestion; often with sweat on the face. In evening; spells of fugitive heat; after eating; with thirst. Hot stage predominates.

Sweat.—Profuse, < at night, but not debilitating; from exertion, with *violent heat;* on face with heat; often attended with or followed by heat; frequent, suddenly ceasing. Better after sweat.

VERATRUM ALBUM.

Characteristic.—Adapted to diseases with **rapid sinking of the vital forces; complete prostration; collapse.**

Cold perspiration on the forehead (over the entire body, Tab.), with nearly all complaints.

Cannot bear to be left alone; yet persistently refuses to talk.

Thinks she is pregnant or will soon be delivered.

Mania with desire to cut and tear everything, especially clothes (Tar.); with lewd, lascivious talk, amorous or religious (Hyos., Mel., Stram.).

Attacks of fainting from least exertion (Carbo v., Sulph.); excessive weakness.

Sinking feeling during hemorrhage (fainting, Trill.).

Sensation of *a lump of ice on vertex,* with chilliness (Sep., Val.); as of heat and cold at same time on scalp; as if brain were torn to pieces.

Face: pale, blue collapsed; features sunken, hippocratic; red while lying, becomes pale on rising (Acon.).

Thirst: intense, unquenchable, for large quantities of very cold water and acid drinks; wants everything cold.

Craving for *acids or refreshing things* (Phos. ac.).

Icy coldness: of face, tip of nose, feet, legs, hands, arms, and many other parts.

Cold feeling in abdomen (Colch., Tab.).

Violent vomiting with profuse diarrhea.

Vomiting: excessive with nausea and great prostration; < by drinking (Ars.); < by least motion (Tab.); great weakness after.

Cutting pain in abdomen as from knives.

Cholera: vomiting and purging; stool, profuse, watery, gushing, prostrating; after fright (Acon., Op.).

Constipation: no desire; stool large, hard (Bry., Sulph.);

in round, black balls (Chel., Op., Plb.); from inactive rectum; frequent desire felt in epigastrium (Ign.—in rectum, Nux); painful, of infants and children, after Lyc. and Nux.

Dysmenorrhea; with vomiting and purging, or exhausting diarrhea with cold sweat (Amm. c., Bov.); is so weak can scarcely stand for two days at each menstrual nisus (Alum., Carbo an., Coc.).

Bad effects of opium eating, tobacco chewing.

Pains in the limbs during wet weather, getting worse from warmth of bed, better from continued walking.

Aggravation.—From least motion; after drinking; before and during menses; during stool; when perspiring; after fright.

Type.—Quotidian; tertian; quartan. Congestive; pernicious; sinking. Yellow fever. Periodicity strongly marked.

Time.—6 *A. M.* **Characteristic—certain.** Fevers of nursing children; coldness predominates.

Prodrome.—Sweat often marks the commencement of paroxysm (Nux).

Cause.—Choleraic. Intermittents occurring during cholera epidemics. Often the genus epidemicus.

Chill.—*With thirst.* Daily chill, with violent shaking, vertigo, delirium, nausea, paleness of the face, and spasms. *Severe, long-lasting, congestive chill, not relieved by external warmth* (**Aran., Camph.**). **Chill, with coldness and thirst,** for half an hour, *without subsequent heat,* with great weakness of thighs and limbs (every other day). **Internal chilliness running from the head to the toes of both feet, with thirst.** Shaking chill, with sweat, at first warm, but soon passes off into general coldness. *Coldness of the whole body, increased by drinking* (**Ars., Caps., Eup., Nux**); *lessened* by getting out of bed (increased by even putting hands from under bedclothes, **Bar., Canth.**). Coldness at times; heat, with profuse sweat at others. *Chill and heat alternating on single parts,* now here, then there (**Puls.**). Great coldness over the back and through shoulders into arms. **Face cold, collapsed. Extremities cold.** Coldness in limbs, shoulders and arms, as if cold air were *streaming through the bones. Skin cold and clammy.* Vomiting and diarrhea (nausea, vomiting and purging, **Elat.**). **Prominent external coldness.** Coldness of the feet, *as if cold water were running into them.*

Heat.—With thirst, mostly internal; with no desire to drink, or continued thirst for cold drinks, the beverages are never cold enough. Heat ascends from extremities to head (chill descends). Heat streaming up the back into the occiput (chill running in successive waves from sacrum to occiput, **Gels.**). Head hot, dull, confused; first *warm,* then **persistent cold sweat on the forehead.** *Redness and heat of the face; burning* and *redness in the cheeks,* with contracted pupils and cold feet (**Op.**—with dilated pupils, **Bell.**). Blood runs cold through the veins (**Rhus**—runs hot, **Ars.**).

Sweat.—*Without thirst,* which is *profuse, cold* and clammy (profuse sweat, *with thirst,* **Ars., Cinch.**). **Sweat always with deathly pale face**; *offensive, bitter smelling, staining yellow. Easily perspires on every motion* (**Bry., Hep.**). **Cold sweat on forehead; after every stool; after vomiting of mucus.** Sweat often begins before the chill and continues through paroxysm until next chill.

Tongue.—Coated white or yellowish-brown; **cold,** *red tip and edges; swollen.* Voracious appetite. *Craves cold fruits, ice water, juicy food, wants everything cold.* Aversion to warm things. Hunger and appetite between paroxysms of vomiting.

Pulse.—Small, weak, slow, and growing continually weaker, often imperceptible. Blood runs like cold water through the vessels.

Apyrexia.—There is great general exhaustion and rapid sinking of strength; oppression of the chest; deep sighing; face pale and cold, *with cold sweat on forehead.* The heart's impulse very weak in the intermission, as well as during the paroxysm; fainting; there are cramps in the stomach, abdomen and limbs; great thirst if much vomiting and diarrhea, and *vice versa;* extremities persistently cold. Skin bluish, cold, inelastic, with deficient reaction.

We may require to compare Elaterium with Veratrum which it resembles in the suddenness of its onset, the profuseness of its evacuations, and its great prostration. But the characteristic predominance of the cold stage will serve to distinguish between them.

Like Camphor, the cold stage is so well marked that it overshadows all the others; the hot stage is light or often wanting altogether. When the hot stage is present the temperature is rarely elevated, and is often diminished during heat. There is such a general lack of vital heat, and slow, defective reaction, that the patient scarcely recovers from one paroxysm ere another begins. The temperature is generally subnormal.

The above makes one of our best pictures of the "sinking," "congestive," or "pernicious" forms of intermittent fever. The patient thinks he will die; and the physician shares his fears. The allopath now resorts to stimulants for the present; and Quinine to prevent the return of future paroxysm. Shall we, on that threadbare plea of psuedo-homeopaths, that "there is no time for homeopathic remedies to act," follow his example? Those are not lacking "in faith," but *in knowledge,* who "desert their colors under fire." The homeopath who knows his Materia Medica will *cure such cases* without resorting to "rational" (?) uncertainty. If he does not know his Materia Medica, he is justified in resorting to anything to try to save his patient; but the treatment should go by its right name, and the failure to cure should be properly credited. Every homeopath is responsible *for not knowing* what he professes to practice.

"Among the great number of intermittent fevers there is a formidable pyrexia called *pernicious,* because it may carry off the patient in the second or third paroxysm; he dies probably from the excess of poisoning. This extremely violent pyrexia forms no exception to the rule; and, like all other pyrexiæ, finds its most prompt and certain remedy in the drug which is most homeopathic to it. But here a delicate question arises which should be solved at once: What shall we do in the presence of a pernicious fever in which we have reason to fear sudden death, in the second or third paroxysm? Find the homeopathic remedy. Without doubt, principles are inflexible, and I know no means more powerful to combat the radicalism of the false than to oppose to it the radicalism of the true.

"We have a law of cure which has always shown itself triumphant when rigorously applied. Why should we be unfaithful to it? I see no reason. The violence of the disease? But the more urgent the haste, the more highly ought we to value the shortest road. Now the most prompt and certain means of curing any disease whatever, however pernicious we may suppose it, consists in opposing to it the homeopathic remedy. Then, instead of renouncing in this emergency the application of our law, it is best to conform to its requirements. The greater the danger, the greater this obligation."—CHARGE.

"When we have to do with an art whose end is the saving of human life, any neglect to make ourselves thoroughly masters of it becomes a crime."—HAHNEMANN.

VERATRUM VIRIDE.

Characteristic.—For full-blooded plethoric persons (Acon.).

Congestions, especially **to base of brain,** *chest, spine and stomach.*

Violent pains attending inflammation.

Acute rheumatism, high fever, full, hard, rapid pulse, severe pains in joints and muscles (Bry., Salyc. ac.); scanty, red urine.

Child trembles, jerks, threatened with convulsions; continually jerking or nodding the head.

Nervous or sick headache; congestion from suppressed menses; intense, almost apoplectic, with violent nausea and vomiting.

Congestive apoplexy, hot head, bloodshot eyes, thick speech, *slow full pulse, hard as iron.*

Convulsions: dim vision; **basilar meningitis**; head retracted; child on verge of spasms.

Cerebro spinal diseases; with spasms, dilated pupils, tetanic convulsions, opisthotonos; *cold, clammy perspiration.*

Sunstroke, head full, throbbing of arteries, sensitive to sound; double or partial vision (Gels., Glon.).

Veratrum viride should not be given simply to "bring down the pulse" or "control the heart's action," but like any other remedy for the totality of the symptoms.

Type.—Remittent; malarial; congestive; malignant; typhoid; continued; yellow. Periodicity not marked; onset sudden and course severe and rapid.

Chill.—Coldness: of whole body; with nausea; with pale face and cold, clammy skin; aching in back of neck and shoulders.

Heat.—Intense fever, with cerebral irritation and tendency to spasms; violent pain in back; sleepy during the day; nausea at stomach, or vomiting and black diarrhea; face hot, flushed; great weakness of lower extremities and marked prostration.

Sweat.—Profuse, cold, clammy; vomiting, with a cold sweat on the pale face.

Yellow fever: fever intense, with pains in nape and occiput, vascular and nervous erethism, with spasms or threatened convulsions; continued gastric nausea; vomiting and cold sweat on face; sudden changes in pulse and violent throbbing in left chest.

Typhoid: temperature, 103-106; pulse, 120-140; violent occipital headache; boring head into pillow, jerking head backward and forward; twitching of facial muscles; dropping of lower jaw; picking of bedclothes; stool and urine involuntary.

Tongue.—White or yellow with **red streak down the middle**; dry, moist, white or yellow coating, or no coating on either side; feels scalded (Sang.).

Pulse.—Suddenly increases and gradually decreases below normal; *slow, soft, weak;* irregular, intermittent (Dig).

Analysis.—*In congestive, pernicious intermittent or yellow fever, with extreme coldness,* thirst; *face cold and collapsed;* skin cold and clammy, great prostration; cold sweat on forehead and deathly pallor on face.

ZINCUM METALLICUM.

Characteristic.—Persons suffering from cerebral and nervous exhaustion; **defective vitality,** *brain or nerve power wanting;* too weak to develop exanthemata or menstrual function, to expectorate, to urinate; to comprehend, to memorize.

Incessant and violent fidgety feeling in feet or lower extremities; must move them constantly.

Always feels better every way *as soon as the menses begin to flow; it relieves all her sufferings,* but they return again soon after the flow ceases.

In cerebral affections: in impending paralysis of brain; where the vis medicatrix naturæ is too weak to develop exanthemata (Cup., Sulph., Tub.); symptoms of effusion into ventricles.

Child repeats everything said to it.

Child cries out during sleep; whole body jerks during sleep; wakes frightened, stares, *rolls the head from side to side;* face alternately pale and red.

Convulsions: during dentition, **with pale face, no heat,** except perhaps in occiput, no increase in temperature (rev. of, Bell.); rolling the eyes; gnashing the teeth.

Automatic motion of hands and head, or one hand and head (Apoc., Bry., Hell.).

Chorea: from suppressed eruptions; from fright.

Hunger: ravenous, about 11 or 12 A. M. (Sulph.); *great greediness when eating;* cannot eat fast enough (Tub.—incipient brain disease in children).

Excessive nervous moving of feet in bed for hours after retiring, even when asleep.

Feet sweaty and sore about toes; fetid, suppressed foot-sweat; very nervous.

Chilblains, painful, < from rubbing.

Spinal affections: *burning whole length of spine;* backache, *much < from sitting* > by walking about (Cobalt., Puls., Rhus).

Spinal irritation; great prostration of strength.

Cannot bear back touched (Chin. s., Tarant., Ther.).

Can only void urine while sitting bent backwards.

Twitching and jerking of single muscles (Agar., Ign.).

Weakness and trembling of extremities; of hands while writing; during menses.

Aggravation.—Of many symptoms from drinking wine, even a small quantity (Alum., Con.).

Amelioration.—Symptoms: of chest, by expectorating; of bladder, by urinating; of back, by emissions (< by Cobalt.); general, by menstrual flow.

Type.—Continued; typhoid; typhus.

Time.—4-8 P. M. (Ars., Lyc., Puls.); forenoon.

Chill.—With cold nose, hands and feet. Begins; after eating dinner; in open air; on approach of a storm; runs down the back; alternate with heat; external with internal heat; from touching anything cold; followed by nausea and much sour saliva.

Shaking chill with pale sunken face, weak, rapid and irregular pulse, often with nausea and vomiting; at last pulse became large, full, with heat, red face, followed by restless sleep, exhaustion and copious sweats.

Chilliness: and coldness of whole body, followed by fever with chilly creeping through the back, with nausea, with constant yawning; over abdomen.

Shivering, with shuddering, nausea, intense headache, followed by cold sweats; down the back, with trembling of the limbs.

Heat.—With thirst; in flushes, with desire to be fanned. Violent throbbing through the whole body, with short hot breath.

Heat; internal, with cold sensation in abdomen; of face, with cool body; with redness of face and burning in eyes; heat in back with coldness in nape of neck; of soles and single parts.

Typhoid; delirium, attempts to get out of bed; complete unconsciousness; sliding down in bed; grasping at flocks; subsultus; decubitus; involuntary stool and urine.

Sweat.—Profuse all night, wants to uncover; easy, during day, from least exertion; offensive, sour smelling; sour, with fine, stitching itching, over body; on head, hands and feet; while walking in open air. Night sweat, with heat, *cannot tolerate any covering.*

Profuse, offensive foot sweat; walks feet sore.

Pulse.—Small and frequent evenings, slow mornings; tense, irregular, small and hard; feeble, easily compressed; wiry, irregular, slow, 40 and intermitting.

REPERTORY

TYPE.

Anticipating: Ant. t., **Ars.**, Bell., **Bry.**, **Chin. s.**, **Cinch.**, Eup., **Gamb.**, Ign., **Nat.**, **Nux.**
every day, two hours: Cham.
every other day: Nat., Nux.
every other day, one hour: **Ars.**
every other day, several hours: Ant. t.
one to three hours, each attack: Chin. s.
two to three hours, each attack: Cinch.
rarely: Bell., Ign., Mer.
or postponing: **Bry.**, Gamb., **Ign.**
converted into a regular: Alst.

Apoplectic: Laur., Nux, Op.

Autumnal: *Æsc.*, Bap., **Bry.**, Carb. ac., *Cinch.*, **Colch.**, *Eup.*, Mal., **Nat.**, **Ver.**

Bilious: *Bry.*, **Chel.**, Hydr., **Ipec.** Nat. s., **Pod.**, Puls., Sep.

Cerebro Spinal: Act., Bell., Bry., Gels., Nat. s., Nux, Tub., Zinc.

Changing: *Elat.*, Eup., **Ign.**, Meny., Psor., **Puls.**
frequently: *Elat.*, Ign., Psor., *Puls.*
no two attacks alike: *Puls.*
after abuse of Quinine: Arn., Ars., *Elat.*, **Eup.**, Ign., *Ipec.*

Congestive: Apis, **Arn.**, Bell., Cac., *Camph.*, Elat., Hyos., *Lyc.*, **Nux**, Op., **Psor.**, **Ver.**

Day: every, at precisely same hour: Anac., *Ang.,* **Aran.,** Bov., Cac., **Ced., Gels.,** Hell., Kali c., *Sabad., Spig.,* Thuja. (see Psor.)

at different times of: Eup. p., Nat.

every other: Ant. c., **Aran., Ced.,** *Chin. s.,* Cinch., *Nat.*

every other, in evening: **Lyc.**

every seven: *Amm. m.,* Canth., *Cinch., Lyc.,* Meny., Plant., Rhus, Sul., Tub.

every fourteen: *Amm.,* **Ars.,** Cal., Chin. s., *Cinch.,* **Lach.,** *Plant.,* Psor., Puls.

every twenty-one: *Chin. s.,* Mag. c., Psor., Sul.

Endemic: Ars., **Ced.,** Chin. s., Cinch., Eup., Gels., *Nux,* **Psor.**

Epidemic: Ant. t., Arn., *Ars.,* Bap., Bry., *Chin. s.,* Colch., Elat., *Eup., Ipec., Mal.,* **Nat.,** Phel., Rhus, Ver.

Epileptic: Cup., Hyos., *Lach.,* **Op., Psor.**

Intermittents, acute: *Ars.,* Bap., *Bry.,* **Chin. s.,** Cinch., *Gels.,* Ign., **Natr.,** *Nux.*

chronic: Alum., Apis, Cal., Carbo v., Graph., Hep., Kali c., Lach., Lyc., Nat., Nux, Phos., **Psor.,** Sep., Sil., **Sul.,** Tub.

of children: **Ars., Cham.,** Cina, Crot., *Gels.,* **Lach.,** *Op.,* **Psor.**

of old people: Alum., Bar., **Op.**

Malarial: Alst., **Arn.,** Cad. s., Canch., Carb. ac., **Chin. s.,** *Cinch.,* Chel., Corn., Eucal., Eup., Eup. p., Gels., Ipec., *Mal.,* Nat. s., Nux, Pod., **Psor.,** Sul. ac., Ter., Ver. v.

tropical: **Ced.,** *Gels.,* Nat. s., **Psor.,** Pyr., Sep., **Ter.,** Tar.

Malignant, tend to: *Anth.,* **Ars.,** Carb. ac., **Crot.,** *Mur. ac.,* Psor. **Pyr.,** Ver. v.

Menses, after the: **Nux, Psor.,** Sep.

Monthly: Nux m., **Nux,** Puls., Sep., Sul.

Paroxysm, irregular: **Ars.,** Eup., Ign., *Ipec.,* Meny., **Nux, Psor., Puls.,** Samb.

irregular, stage irregular: **Ars.,** *Ipec.,* **Nux.**

Paroxysm, irregular, stage irregular, *long chill, little heat, no thirst*: **Puls.**

irregular, stage irregular, short chill, long heat, no thirst: *Ant. t.,* **Ipec.**

irregular, one stage wanting: *Apis,* Aran., **Ars.,** Bov., Camph., Dros., Led., Lyc., Mang., Meny., Mez., Ver.

of only heat and sweat: Mang.

regular: Chin. s., Cina, Cinch.

regular, stages irregular: *Opium,* Oleand.

regular, stages, first two irregular: *Rhus.*

regular, stages, regular: **Chin. s.,** Cina, Cinch.

regular, stages, regular, apt to run into each other: Ars., Nux, Puls., Pod.

increasing in severity: Ars., **Bry.,** Eup., *Nat.,* Nux, Puls., **Psor.**

Periodicity, marked: Æsc., Ang., **Aran.,** Cac., Caps., **Ced., Chin. s.,** Cinch., *Cina,* **Gels.,** Pod., Sabad., Spig., Sul. ac.

not marked: Acon., Amb., Amm. m., Bell., Camph., Canth., Carbo an., Carbo v., Caust., Chel., Cic., Col., Mag. c., **Psor.,** Ver. v.

Pernicious: *Apis, Arn.* **Camph.,** *Cur.,* Lyc., **Nux,** Op., **Psor.,** Sul., Sul. ac., Ver. v., **Ver.**

long lasting chill passing off without heat or sweat: Lyc.

Perspiration, when checked by draft of air: Cad. s.

Postponing: Alst., Cina, Cinch., **Gamb.,** Ign., *Ipec.*

Quartan: Acon., Anac., Ant. c., *Arn.,* **Ars.,** Bell., Bry., Carbo v., Cinch., Cina, Clem., Cof., Coral., Elat., **Hyos.,** Ign., **Iod.,** Ipec., Lach., Lyc., **Meny.,** *Nat.,* Nux m., *Nux,* Plant., Pod., **Puls.,** Rhus, **Sabad., Ver.**

double: *Ars.,* Cinch., **Dul.,** Eup., Eup. p., Gamb., Lyc., Nux m., Puls., Rhus.

Quotidian: Acon., Æsc., Anac., Ant. c., Ant. t., Apis, *Aran., Ars.,* Bap., Bar., Bell., Bry., *Cac.,* Cal., *Cap.,* Carbo v., *Ced.,* Cham., Cic., *Cina,* Cinch., Con., **Cur.,** Dros., Elaps, Elat., Gamb., *Gels.,* Graph., Hep., Hydr., Ign., Kali bi.,

Kali br., Kali c., Lach., Lob., Lyc., Mag. c., *Nat.*, Nit. ac., **Nux,** Petros., Phos., Plant., *Pod.*, Polyp., *Puls.*, *Rhus,* Sabad., Sarr., Spig., Stan., Staph., Stram., Sul., Ver.

double: Ant. c., Apis, Bap., *Bell.*, *Cinch.*, Dul., **Elat.**, *Graph.*, Led., *Stram.*, *Sul.*

Relapsing: Ars., Eucal., **Psor.**, **Sul.**

after abuse of Quinine: **Ars.**, Ipec.

Remittent: **Ars.**, Arg. n., Ant. t., Bap., Carb. ac., Chel., Chin. s., Clem., Crot., Eup., Ipec., Nat. s., Nux, Pod., *Psor.*, Tar., Ver. v.

of children: Ant. c., Gels.

resembling: Bap., Ced., Pod.

prone to become: Ant. t., Eup. p., Phos. ac., Phos., *Psor.*

intermittent becomes: Eup., *Gamb.*, *Pod.*

becomes intermittent: Gels., Phos., *Psor.*

becomes intermittent or typhoid: Ant. t., Phos. ac., **Psor.**

prone to become typhoid: *Ant. t.*, **Ars.**, **Bap.**, Carb. ac., Mez., **Mur. ac.**, Phos., **Psor.**, **Rhus,** *Sec.*, Ter., Tub.

prone to become typhoid and typhus, after abuse of Quinine: **Ars.**, Bry., Lach., Rhus.

Septic: Acet. ac., *Anth.*, **Ars.**, *Carb. ac.*, **Crot.**, **Lach.**, **Pyr.**, Sul. ac., Tar., Ter.

Septimania: *Amm. m.*, *Psor.*, Sul.

Sinking: (See Pernicious.)

Spasmodic, with epidemic pertussis: Dros., Kali c., Hyos., Tub.

Spring: *Ars.*, *Canch.*, Carbo v., *Gels.*, **Lach.**, **Psor.**, Sep., Sul.

and Autumn: Lach., **Psor.**, Sep.

early: **Ant. t.**, *Lach.*, Sul.

Summer: Caps., Casc., Ced., Lach., Nat., Polyp., **Psor.**

excessive heat of: **Bap.**, Nat.

Suppressed, by Quinine or anti-periodics: Stan.

Tertian: Æsc., Alum., Anac., Ant. c., *Apis,* **Aran.**, Arn., **Ars.**, Bar., Bar. m., **Bell.**, Brom., **Bry.**, Calc., **Canth.**, Caps.,

Carbo an., Carbo v., **Ced.**, Cham., **Chin. s.**, Cic., Cina, **Cinch.**, Coral., Dros., Dul., Elat., **Eup.**, Fer., Gamb., Gels., Hydr., Hyos., Ign., Iod., **Ipec.**, **Lach.**, **Lyc.**, **Mez.**, **Natr.**, Nux m., **Nux**, Plant., Petros., *Pod.*, *Polyp.*, *Puls.*, **Rhus**, *Sabad.*, Sarr., Staph., Sul., Ver.

fever, with no chill: **Gels.**

double: Æsc., Ars., Cinch., Dul., Elat., Eup. p., Gamb., Lyc., Nux, Rhus.

Typhoid: Acet. ac., Anth., Apis, Arn., **Ars.**, **Bap.**, **Bry.**, Carbo v., Carb. ac., Coc., **Crot.**, *Elaps*, *Gels.*, Ham., **Hyos.**, **Lach.**, Lyc., **Mur. ac.**, Naja, Nit. ac., Nux, *Op.*, *Phos. ac.*, Phos., **Psor.**, **Pyr.**, **Rhus**, Sec., Sil., *Stram.*, Sul., *Sul. ac.*, Tar., **Ter.**, Tub., *Zinc.*

Typhus: Arn., *Aran.*, Arg. n., **Ars.**, **Lach.**, **Mur. ac.**, **Op.**, *Phos. ac.*, **Psor.**, **Pyr.**, *Sul. ac.*, *Sec.*, *Ter.*, Zinc.

Vernal: Canch., *Gels.*, **Lach.**, **Psor.**, **Sul.**, Staph., Sul. ac.

Weather, change of: Mer., Psor., Thuja, Tub.

Weekly: (See days, every seven.)

Winter: Ant. t., Natr., Polyp., **Psor.** (Cough.)

Yearly: *Ars.*, *Carbo v.*, **Lach.**, *Natr.*, **Psor.**, *Sul.*, Thuja, Tub.

half: Lach., *Sep.*

Yellow Fever: Act., **Ars.**, Arg. n., **Cad. s.**, Calad., *Camph.*, **Canth.**, **Carbo v.**, *Carb. ac.*, Colch., **Crot.**, Gels., Hydr., Ipec., Lach., Mur. ac., **Natr. s.**, **Nux**, **Psor.**, Phos., Rhus, Staph., Sul. ac., **Ter.**, *Ver.*, Ver. v.

Zymotic: Anth., Apis, **Arn.**, **Ars.**, *Bell.*, **Bar.**, **Bry.**, *Cad. s.*, Carbo v., **Crot.**, *Cur.*, *Hyos.*, **Lach.**, **Lyc.**, Mer., **Mur. ac.**, Nux m., Nux, Op., Phos., **Pyr.**, Rhus, Sec., Staph., Sul., *Sul. ac.*, Tar., Ter.

TIME.

Autumn: Æsc., *Ars.*, Bap., Carb. ac., **Colch.**, *Eup.*, Mal., *Nux*, **Psor.**, **Sep.**, *Ter.*, Tub.
hot days and cool nights in: Acon., Colch., Mal., Mer.
and Spring: Lach., **Psor.**, **Sep.**, Tub.

Bed, in: *Alum.*, Amm. m., Ars., Bov., Bry., Calc., Carbo an., Chin. s., Dros., Fer., *Hep.*, Laur., *Mer.*, Nux, **Phos.**, Sil., Sul.
in morning: Chin. s., Graph., Nux.
at night: Canch.

Day, all: *Alum.*, Sab., **Sil.**, Tub.
during, fever at night: Alum.
during: Asar.
during, at any time: **Ars.**, Camph., Hell., Kali c., *Plant.*, Sars.
and night: Sars.

Evening: Acon., Æsc., **Alum.**, Agar., Amm. c., *Amm. m.*, Aran., **Arn.**, **Ars.**, Bell., *Bov.*, Bry., *Calad.*, *Calc.*, Carb. ac., Carbo v., Ced., Cham., Chel., Chin. s., **Cina**, Coc., Cyc., Dul., Fer., *Gamb.*, Graph., **Hep.**, Hyd., *Ign.*, Kali bi., *Kali c.*, *Lach.*, Lachn., *Lyc.*, Mag. c., *Mag. m.*, Mer., Mez., *Nit. ac.*, *Nux*, *Petr.*, **Phos.**, Phos. ac., Plat., Prun., *Psor.*, **Puls.**, **Rhus**, Sab., Samb., Sarr., **Sep.**, Sil., Stan., Staph., Stron., **Sul.**, Tab., Tub.
at sunset: *Ign.*, Puls., Thuja.
in bed: Alum., Amm. c., Bov., Carbo an., Chin. s., Fer., *Dros.*, Hep., *Nat. s.*, Nux, **Phos.**, Sil., *Sul.*
in bed, going off in bed: *Natr. s.*
with the pains: *Cyc.*, Ign., **Puls.**

Forenoon: Alst., Amb., Ang., *Arn.*, Asar., Calc., Con., Cyc., **Eup.**, Euph., Led., **Natr.**, **Nux**, Sil., Stan., Stron., Zinc.

Midnight: Ars., Canth., Caust., **Sul.**
before: Cad. s.
after: Ars., Kali c., Op., Thuja.
heat before, chill after: Calad.

Morning: Ang., Apis, Arn., **Bry.**, Calc., Con., Cyc., Dros., **Eup.**, Euphor., *Fer.*, Gels., Graph., *Hep.*, Hydr., Kali c., Led., *Lyc.*, Mer., **Natr.**, **Nux**, Phos., **Pod.**, **Sep.**, Sil., *Spig.*, *Sul.*, Thuja, Ver.

Morning, early in: Arn., *Chin. s.*, Graph., Lyc., *Natr. m.*, **Nux**, **Ver.**

to noon: *Eup.*, **Natr.**

Night, at: *Alum.*, Amb., Arg., **Apis**, Bell., Bov., Carbo v., Caust., Fer., Gambo., Hep., Iris, *Kali iod.*, Mag. s., **Mer.**, Mur. ac., Nat. s., Nit. ac., **Nux**, Op., **Phos.**, *Sars.*, Sil., Staph., *Sul.*, Thuja.

in bed: Canch.

never at: Cinch.

Noon, at: *Ant. c.*, *Elat.*, Elaps, *Eup.*, *Lach.*, *Lob.*, Mer., Nux, Psor., Sil., *Sul.*, Tub.

Noon, after: Alum., Anac., Ant. c., Arg., *Arn.*, **Ars.**, Bap., Bar., *Bor.*, Bry., Chel., Chin. s., Cic., Cina, Coc., Croc., Crot., Dig., Eup., Gels., Graph., Kali bi., Lach., **Lyc.**, Mercurialis, *Natr.*, Nat. s., Nit. ac., *Nux*, Op., Petr., Phos. ac., Phos., **Puls.**, Ran., Rob., Sab., Samb., Sarr., Sil., Staph., Sul., Thuja.

Paroxysm returning at:

1 A. M.: **Ars.**, Canth., Puls., Sil.

1 to 2 A. M.: Aloe, Ars.

2 A. M.: **Ars.**, Benz. ac., Canth., Hep., Lach., Puls., Sil.

2 to 4 A. M.: Bor., Kali c.

3 A. M.: Amm. m., Canth., Ced., Eup., Led., Lys., Natr., Sil., **Thuja.**

4 A. M.: *Alum.*, Amm. m., Arn., **Ced.**, Con., Dios., Natr., Sil.

5 A. M.: Apis, *Bov.*, Chin. s., *Cinch.*, Cof., Con., Dros., *Natr.*, *Polyp.*, Sep., Sil.

5 to 8 A. M.: Sul.

5.30 to 6.30 A. M.: Hura. (Brazil.)

6 A. M.: *Arn.*, *Bov.*, Chin. s., Eup., **Fer.**, Graph., *Hep.*, Natr., *Nux*, Stram., **Ver.**

Paroxysm returning at:

6 to 9 A. M.: Bov., Chin. s., Eup., Nux.

7 A. M.: Amm. m., *Bov.,* Dros., Elat., **Eup.,** Fer., Graph., Hep., Hura, Natr., *Nux,* **Pod.,** Sil., Stram.

7 to 8 A. M.: Fer.

7 to 9 A. M.: **Eup.,** Natr., *Pod.*

7 to 9 A. M.: one day, 12 M. next day: Eup.

8 A. M.: *Bov.,* Chin. s., Coc., Dros., **Eup.,** Lyc., Mez., Natr., Pod., Puls., Sul.

8:15 A. M.: Hura.

8 to 9 A. M.: Asaf., Eup.

8 to 10:30 A. M.: Arn., Eup., Ipec., Natr.

8:30 to 9 A. M.: Asaf.

9 A. M.: Alst., Ang., Ant. t., Asaf., Carb. ac., **Eup.,** Hura, Hydr., Ipec., Kali c., Lyc., Mag. c., Mez., *Natr.,* Phos. ac., Polyp., Sep., Sul.

9 to 10 A. M.: Eup., Fer. i., Rhus.

9 to 11 A. M.: *Alst.,* **Natr.,** Polyp., *Stan.*

10 A. M.: Act., Alst., Ars., Berb., Bap., Cac., Carbo v., Chin. s., Eup., Fag., Fer. i., Hipp., Ipec., Led., Med., **Natr.,** Petr., Phos. ac., *Polyp.,* Rhus, Sep., Sil., **Stan.,** Sul., Thuja.

10:30 A. M.: Cac., Caps., Hura, *Lob., Natr.*

10 to 11 A. M.: Agar., Ars., Chin. s., Med., **Natr.,** Nux.

10 A. M. to 2 P. M.; Chlor., Mer., Sul.

10 A. M. to 3 P. M.: Sil., Sul., Tub.

11 A. M.: *Bap.,* Berb., **Cac.,** Canth., Carbo v., Cham., *Chin. s.,* Coc., Hydr., Hyos., *Ipec.,* Lob., Med., **Natr., Nux,** Op., Pod., *Polyp.,* Puls., *Sep.,* Sil., Sul., Tub.

11 A. M.: one day, 4 P. M. next: Calc.

11 A. M. to 12 M.: Act., **Cac.,** Kali c., Kob., Sul.

1 A. M. to 2 P. M.: Cac., Lach., Med.

11 A. M. and 4 P. M.: **Cac.,** Gels.

12 M.: Ant. c., Chin. s., Elat., Elaps, Eup., Fer., *Kali c., Lach.,* Lob., Mer., Nux, *Sil., Sul.*

12 M. to 1 P. M.: Ars., Fer. i., Lach.

12 M. to 1:30 P. M.: Mer., Sul.

12 M. to 2 P. M.: *Ars.,* Kob., *Lach.,* Sul.

Paroxysm returning at:

1 P. M.: **Ars.**, Cac., Canth., *Cina,* Chel., Elat., Eup., Fer. p., Ipec., *Lach.,* Mer., Nux, Phos., Polyp., **Puls.**, Sil., Sul.

1 to 2 P. M.: **Ars.**, Eup., Natr., Puls.

2 P. M.: **Ars.**, *Calc.,* Canth., Cic., Cur., *Eup.,* Euph., Gels., Ipec., Plant., Sil., Sul.

2 to 3 P. M.: Cur.

2 to 4 P. M.: Gels.

2 to 6 P. M.: Bor.

2:30 P. M.: Led.

3 P. M.: **Ang.**, **Ant. t.**, **Apis**, Ars., Asaf., Calc., *Canth.,* **Ced.**, **Chin.** s., Cic., Cof., Con., Cur., Fer., Ipec., Lyc., Med., Nux, Petr., Polyp., Sabad., Samb., Sil., **Staph.**, *Thuja.*

3 to 4 P. M.: Apis, Asaf., Canth., Med., Lach., Polyp., Puls.

3 to 5 P. M.: Coc., Con.

3 to 6 P. M.: Ars., Eup., Fer.

4 P. M.: Æsc., Anac., **Apis**, Asaf., Bov., Canth., Caust., **Ced.**, Cham., Chin. s., Chel., Eupion, Gamb., Gels., Graph., Hell., *Hep.,* Ipec., Kali i., **Lyc.**, Mag. m., Med., Natr., Nux, Petr., Phel., Phos. ac., Polyp., **Puls.**, Samb., Sep., Sil.

4 to 5 P. M.: Graph., Kob., Lyc., *Puls.,* Stan.

4 to 7 P. M.: Kali i., Natr., Rhus.

4 to 8 P. M.: **Bov.**, Graph., Hell., *Hep.,* Kali i., **Lyc.**, Mag. m., Nat. s., Sab., Zinc.

4 to 10 P. M.: Phel.

5 P. M.: Act., Alum., Amm. m., Apis, Ars., Bov., Canth., Caps., Carbo an., Castor., *Ced.,* Chel., Cinch., Con., Elat., Eup., Gamb., Gels., Graph., Hell., Hep., **Kali c.**, Kali i., Mag. c., Med., Natr., Nux m., Nux, Phos., Puls., *Rhus,* Sabad., Samb., Sarr., Sep., Sil., Sul., **Thuja.**

5 to 6 P. M.: Caps., Kali c., Phos., Sul., Thuja.

5 to 8 P. M.: Alum., Arn., Carbo an., Gamb., Natr., Rhus.

6 P. M.: Amm. m., *Ant. t.,* Arg. n., Ars., Bell., Bov., Canth., Caps., Carbo an., Ced., Cham., Chel., Gamb., Graph., Hell., **Hep.**, **Kali. c.**, Kali. i., Lyc., Mag. m., Natr., Nux m., Nux, Petr., Phel., Phos. ac., Phos., *Rhus,* Samb., Sep., *Sil.,* Sul., Thuja.

Paroxysm returning at:

6 to 7 P. M.: Hep., Rhus.

6 to 8 P. M.: Gamb., Hep., Kali i., Sul., Rhus.

6 to 7:30 P. M.: Clem.

6 to 12 P. M.: Lachn.

6:30 P. M.: Canth., Rhus.

7 P. M.: Alum., Amm. m., *Bov.,* Calc., Canth., Carbo an., Carbon sul., Castor., Caust., Ced., Gamb., Graph., Hell., **Hep.,** Kali i., **Lyc.,** Mag. c., Mag. s., Med., Natr., Natr. s., Nux, Petr., Phel., Phos. ac., Phos., **Rhus,** Sil., *Sul.,* Thuja.

7 P. M.: Thuja.

8 P. M.: Alum., Ars., Bar., *Bov.,* Canth., Carbo an., Chel., Cof., Elaps, Gamb., Gels., Graph., Hell., Hep., Kali i., Mag. c., Mag. m., Nux, Phel., Phos. ac., *Rhus,* Sil., *Sul.,* Tarax.

8:30 P. M.: Chin. ars.

9 P. M.: **Ars.,** *Bov.,* Canth., Carbo an., Castor., Cac., Coc., Croc., Cyc., Gamb., Gels., Hydr., Mag. c., Mag. s., Mercurialis, Nux m., Nux, Phel., Phos. ac., Polyp., San., Sul.

10 P. M.: *Ars., Bov.,* Cac., Canth., Carbo an., *Chin. s.,* Elaps, Euphorb. amyg., Hydr., *Kali i.,* Mag. c., Phel., Phos. ac., Sabad.

11 P. M.: Ars., **Cac.,** Canth., Carbo an., Euphorb. amyg., Sul.

12 P. M.: *Ars.,* Canth., Caust., Sul.

Anticipates, 2½ hours every day: Aranea sciencia, Chin. s.

1 hour every other day: Ars., Cinch., Ign., Natr., Nux.

Regular intervals: Aran. s., Chin. s.

intervals of two days: Brom.

intervals of seven days: **Amm. m.**

intervals of fourteen days: Ars.. Calc., Cinch., Puls.

Sunset: Puls.

Yearly: Ars., Carbo v., Lach., Sul.

Fever, without chill, returning at:

midnight: Stram., Sul.
12 to 3 A. M.: **Ars.**, Kali c., Med.
12 to 2 A. M.: Ars.
1 to 2 A. M.: Ars.
2 to 4 A. M.: Kali c.
3 A. M.: **Ang.**, Thuja.
4 A. M.: Arn.
6 to 10 A. M.: Rhus.
7 A. M.: Pod.
8 A. M. to 2 P. M.: Doryph.
9 A. M.: Kali c., Meny.
9 A. M. to 12 M.: Cham.
9 A. M. to 3 P. M.: Meny.
10 A. M.: **Natr.**, *Rhus,* Thuja.
10 to 11 A. M.: Bap., Gels., **Natr.**, *Thuja.*
11 A. M.: *Bap.,* Cac., Calc., Med., **Natr.**, Thuja.
12 M.: Spig., *Stram., Sul.*
12 M. to 1 P. M.: Sil.
1 to 2 P. M.: **Ars.**
1 to 4 P. M.: Lac. ac.
2 P. M.: **Puls.**
2 to 3 P. M.: Cur.
3 P. M.: Ant. t., Ars., Cof., Cur., Fer., Lyc., Nicc.
3 to 4 P. M.: **Apis,** Clem., Lyc.
4 P. M.: **Anac.**, *Apis,* Ars., Graph., Hep., Ipec., Kali bi.
4 P. M., lasting all night: Ars., Hep., Puls., Stan.
4 to 8 P. M.: Lyc.
5 P. M.: Con., Kali bi., Kali c., Petr., Sab., Stan.
5 P. M. and 5:30 P. M., pricking in the tongue: Ced.
5 to 6 P. M.: Hell.
5 to 6 P. M., very ill humored: Con.
6 P. M.: Ant. t., Bor., Calc., Carbo v., Caust., Ced., Coc., Hep., Kali c., Lac. ac., **Nux**, Petr., Rhod.
6 to 7 P. M.: Calc., Nux.
6 to 12 P. M.: Lachn.
6 P. M., lasting all night: *Nux,* Lyc., Rhus.

Fever, without chill, returning at:
6 to 8 P. M.: Ant. t., Caust.
6:30 P. M.: Ced., Hura.
7 P. M.: Æsc., Bov., Lyc., *Calc.*, Mag. m., Mag. s., **Nux**, Petr., *Rhus.*
7 to 8 P. M.: Amb.
7 to 12 P. M.: Æsc.
8 P. M.: Ant. t., Cof., Fer., Hep., Mur. ac., Sul.
9 P. M.: Mag. s.
9 P. M. to 10 A. M.: Mag. s.
9 to 12 P. M.: Amm. c.
10 P. M.: *Ars.*, Hydr., Lach., Petr., Sab.
11 P. M.: Cac., **Calc.**
twice a day and 3 to 4 P. M.: Apis.
different times of day: Eup., Tub.

CAUSE.

ATTACK BROUGHT ON BY:

Air, in open: Zinc.

Acids, abuse of, or after taking: Lach.

Alcohol, abuse of: Crot., Led., *Nux.*

Anger: Bry., Cham., Coc., **Nux.**

Animal, heat, want of: Led., Mar. v., Sep., Sil., Tub.
tissue, decayed: Anth., Ars., Pyr.

Anthrax: Anth., Ars., Carb. ac., Crot., Lach., Pyr.

Anxiety: Ars., *Gels.*

Arsenic, abuse of: *Ipec.*

Choleraic, occurring during cholera epidemics: Elat., Ver.

Coffee, abuse of: Cham., Nux.

Diet, indiscretions in: Ant. c., Çyc., *Ipec.*, Puls.
indiscretions in, may produce relapse: Ant. c., *Ipec.*
indiscretions in, eating pork; rich fat food: **Puls.**

Diet, indiscretions in, eating pastry, sweets: Cina, Ipec.
indiscretions in, eating late suppers, irregular, unseasonable: *Nux*.

Dissecting wounds: *Anth.*, **Ars.**, Carb. ac., **Lach.**, **Pyr.**

Drinking, after: Ars., Asar.

Eating, after: Ars., Asar., Bell., Carbo an., Kali c., Mar. v., Nux, Tarax., Zinc.
after, and drinking: Asar., Tarax.
beginning to: Bell., Euphor.

Exertion, physical: Ars., Eup., Mer., Sil., Sul.
too much mental, too little physical: Nux.

Exposure: *Acon.*, Ang., Ant. c., Ant. t., *Aran.*, Arn., Ars., Bar., Bry., Cac., *Calc.*, Canth., Carbo v., *Ced.*, *Chin. s.*, Cinch., Dros., Dul., Eucal., Hep., Kali c., Led., Lach., Natr., Nat. s., Rhus, Sep., Spig., Zinc.
basements, cellars, living in: *Ant. t.*, **Aran.**, *Ars.*, Ars. i., Carbo v., *Nat. s.*, **Ter.**
bathing while warm: Clem.
bathing, cold, too frequent: Ant. c., *Rhus.*
cold sheets, soon as he touches: **Aran.**, Pyr.
cold drinks when overheated: Acon., Bellis.
cold vegetables or fruit, handling: Calc., Val., Zinc.
draft, to a: *Acon.*, Bar., Canth., Hep.
draft, to a, when heated: **Acon.**
margins of streams or ponds, from living on: **Natr.**
malarial influences, to: *Arn.*, Cad. s., Carb. ac., **Ced.**, **Chin. s.**, Cinch., Cur., *Eucal.*, Eup., Natr., Nat. s., Ter.
marshy regions: Ced., Chin. s., Eucal.
swamps, in; Ang., Ced., *Chin. s.*, *Natr.*
swamps, in, tropical countries, in: *Ang.*, **Ced.**, Chin. s., *Eucal.*, **Natr.**, Ter.
sleeping in damp rooms or beds, from: Ant. t., *Aran.*, *Carbo v.*, Nat. s., *Rhus*, Ter.
rheumatic, and living or working in basements: Ant. t., Aran., *Ars.*, Carbo v., **Nat. s.**, *Ter.*

Exposure, soil freshly turned, to: **Natr.**
water, standing in: Aran., *Calc.,* Led., Rhus.
water, living near: Nat. s.
water, working in: *Calc.,* Rhus.
wet, from getting: Acon., Aran., Bellis, *Bry.,* Clem., Dul., **Rhus,** *Sep.*
wet, from getting, when overheated: *Acon.,* Bellis, Clem., **Rhus.**
working in clay: **Calc.**
working in the rain, from: *Aran.,* Clem., **Rhus.**
rains, during: Aran., Ced., Cur., Fer., Dul., Zinc.
seashore, residing at: Natr., Nat. s.
seashore, visits to: *Ars.,* Nat. s.
sun to: Ant. t., *Cac.,* **Glon.,** Lach., Nat. c.
sun to, heat of: Ant. c., *Cac.,* Glon., Lach., Ter.
dry, cold, north or west winds: **Acon.,** *Bry.,* Hep.

Fright: Acon., Gels., Op.

Gonorrhea: Clem., Med., Nat. s., Thuja.

Grief: *Gels.,* **Ign.**

Ground: (See exposure, soil freshly turned.)

Heated, after getting: Ant. c., Carbo v., Glon.

Hemorrhagic diathesis: Crot., Lach., Phos., Sec.

Infection, septic: Anth., Crot., Lach., Pyr.

Joy, excessive: **Cof.**

Malarial: (See exposure.)

Mechanical injuries, from: Arn., Bellis, Calend., Ham., Hep., Mill., Rhus.

Organic lesion: Anth., Ars., Hydr.

Overheated, from becoming: *Ant. c.,* **Carbo v.,** Glon.

Paludal: **Arn.,** Carb. ac., Casc., *Ced., Chin. s.,* Cinch., **Eucal.,** Eup., *Natr.,* Ter.

Perspiration, suppressed, from: Acon., Cup., *Sil.*
suppressed, from a draught: **Acon.**
suppressed, of feet: *Cup.*, **Sil.**

Post mortem infection: *Anth.*, **Ars., Lach., Pyr.**

Pus, absorption: Anth., Ars., Lach., Pyr.

Quinine, abuse of: Alst., Arn., Ars., Carbo v., Ipec., Lach., Natr., Puls., Stan.

Rheumatic: Acon., *Aran., Bry.*, Led., **Rhus,** *Spig.*, Sul.

Room, when in a: Ars.
warmth of: *Apis, Ipec.*, Puls.

Sewer gas: Anth., Bov., Op.

Sycosis: Med., *Thuja,* Sars.

Tobacco, abuse of: Bell., Gels., Ign., Ipec., Nux, Phos., Sec.

Touched, from being: Spig.

Underground, living, working: Ant. t., Aran., Carbo v., Nat. s., Ter.

Undressing, when: Euphorb. amyg., Hep.

Unpleasant things, after talking about: Cham., Mar. v.

Vital forces exhausted: Ars., Carbo v., Crot., Psor., Sec.

Weather, cold, damp, rainy: Aran., Dul., Rhus, Mer., Nat. s.
damp, suddenly becoming cold: **Dul.**
dry, whether hot or cold: *Bry.*
dry and cold: Acon., Hep.
storm, approach of: Phos., Psor., Zinc.
every change from dry to wet: Nat. s.
hot days and cool nights: **Acon.,** Colch., Mer.
hot days and cool damp nights in autumn: Colch., *Mer.*
warm, during: *Ant. c., Ars., Bell.*, Bry., *Calc.*, **Caps.,** Carbo v., Ced., *Cina, Ipec.*, **Lach.,** Natr., Puls., **Sul.,** *Thuja.*

Whooping cough, during epidemic: Dros., Kali c.

Worms, or intestinal irritation: Cina, Spig., Sil.

Wounds, dissecting: *Ant. t.,* **Ars.,** Carb. ac., **Lach., Pyr.**

Yellow fever, during epidemic of: Cad. s.

PRODROME.

CONDITIONS OCCURRING DURING:

Abdomen, distention of: Ars. h.

Anguish: Cinch.

Anticipation of any unusual ordeal may hasten chill: Gels.

Anxiety: Ars., Ars. h., Cinch.

Appetite, loss of: Hydr.

Back, aching in: Aran., Carbo v., *Eup.,* Ipec., **Pod.,** Rhus.
pain in, above right ilium: Eup.
pain severe in lumbar region: *Æsc.,* **Pod.**
pain in lumbar region: Lac. ac.

Bilious, symptoms strongly marked: **Pod.**

Bones, pains in: Cinch., *Eup.,* Eup. p., Natr.
pains in, of extremities: Eup. p.
pains in, of extremities, as if broken: **Eup.,** Tub.

Bowels, pain in: Ars., Elat., Eup.
pain in, cutting like knives: Ars.

Chest, pain in: Ars., Plant.
pain in, cutting: Ars.
pain in, erratic: Plant.
oppression of: Ars. h.

Chilliness: Elat., Thuja.
and weakness some time before: *Thuja.*
and crawling after drinking: Ars.

Colic: Cinch., Eup.
pain in upper abdomen: Eup.

Cough: Apis, **Rhus,** Rum., Samb.
dry, teasing for hours: **Rhus.**
dry, hacking, in spells: *Eup. p.*
deep, dry, for half an hour with nausea, thirst: Samb.

Covered, desire to be: **Eup.,** Nux, Tub.

Debility: Anth., *Ars.,* Cinch., Corn. fl.

Dreads the attack: Coc., **Natr.**

Diarrhea: *Ars.,* Cina, *Puls.,* Ver.
mental emotions, from: Arg. n., Calc. ars., *Gels.,* Psor.
mucous, at night: **Puls.**
in early morning: **Fer.,** Sul.
previous night without thirst, if morning chill: *Puls.*

Drink, can *now:* Cimex.
can not, enough: *Eup.*
desire to, some time before: *Caps.,* Cinch., *Eup.,* Natr.

Drinking causes nausea and hastens chill: *Eup.,* Nux.
chilliness and crawling immediately after: Ars.
creeping over the back, after: Ars.
vomiting after: Ars., **Eup.,** *Natr.*
refreshes: *Arn.*

Excitement, mental: **Ced.**

Emotion, sudden mental, may hasten chill: Gels.

Emptiness, in head: Ars.

Epigastrium, entire goneness five days before attack: **Hydr.**
bloats, sensitive to touch: Coc.

Eruption, miliary, worse on forehead and face: Ailan.

Eyes, blue margins around: **Cina,** Phos.
burning in: Rhus.
pain over, in forehead: Lac. ac.

Eyeballs, painful soreness of: Eup., Pyr.

Face, heat of: Stram.
florid, animated: Ced.
pale: Ars., Cina, Fer.

Face, heat of, with blue margins around eyes: **Cina.**
yellow, sallow: **Ars. h.**

Feet, cold: Carbo v.

Fever: **Ced.,** Lyc., Nux, *Sul.*
evening, without chill: *Sul.*

Fright may hasten chill: Gels.

Gaping: (See yawning.)
and quivering: Elat.

Gastric disturbances: *Ant. c.,* Cyc., *Ipec.,* Puls.
disturbances, may bring on a relapse: *Ant. c., Ipec.*
disturbances, eating pork, fat, rich food, from: **Puls.**

Grief may hasten chill: **Gels.,** Ign.

Head, heat of: Ced., **Stram.**
heaviness of: *Calc.*
heaviness of, and body: Calc.
pain, violent in, and in back: Eup.
pain, pressive in: Ced.
throbbing in temples: Carbo v.
throbbing and dullness in: Plant.

Headache: *Æsc.,* Ars., Ars. h., **Bry.,** Carbo v., Chin. ars., Cinch., Ced., Corn., Elat., Ipec., *Natr.,* Plant., Rhus, *Thuja.*
bursting: Æsc., *Bry.*
stitching, jerking, throbbing from before backward, as if head would burst: **Bry.**

Heat: Ced., Lyc., *Nux, Sul.*
in evening: *Sul.*
general: Ced.
flushes of: Lyc., Sul.

Heart, palpitation of, with anxiety: Cinch.

Hunger: Cina, Cinch., Eup., **Staph.**
canine: Cinch.

Illness, a general feeling of: Cinch.

Ilium, pain above: Eup.

Irritable, irascible, peevish: Cham.

Joints, drawing pain in: Calc.
aching in large: Polyp.
aching in knees, ankles, elbows and wrists: Cham., ***Pod.***

Languor: Ars., *Bap.,* Natr., Polyp., Tub.
wants to lie down: *Bap.,* Tub.

Limbs, drawing in: Ars., Bry., ***Nux.***
drawing in, upper: Ars. h.
drawing pain in thighs and legs: **Nux.**
drawing up and stretching out: Ars., **Nux.**
drawing pain as if in periosteum: *Arn.,* Pyr.
heaviness of lower: Cimex.
pain in: Carbo v., Elat., *Eup.,* Natr., ***Nux, Rhus.***
pain, tearing, in: *Carbo v.*
pain, tearing, in hands, feet, and kidneys: ***Natr.***
paralytic weakness of: Nux.
soreness of: Elat.

Lip, upper, excoriated: Ars. h.

Liver, constant pain in region of, with nausea and vomiting: Tar.

Malaise: Ars., Bap., Tub.

Melancholy: **Ant. c.,** Ced., Puls.
spirits depressed, senses dull: Ced.

Neck, pain in: Ars. h.

Nose, excoriated: Ars. h.

News, bad, may hasten chill: *Gels.*

Nausea: Amm., Cina, *Cinch., Eup.,* **Ipec.,** Lyc., Natr., Puls., Samb.
and thirst, night before: **Eup.**
and vomiting: Lyc., Natr.
and retching: Ipec.

Paroxysm, always better before the: **Psor.**

Periosteum: (See limbs.)

Retching, violent: Ipec.

Sadness, great: **Ant. c.**

Saliva, flow of: Ipec., Rhus.

Shuddering: *Ars.,* **Ign.,** Lach.
after thirst: Lach.
after drinking: **Caps.**

Skin, blue: Arn.

Sleep, restless: Anth., Arn., *Cinch.*
restless, night before paroxysm: **Cinch.**

Sleepiness: Ars., Corn., Puls.
and drowsiness all day: Puls.
night before: **Ars.**
preceded for days by: Corn.

Sleeplessness: Amm. m.
night before: Cinch.

Sneezing, when exposed to cold air: Cinch.

Sore, bruised feeling: Arn., Bap., Pyr.
bruised feeling of limbs: Elat.
bruised feeling of parts lain on: Bap., Pyr.

Stomach, cramp in: Aran.

Stretching: Æsc., Amyl, Ant. t., Aran., Arn., *Ars.,* Bry., Chin. ars., *Eup.,* Ign., *Ipec., Natr.,* Rhus.
of limbs: Ars., *Nux,* Plant., Rhus.
and drawing in limbs: Bry.
and aching in limbs: Rhus.

Sweating: Corn., Nux, Samb., *Ver.*
after exercise: Bry., Corn., Psor.

Taste, bitter, in mouth, hours before: Hep.

Thirst: Alst., Amm., Ang., **Arn.,** Ars., Bor., *Bry.,* Cimex, Cina, **Cinch., Eup.,** Lach., Lob., *Puls.,* Samb., *Sul.*
and bone pains for some time before: **Eup.,** *Natr.*

Thirst, but hurts to swallow: Gels.
some time before: **Caps.**, Cinch., Natr.
for large quantities of cold water: **Arn.**, Eup., Bry.
for warm drinks: *Eup.*, Casc., Ced.
then shuddering: Lach.

Tonsils, pressure in: Ars. h.

Trembles, as after severe illness: Bap.

Toothache: Carbo v.

Uneasiness: Caps.

Urine, incontinence of, sets in before: Gels.

Urticaria, itching, stinging: *Hep.*

Vertigo: Ars., Bry., Natr.

Vomiting: Apis, Arn., Cina, *Eup., Fer.*, Lyc., Natr., Puls., Sec.
of bile: Cina, **Eup.**
of ingesta: Cina, *Eup.*, **Fer.**
of mucus: Puls.
of ingesta, water: *Natr.*
sudden: Apis.
sour: Lyc., Rob.

Weakness: *Ars.*, Ars. h., Bap., Natr., Thuja, Pyr.
weariness and inclination to lie down: Ars., *Bap.*, Rhus.

Wrists, aching in: Arn., Polyp., Pod.

Woeful mood: **Ant. c.**

Yawning: Æsc., Ant. t., Aran., Arn., Ars., Ars. h., Chin. ars., Cinch., Elat., *Eup.*, Ign., Ipec., Natr., Nicc., Nux, Rhus.
mouth remains open for a time, when: Ant. t.

COMMENCEMENT OF CHILL.

CHILL BEGINS IN:

Abdomen: Apis, *Bry.,* Col., Cur., *Ign.,* Ver.
and extends to fingers and toes: Calad.
which spreads out as if from: Mar. v.

Ankles, between knees and: Cinch., Lach., Puls.

Arms: Bell., Dig., **Hell.,** *Ign.,* Mez., Plat.
both, in: *Bell.,* Hell., Mez.
both, at once, in, thence over the body: **Bell.**
front of: Chlor.
upper, and spreads to chest and back: **Ign.**
upper and thighs: Psor.

Arm, right: *Mercurialis.*
right and leg: Apis, Kreos., Rhus.
right, right side of chest: Mercurialis.
left: Carbo v., *Nux.*
left, and lower limbs: **Nux m.**
left, and hand: Carbo v.
on which he lies: Carbo v.

Back: Ang., Arg. m., Ars. h., Bap., Benz. ac., Bov., Cac., Canth., Calc. ars., **Caps.,** Ced., Chlor., Chin. s., Cim., Crot., Dul., **Eup., Eup. p.,** *Gamb.,* Gels., Hipp., Jatrop., Kali i., Kali m., **Lach.,** Led., *Lyc.,* Natr., **Polyp.,** Rhus, Sarr., *Sep.,* Spong.
running up the: **Canth.,** Mer., Sul.
passing up and down, thence over the body: Eup. pur., **Gels.**
dorsal region: *Eup.,* Gels., **Lach.,** Med., Natr., Tub.
interscapular region: **Caps.,** Eup. p., Led., **Polyp.,** Rhus, Sarr., *Sep.*
lumbar region: **Eup. p., Lach., Natr.**
spreads from the: Act., Cup. s., *Eup., Gels.*
spreads from the, towards arms and chest: Calc. ars.

Back, spreads from the, all over body, to left leg, then to right leg: Cup. s.
spreads over, and on left scapula: Dios.
over entire: Stan.

Body, left side: Caust.
right side: Bry., Natr., Rhus.

Chest: *Apis,* Ars., *Carbo an.,* Cic., Cina, Kreos., Lith., Mercurialis, Nux, Rhus, *Sep.,* Spig.
and extends down the legs and into the arms: Cic.
and extends from face downward: Lil. t.
front of, in: **Apis.**
right side of, in: **Mercurialis.**

Ears, in: Cyc.

Face: Bar., Berb., *Caust.,* Kreos., Petr.

Feet: Apis, Arn., Bar., *Chel.,* Cimex, Gels., Hyos., Kali bi., Mag. c., Med., **Natr.,** Nux m., *Nux,* Sabad., Sarr., *Sep.,* Sul.
and legs: Kali bi.
soles of: Dig.

Fingers: *Bry.,* Cof., Dig., Med., **Natr.,** Nux, *Sep.,* Sul.
and toes: Med.
tips of: **Bry.,** Cyc., Natr.
tips and toes: **Bry.,** Cyc., Dig., Meny., Natr., Nux, **Sep.,** Stan., Sul.
tips, toes and nose: Cyc.

Foot, right: Chel., Lyc., Sab.

Hands: **Chel.,** Bry., Benz. ac., Dig., Eup., **Gels.,** *Nux,* Rhus, Sabad., Sul.
with clenching of: Cimex.
palms of: Dig.
palms of, and soles of feet: *Dig.*
and feet: Apis, Bry., Calc., Carbo v., Chel., Calend., Dig., Gels., **Natr.,** Nux m., Op., Sabad., Sul.

Hand, left: **Carbo v.,** Nux m.
right: **Mercurialis.**

Heart, region of: Spig.

Head: *Bar.,* Natr., Stan.

Knees: **Apis,** Benz. ac., Thuja.
and thighs: *Thuja.*

Legs: Ced., *Cinch.,* Kali bi., *Nux m.,* Thuja.
below the knees: Cinch.
lower: Nux m.

Lips: **Bry.**

Mouth, around the: Bry.

Neck: Staph., Val.
and back: Kali m.
nape of, running down the back: Val.
nape of, and running along the spine between the shoulders: Polyp.

Nose: Sabad., Zinc., Tub.

Shoulders, begins on: Lach.
between: Sarr.

Scalp, in: Mosch.

Scapulæ, sometimes between the: Rhus.
begins over left: Dios.

Scrobiculus cordis: Bell., Bry., *Calc.,* Helon.
with spasms, or fixed cold agonizing weight: **Calc.**

Stomach: Berb., Bry., Cahinca.
from pit to abdomen: Spig.

Thighs: Ced., Ther., **Thuja.**
in one: Rhus.

Thorax, shudder starting from: Lith.

Touching, anything cold, begins from: Zinc., Zinc. val.

Vertex: Arum t.
to chest: Ol. an.

CHILL, LOCATION OF.

CHILL; PART AFFECTED, LOCATION OF.

Abdomen: **Æth.**, Agar., *Apis,* Ars., **Calc.**, Cham., Chel., Cist., Colch., Cur., *Ign.,* Mar. v., **Meny.**, *Mer., Mercurialis,* **Mez.**, **Op.**, *Par.,* Phos. ac., *Puls., Sec.,* Sul., Ter., Ver., Zinc.
coldness and chill in: Ter.
coldness, objective and subjective: Agar.
and chest: *Apis,* Spig.
to fingers and toes: Calad.

Arms: **Bell.**, *Camph., Caust.,* Cham., Cic., Dig., Euph., *Hell.,* Ign., Kali bi., **Mez.**, Op., *Puls.,* Sec., *Sil.,* Sul., Ver.
upper and spreads to back and chest: **Ign.**
backs of: Berb.

Arm, left: **Carbo v.**, *Nux m.,* Rhus, Stan.
right: Lyssin, **Mercurialis.**

Ascends: **Acon.**, Amm. m., *Ars.,* Benz., Caust., Cina, Coff., Eup., *Gels.,* **Hyos.**, Kali bi., *Sabad.,* Sul.
feet to chest, from: *Acon.,* Benz.
extremities of fingers and toes to chest, head and vertex, from: *Benz.,* Coff.
upper part of body to head, from: *Cina.*

Axilla: Astacus.

Back, in or on the: Æsc., Agar., Amyl, Alum., Ang., Apis, Ars., Ars. h., Asaf., Bell., Bov., Benz. ac., Berb., **Cac.**, Calc. ars., *Camph., Canch., Canth.,* Caps., Carbo an., Ced., Cham., Chel., Cim., Coc., Coff., Con., Croc., Crot. t., Cup. s., Dios., Dul., **Eup.**, **Eup. p.**, *Gels.,* Ham., Hydr., Hyos., Ign., Ipec., Kali bi., Kali m., Kalm., Lac. ac., **Lach.**, *Led., Lob., Lyc.,* Mag. c., Meny., Nit. s. d., **Natr.**, Sep., Stan., Staph., *Stram.,* **Sul.**, Val., Ver.

Back, creeping up and down the: *Æsc., Crot.*, Gels., Med.
and abdomen: Cham.
from small of, to lower limbs: Nit. s. d.
extending to hips: Berb.
water were running down, as if: Agar.
running down the back and through the limbs: Colch., Mag. c., Nit. s. d.
running down the back, body and in a zigzag course: Med.
running down the: Act., *Agar.*, Apis, Bell., Canch., **Canth.,** Carbo an., *Caust., Chel., Cina, Coff., Croc., Eup.*, **Eup. p.,** Ipec., Lob., Med., Phos., Staph., **Stram.,** Val., Zinc.
running down the, and terminating in the pit of stomach: **Bell.**
running down the, and right arm: Lept.
running down the, with heat in stomach: *Lob.*
and sides, over: **Meny.**
runs up the: Æsc., Amm. m., Arg. n., Ars., Eup., *Eup. p.*, **Gels.,** Hyos., Ipec., Kali bi., Kali i., **Lach.,** Mag. s., Mer. s., Nat. s., Puls., *Sabad.*, Sul.
runs up and down the: Amyl, **Eup. p., Gels.**
runs up from sacrum to occiput in rapid successive waves: **Gels.,** Lach., Lachn., *Sul.*
runs up with shaking and chattering of teeth without external coldness: Nat. s.
constantly creeps up the, from sacrum: **Sul.**
interscapular region, in the: **Caps.,** Eup., Led., **Polyp.,** Sarr., *Sep.*, Sul.
interscapular region like a piece of ice: **Lachn.**
lumbar region, in the: Asaf., **Eup. p., Lach.,** Led.

Body, all over the: Agar., Alum., Anac., Ant. t., Arn., Ars., Calad., **Camph.,** Canch., Canth., Carbo an., **Carbo v.,** Ced., Chel., **Chin. s.,** Cic., Cim., **Cinch.,** Coc., Con., Cup., Cur., Dig., Dul., Eup., Eup. p., Euphor., Fer., Gamb., Gels., Graph., Hep., Hyos., **Ign.,** Iris, Kali i., Kali m., *Lach.*, Lachn., Lys., *Lyc.*, Mar. v., *Meny.*, Mer., *Mercurialis,* **Mez., Nux m., Nux,** Op., *Petr.*, Phel., Phos. ac.,

Puls., **Rhus**, *Sec.*, *Sep.*, Spig., **Staph.**, *Stram.*, *Sul. ac.*, Stan., **Ver.**, *Ver. v.*, Zinc.

all over the, and head, with heat and redness of face: **Arn.**, Can. s., Cham.

all over the, alternating with heat of face: *Cham.*

all over the, with burning heat of face, which comes out of the eyes like fire: **Cham.**

all over the, with a stretched sensation: Calad.

all over, except face, neck and genitals: *Amb.*

anterior parts of: Cham.

lower parts of, face hot: Calc. p.

posterior parts of, only: Cham., *Ign.*

posterior parts of, with heat of anterior: **Cham.**

upper parts of: **Meny.**

one side of: Arn., Bar., **Bry.**, **Carbo v.**, **Caust.**, Chel., Dig., Elat., Fer., *Lach.*, **Lyc.**, Nat. c., Natr., Nux, Par., *Phos.*, Puls., Rhus, *Sep.*, **Sil.**, Thuja, **Ver.**

left side of: **Carbo v.**, **Caust.**, Elat., Fer., *Lach.*, **Lyc.**, Nat. c., Rhus, **Thuja.**

right side of: Arn., **Bry.**, Natr., **Par.**, *Rhus*, **Thuja.**

right side of, from head to feet, the other half natural warmth: **Par.**

right side of, with heat of left: Par., **Rhus.**

on side on which he lies: **Arn.**

on icy cold spots here and there: *Par.*, Ter.

Bowels: Gymno.

Cheeks: Colch.

Chest: **Apis**, Carbo an., Cham., Cic., Cina, Hydr., *Ign.*, *Mercurialis*, Nat. p., Par., Sep., **Sul.**, Sul. ac., Zinc.

and abdomen: **Apis**, Par., *Sul.*, Spig.

and extends to legs and arms: *Cic.*

right side of: **Mercurialis.**

Coldness, external: Agar.

internal, as if frozen: Aran.

internal, organs of: **Cal.**

Coldness, with external heat: Rheum.
external, with internal heat: Zinc.

Descends: Agar., Bar., Bor., Canch., Carb. ac., Caust., Cic., Lil., *Phos.,* Val., **Ver.**
from head to toes of both feet: **Ver.**

Epigastrium: *Arn.,* Bar., **Bell., Calc.**

Extremities: Colch.
to face and head: *Acon., Benz.,* **Gels.**
of fingers and toes, to chest, head and vertex: *Benz.*

Face, of: Aster., **Bar.,** Berb., Cann. I., Caust., Cham., Ign., Lil., Mer. c., *Petr.*
left side of, after midnight: *Dros.*

Feet, of: Alum., Aur., Benz. ac., Chel., Hyos., Ign., **Meny., Mez.,** Nux, Op., *Sep.,* **Sil.**
extending to calves: Crot. t.
soles of: Col., **Dig.,** Lith., Manc., *Meny.*
as if in cold water: Mag. c., Mer., **Meny., Sep.**

Genitals, icy coldness of: **Sul.**

Glands, cervical, painful swelling of: Cist., Tub.

Fingers, on the: *Bry., Meny.,* Natr., **Phos. ac.**
tips of, on the: *Bry.,* **Phos. ac.**

Hands: Aur., Benz. ac., **Cac., Camph.,** Can. I., *Canth.,* **Carbo v.,** *Chel.,* Colch., Col., Dros., Fer., *Hep., Hyos.,* Ipec., Led., *Lyc.,* Manc., **Meny.,** Mer., Mer. c., **Mez.,** *Natr., Nux,* **Op.,** Polyp., **Phos., Sec., Ver.**
and feet cold with warmth of rest of body: Col., **Meny.**
cold, mouth and throat hot: Jatr.
and feet cold, head hot: Nat. c.

Head: Chlor., Lac. ac., Mer. c.
occiput in: *Dul.*
to extremities: **Ver.**

Hips: Ham., Mez.

Hip, right: Bry., *Mercurialis,* Rhus.
left: Carbo v., Caust., Thuja.

Knees: Apis, Carbo v., China, Ign., **Phos., Sil.,** Stan.
icy coldness of right: *Chel.*

Larynx, cold sensation in: Cist.

Legs: *Caust.,* Cic., Cocc., Coff., Colch., Ign., Kalm., Lac. ac., **Meny.,** *Nux,* Op., Par., Puls., **Rhus,** *Sec., Sil.,* **Stram.,** *Sul.,* Ter.
to knees: Aur.
running up to back: Caust.
running up: Ham.

Leg, left: Carbo v., Caust., Ol. an., Stan., Thuja.
right, icy coldness of: *Chel., Sab.,* **Sep.**
right as if standing in cold water: *Sab.,* **Sep.,** Tub.

Limbs: Chlor.
very cold, body hot: Ter.

Loins: Asaf., Camph., *Puls.,* Thuja.

Mouth and throat hot with cold hands: Jatr.

Neck, running down from: Par., Val.
nape of: Chin. s.

Nose: Can. I., Colch.

Parts, single, of: **Amb.,** Ars., Asar., Bar., Bell., Benz., Bry., Calad., *Calc.,* **Caust.,** *Cham.,* Col., Hep., Hydr., **Ign.,** *Led.,* Lyc., **Mez.,** Nux, Par., **Puls.,** Rhus, **Sep.,** *Sil., Spig., Thuja,* Ver.

Sacrum: Æsc., Asaf., Eup. p., Puls., Sul.

Shoulders: Clem., Hydr., *Kali bi.,* Lach., *Polyp.,* Ver.
across: Chin. s.
between: Lachn., Sarr.

Solar plexus, radiating from: Helon.

Soles and hands, rest of body warm: Col.

Spots, isolated, as from cold substances: Berb., Par.

Stomach, pit of: **Arn.,** Bar., *Bell., Calc.*
pit of, most severely felt in: **Arn.**
chilly shivering in: *Colch.*

Thighs, with aching in: Hydr.
Chlor., Thuja.

Vertex to chest, shuddering from: Ol. an.

CHILL AGGRAVATED.

Air, in a draft of: Caps., Carbo an., Dulc., **Nux.**
in open: Anac., Agar., Ant. t., **Ars.,** *Bar.,* Bufo, Canth., Carb. ac., Calc. p., Calend., Cham., Chel., Cinch., Dulc., **Hep.,** Kali chl., Lil., *Mer.,* Mer. c., Mosch., Myr., Nit. ac., *Nux m.,* **Nux,** Ol. an., Petr., Plat., Polyp., *Puls.,* Ran., Rhus, Seneg., Sep., Sul., Zinc.

Arms, motion of: Helon.

Awakes, as often as he: *Amm. m.*

Bed, by getting out of: Bar., *Canth.,* **Nux,** *Sil.*
by getting into: Aran., Bov., Pyr.
as long as he is out of: Hell.

Dampness, exposure to: **Aran.,** *Calc.,* Dul., *Rhus.*

Days, cold during: Acon., *Aran.,* Cham., Ign.
rainy, during: *Aran., Cur.,* Dul., **Rhus.**

Drinking, by: Alum., *Ars.,* Arn., Asar., Cad. s., Can., **Caps.,** Cinch., Coc., Croc., *Elaps, Eup., Lob.,* Lyc., Mez., **Nux,** *Rhus,* Sil., Tarax., **Ver.**

Drinks, warm, after: *Alum.,* Cham.
cold, after: Calend.

Eating, after: Arg. n., **Bell.,** Carbo an., Coc., Euph., **Graph., Kali c.,** Mar., *Rhus,* Tarax.
and drinking, after: Asar., Tarax.
during: Euph., Lyc., *Rhus.*

Evening, in the: Carbo v., Cyc., **Kali c.,** Lyc., *Puls.*

Exercising, when: *Ars.,* Bar., Mer., Nux, Sil., Sul.
when in open air: Sul. ac.

Motion, by: *Acon.,* Agar., Alum., *Ant. t., Apis,* Arn., **Bry.,** Camph , *Canth.,* Ced., Chin. ars., Cinch., Cof., *Cur.,* Eup., *Hep., Kali c.,* Kali n., Mer. c., *Nit. ac.,* **Nux, Rhus, Sep., Sil.,** Spig., Sul., Thuja.

Moving hands and feet to cool part of bed: Chin. ars.

Pains: Aur.

Rest, during: Dros., Rhus.

Rising from stooping: Mer.

Room, in a: **Apis,** Bry., **Ipec.,** Sul. ac.
warm: Arg. n., Croc., Grat.
coming in from open air: Arg. n.

Smoking, by: Coc., *Ign.*

Stove, near a warm: Alum., **Apis,** Cinch., Ipec., Nux, Sep.

Thinking of it: Chin. ars.

Touched, when: **Acon.,** Arg. n., Spig.

Touching anything cold: Zinc.

Uncovered: *Acon.,* Agar., *Amm. m.,* Arg. n., Arn., Bell., Bor., Card. m., Carbo an., Cham., Clem., *Cyc.,* Mercurialis, *Nit. ac.,* Nux m., **Nux,** Stram., *Thuja.*
returns when: Arg. n.

Undressing, when: Cham.

Walking in the open air: Alum., Amm. c., *Ars.,* Cad. s., Caust., Chel., Cinch., Kali chl., Mer., Nit. ac., **Nux, Petr., Puls.,** Rhus, Tab.

Warmth, in: Alum., Anac., Ant. c., **Apis,** Ars., Bell., Bry., Bor., Canth., Caust., Cic., Cina, Cinch., Coc., Dulc., Grat., Guaj., Iod., **Ipec.,** Kreos., Laur., Mag. m., Meny., Mer., Mez., Natr., Nux m., Phos., Puls., Rhus, Ruta, Sep., Sil., Staph., Spong.

Water, by bathing with cold: Ant. c., Aran., Phos., Rhus.
washing hands in cold: Lac d., Phos.

Weather, in damp: Cur., Dul., **Rhus.**

Wind, in cold: *Acon.*, Cur., Hep.

CHILL AMELIORATED.

Air, in open: *Graph., Ipec.*, Phos., Puls., Sul. ac.

Bed, covering up in, by: *Kali i.*, Mag. s., **Pod.**, Rhus.
covering up warmly in, by: Hyp., **Pod.**
getting out of, by: Aur., Lyc., *Ver.*
warmth of, by: Kali i.

Covering, by: Mercurialis, *Pod.*, Rhus.

Dinner, before: Berb.

Drinking, after: **Caust.**, *Graph., Ipec.*

Eating, after: Amb., *Cur.*, Ign., Nat. c., Phos.

Exercise in open air, by: **Caps.**, Mag. c., *Puls., Staph.*, Sul. ac.

Heat of hot irons: **Caps.**, *Lachn.*

Held, by being: *Gels.*, Lach.
firmly, by being: **Lach.**

Lying down, after: Kali c., Kali n., Mag. m., Mercurialis, Rhus, Sul.

Motion, on: Apis, Arn., Asar., Bell., **Caps.**, Cyc., Mer., Mez., Nit. ac., Nux, Pod., Rhus, Sil., Spig.

Pressed down upon, by being: *Lach.*

Rising, on: Rhus.

Room, disappears when in: Chel.

Sitting, by: Ign., Nux.

Sleep, after: Bry., Nux.
during: Rhus.

Sunshine, by exposure to: Anac., Con.

Uncovering, by: Camph., Med., Sec.

Walking in the open air: **Caps.**

Warmth, external: **Ars.**, Bar., Camph., Caps., Carbo an., Cic., *Cinch.,* Con., Coral., **Ign.,** *Kali c., Lach., Meny., Mez.* Nicc., Nux m., Nux, Ptel., *Sabad.,* Sul.

Wrapping up, followed by severe fever and sweat: **Sil.**

SYMPTOMS DURING THE CHILL.

Chill absent: *Anac., Ars., Apis, Calc.,* Caust., Cham., Cina. Cof., Eup., Fer., Fl. ac., *Gels.,* Hep., Ipec., Kali b., Kali c., Lachn., Lyc., Natr., Nux, Petr., Rhus, Stram., Sul., *Thuja.*

Chill predominates: *Alum., Amm. m.,* **Ant. c., Aran., Arn.,** *Bov.,* **Camph., Canth.,** Caps., Carbo v., *Ced.,* **Chin. s.,** Cim., Cina, **Cinch.,** *Coc.,* Dig., *Dros.,* Elaps, Hep., Laur., Led., *Lyc.,* **Meny.,** Mercurialis, **Mez., Nux,** Petros., Petr., *Polyp., Rob.,* Rhus, **Sabad.,** Sec., Sep., **Staph.,** Tar., Thuja, **Ver.**

predominates, afternoon, in the: Apis, Arn., **Ars., Lyc., Puls.,** *Rhus,* Thuja.

predominates, at noon: *Ant. c.,* Elat., **Sul.**

predominates, morning, in the: *Bry.,* **Eup., Natr., Nux,** *Pod., Sep.,* Ver.

predominates, evening, in the: Alum., Arn., *Cina,* Cyc., Hep., *Phos.,* **Puls., Rhus, Sul.**

predominates, night, at: Apis, *Mer.,* Phos.

Chill in General: Acon., Æth., *Agar., Alum.,* Alst., Amb., Amm. c., Amm. m., *Anac.,* Ang., **Ant. c.,** *Ant. t., Apis,* **Aran.,** Arg., **Arn.,** *Ars.,* Asaf., Asar., Bap., Bell., Benz., Berb., Bov., Bry., Cac., Calad., Calc., **Camph.,** Canch., **Canth.,** *Caps.,* Carbo an., *Carbo v.,* Caust., **Ced., Cham.,** Chel., **Chin. s.,** Cic., *Cim., Cina,* **Cinch.,** Coca, Cof., Colch., Col., Con., Corn., Croc., Cup., Cyc., Daph., *Dig.,* Dros., Elat., *Elaps, Eup., Eup. p.,* Euphor., Euon., Fer., Gamb.,

Gels., Graph., Guaj., Hell., *Hep.*, *Hyos.*, *Ign.*, Iod., *Ipec.*, Kali b., *Kali c.*, *Kali i.*, Kali n., *Kreos.*, *Lach.*, Lachn., Laur., *Led.*, *Lob.*, *Lyc.*, Mar., *Meny.*, Mag. c., Mag. m., Mag. s., Mercurialis, Mer., **Mez.**, Mur. ac., Natr., Nat. c., *Nit. ac.*, *Nux m.*, **Nux, Op.**, Par., *Petr.*, Phos. ac., Phos., Plant., *Pod.*, Polyp., Psor., *Puls.*, **Rob.**, **Rhus**, Ruta, **Sabad.**, Sab., Samb., Sarr., Sars., **Sec.**, *Sep.*, *Sil.*, Spig., Stan., *Staph.*, *Stram.*, *Sul.*, **Tarax.**, Ther., **Thuja**, Val., Ver.

CHILL, CHARACTER OF.

Alternating with heat or sudden cold sweat: Croc.
- heat and chill: **Amm. m.**, **Ars.**, *Bap.*, Bar., **Bell.**, *Bry.*, **Calc.**, Cham., **Cinch.**, Dig., *Cyc.*, *Elaps*, Hell., **Hep.**, Hyos., **Ign.**, Laur., *Lyc.*, Mag. m., **Mer.**, **Nux**, Phos., **Psor.**, **Rhus**, Sec., *Sep.*, **Sul.**, Ver., Zinc.
- with heat, not perceptible to touch: **Mer.**
- with dry, burning heat: *Bell.*, **Mal.**, *Pyr.*, Sanic.
- with thirst then sweat: Sabad.
- with flushes: Lachn.
- with pain in joints: Hell.

Coldness, icy: Bis., Cad. s., Nat. s., **Tar.**
- and trembling, then general rigor: Sul. ac.
- intense, of limbs, body hot: Ter.
- intense, with shaking: Tar.
- running downwards: Sul. ac.
- even when near the fire: Cad. s.
- not > by warmth: Asar.

Fright, from, during menses: Amm. c., Psor., Thuja.

Irregular, and flushes of heat: Ter.

Long-lasting, passing off without heat or sweat: Hep., Lyc., Tar.

Severe, as if frozen: Aran., Camph., Ver.

Shaking: Aran., **Chin. s.**, Zinc.

Shaking, with pale, sunken face: Zinc., Ver.

Waves, chill comes in: Chin. ars., Gels.

CHILL, SYMPTOMS DURING.

Abdomen, bloated: Cina, *Kali c.*
cold: Æth., Apis, *Ars.,* Cham., Chel.. *Cinch.,* Cist., **Meny.,** Phos. ac., Puls., Sec.
restlessness and heaviness in: Mer. s.
coldness in from pressure with the hand: **Meny.**
pain in: Aran., Ars., Bov., Bry., Calad., Calc., Cal. p., Cinch., Cof., Eup., Ign., Lach., Meph., Mercurialis, Mer., Nit. ac., Nux, Phos., Pod., Puls., Rhus, Rumex, Sep.
pulse beat in: Card. m.

Air, sensation of being too hot: *Puls., Sep.*
of room seems too hot: *Apis,* **Puls., Sep.**
sensitiveness to cold: *Bar.,* **Camph.,** *Canth.,* Caps., Carbo an., Caust., Chel., Cof., Cyc., *Dig.,* Elaps, **Hep.,** Kali c., Kalm., Mer., *Mez.,* Nux, *Petr.,* Plumb., **Sil., Stram., Thuja.**
open, sensitive to: Ars., *Bap.,* Camph., *Caps.,* Chel., **Hep.,** *Mer.,* Mez., *Nux,* Polyp., Sul., Thuja.
warm, feels cold: **Thuja.**

Ankles, swollen: Chin. s.

Ants, as if biting over whole body, at night: Gamb.

Alternate flushes and chilliness: Lachn.

Anxiety: Acon., Anth., Ars., Camph., Caps., Nux, Puls., Ver.

Appetite good: *Chin. s.*
loss of: Anth.

Arms, cold: Bell., Dig., Hell., Mez.
paralytic weakness of: Phos. ac.
distention of the veins of: **Chel.,** Meny. (See veins, distended.)

Back, small of the, lameness of the: Coc.
small of the, lameness of the, and sore: Lept.
craves heat to: Caps., Eup. p.
craves heat to, without relief: Eup.
cold water poured down, as if: Alumen.
lumbar region, aching in: Myr.
pain in: Anth., Apis, Ars., Bell., Calc., *Caps.*, Carbo v., Caust., **Chin. s.**, Dios., Elat., *Eup.*, Gamb., Hyos., Ign., Lach., Lys., Mosch., Natr., **Nux,** Pod., **Polyp.**, Puls., Zinc.

Blood, feeling as though it did not circulate: **Lyc.**, Rōb.
feeling as though cold: Acon., Ars., *Lyc.*, **Rhus.**

Body cold, internal burning heat: Euphor.

Bones, pains in: Aran., Arn., Ars., Eup., Eup. p., Natr., Nux, Polyp., Rhus, Sabad., Tub.
aching in: **Arn.**, Dios.

Bowels, aching in: Æth.
pain in: Gym.

Breath cold: **Carbo v.**, *Ver.*
desire to take a long: Cimex.
hot: Anac., Camph., Cham., **Rhus.**

Breathing, oppressed: Apis, Ars., Bry., Natr., Nux.

Bruised, feeling as if: **Arn.**, **Bap.**, Pyr.

Cheek, heat in one: *Acon.*, Arn.
redness of one: Acon., Arn., *Cham.*, Ipec.
heat and redness of one: **Arn.**
redness of one, the other pale and cold: *Acon.*, Cham., Ipec.
one pale and hot, the other red and cold: Mosch.

Cheeks, cold: Chel., *Cina, Petr., Rhus,* Rheum, Sec.
hot: *Acon.*, Bry., Calc., Cham., *Cina, Cinch.*, Led., Puls., Staph.
red: Alum., *Ars., Cinch.*, Kreos., Mercurialis.
red, dark: *Alum.*

Chest, oppression of: **Apis,** *Bry.,* Cimex, Ipec., Lach., Mercurialis, *Mez., Natr., Puls.*
fullness of: Ant. t.
pains in: Ars., Bell., Chin. s., Lach., *Sabad., Rhus,* Senega.
pains in, boring: Med.
panting, beating in: Calad.
soreness of: Lach.
stitches in: **Bry.,** Eup., Kali c., Lach., *Rhus, Rumex,* Sabad.

Coldness, chill severe with little: Eup.
alternating with heat on different parts of the body: Arundo.
deathly, of whole body: Bis., Camph.
great, of single parts: Asar.

Colic: Coc., Eup., *Led.,* Mer. c.
one day, chilly the next: Eup.

Coma: Bell., *Hep., Natr.*

Convulsions: *Lach.,* Mer., Nux.
choreic: Tar.
choreic aggravated after punishment: Ign., Tar.

Coryza: Calad., Calc. p., Elat.

Cough: Apis, **Bry.,** Calc., Calc. p., Cina, Kreos., Phos., *Psor.,* **Rhus,** Rum., **Sabad.,** *Samb.,* Sul.
drinking causes: **Psor.**
drinking, dry, uninterrupted, with tickling in the larynx, after: Cimex.

Covered, cannot bear to be: **Camph.,** Med.
desire to be: Arn., Camph., *Eup.,* Hep., Natr., Nat. ars., **Nux,** Phos., **Stram.,** Tub.

Covering, not relieved by: Asar., Cac., **Nux,** *Phos.,* Pyr., Rhus.

Cramps: Mag. p., *Sil.*

Crawling of single parts: Calad.

Debility, with: Anth.

Delirium: Agar., *Arn.,* Astacus, Bell., **Natr.,** Nux, Sul., Ver.

Depression of spirits: Mer. s.

Diarrhea: Ars., Elat., Phos., Rhus, Ver.

Diseased parts, coldness of: Caust.

Dyspnea: **Apis,** Arn., Cina, *Natr.,* Nux, Puls.

Earache: Graph., Gamb.

Ears, Cold: Cic., Natr.
hot: Acon., **Ign.,** Ran.
buzzing in: Glon.
red: *Bell.,* Ign.
ringing in: Ced., **Chin. s.**
stitches in: Gamb.
swelling of glands below and in the throat: Cist.

Elbows, pain in: Ang., **Pod.**
lacking in: Hell.

Empty feeling in stomach: Ailant.

Epistaxis: Kreos.

Eructations, empty: Gamb.

Exhaustion: Amb., Aran., Ipec., Mercurialis.

Extremities, cold and blue: *Camph.,* Stram., Nux, **Ver.**
cramps in: Ced., Cup.
icy cold: **Camph.,** *Canth.,* Carbo v., *Ced.,* Colch., Con., Hep., Ipec., Lyc., **Meny.,** Mur. ac., *Natr.,* Nux m., **Nux, Phos.,** Samb., *Stram.,* **Ver.**

Eyes, fixed: Acon.
pain in: Lac. ac., Senega.
sensation of foreign substance in right, then in left eye: Med.
sensitiveness to light: Nux.
smarting of: Ced.

Eyelids, tumefied: Astacus.

Face, bloated and red: *Amm. m., Bell.*
burning: Mur. ac.

Face and hands bloated: *Lyc.*
blueness of: Natr., **Nux,** Petr., **Stram.,** Tar.
cold: *Camph.,* Chel., *Cina, Dros., Hep.,* Ign., Iris, **Nux,** Mer. c., *Petr., Puls.,* Rhus, *Sec., Stram.,* **Ver.**
cold and collapsed: *Camph., Ver.*
flushed: Glon.
hot: Acon., Agar., Alum., Amb., Anac., *Apis,* **Arn.,** Bell., Berb., Bry., Calc., Calc. p., Ced., Cham., Cinch., Col., Dig., *Dros.,* Euph., *Fer.,* Gels., Hell., *Hyos.,* Jatr., Kreos., Lach., Led., Lyc., Mer., Mercurialis, Mez., Mur. ac., Nat. c., **Nux,** Oleand., Puls., Ran., *Rhus,* Sab., Samb., Senega, Staph., *Stram.,* Sul.
hot and red: Arn.
heat and redness of the, rest of the body cold: **Arn.,** Dig.
hot alone, rest of body cold: *Arn.*
pale: Ant. t., Bell., *Camph.,* Canth., Cinch., Chin. s., *Cina, Dros., Hep.,* Ign., *Nux m.,* Nux, *Puls., Sec.,* Sul., **Ver.,** Ver. v.
pale when lying down, red when sitting up: **Bell.**
pain (sticking) in left side of: Dros.
right half of, hot and dry: **Dros.**
red: Agar., *Acon.,* **Amm. m.,** Arn., Ars., Astac., **Bell.,** Bry., Cham., Cinch., Dig., Fer., *Hyos.,* **Ign.,** Kreos., Led., Lyc., Mercurialis, Mer., Nux, Plumb., Puls., *Rhus,* Stram., Sul.
red, and pale alternately: Rhus.
red, while sitting up: **Bell.**
twitching of, worse on left side: Tar.

Fainting: *Val.*
death like: Alumen.

Fanned continually, desire to be: Carbo v.

Feet, burning and cold alternately: Graph.
cold: Acon., Alum., Ang., Ant. c., *Apis,* Asaf., Ascl., *Bar., Bell.,* Berb., Brom., Calad., Camph., *Canth.,* Carbo an., *Carbo v., Caust.,* Ced., Chel., Cim., *Cinch.,* Cof., Cup.,

Dig., Doryp., Dros., Eup. p., *Fer.*, Gels., Graph., *Hep.*, Hipp., *Hyos.*, Iod., Ipec., Kali i., Kreo., Lach., Lac. ac., *Lyc.*, Mag. c., Mag. s., **Meny.**, Mer., *Mez.*, Natr., *Nit. ac.*, Nux m., *Op.*, Par., Petr., **Phos.**, Plant., Plumb., *Polyp.*, *Psor.*, *Puls.*, Rhus, Sabad., *Samb.*, Sarr., *Sec.*, **Sep.**, **Sil.**, Stan., *Stram.*, Sul., *Thuja*, **Ver.**

cold, sweat on rest of body: Ant. c.

cold sweat on: Mur. ac.

cold stinging or pricking: Eup.

cold with oppressed breathing: *Apis.*

cramps in: **Cup.**, Elat., *Nux.*

dead feeling of: Cim., Ced., **Puls.**, Stram.

dropsical swelling of: Eup., Kali i.

heat of: Calad., Kali ch., Kali m., Med.

heat of, soles of: Mang., Mer.

icy coldness of: *Ant. c.*, *Calad.*, **Meny.**, *Phos.*, Stan., Sep., **Ver.**

icy coldness of soles of: *Nit. ac.*

icy coldness of soles of, as if put in cold water: Mer.

icy coldness of, and hands: Canth.

icy coldness of, as if in snow: Fer., Petr.

icy coldness of right limb, as if standing in ice water: Sab.

livid: Stram.

numbness of: Fer., Lyc., Lept., Nux m., Puls., Sep., Stan.

one cold, other hot: Cinch., Dig., Ipec., Lyc., *Puls.*

pain in: Cup.

pain in dorsum: Cop., Cup.

pain, cutting in: Chin. s.

soles of, cold: Lith., Phyt.

wet, feeling as though: Ipec., **Sep.**

water, feeling as though in cold: Gels., Mer., **Sep.**

Fingers, blueness of: Natr., Nux, Petr., Tar.

drawing pain in left little, as if full and gone to sleep: Calad.

cold and hot alternately: Par.

cold: Ang., *Apis*, *Cac.*, *Calad.*, Ced., Dig., Meny., *Natr.*, Nux, Par., Phos. ac., Plant., **Sep.**, **Sul.**, **Tarax.**

Fingers, deadness of the: Par., Sep., Stan.
shriveled like a washerwoman's: **Canch.**
stiffness of: Fer., Stan.

Flushes alternate with chilliness: Lachn.

Food, aversion to: Coc., Kali c.
tasteless: Ars.

Forehead, cold sweat on: Cina, Cinch.
hot: *Acon.,* Calc., Cinch., *Led.,* Nat. s.
pain in: Eup. p., **Nat.**
stinging in: Mang.
sweat on: Bry., Cina, Cinch., Dig.

Formication, in right side of face: Plat.

Frozen, feeling as though: Aran., *Rob.,* Ver.

Gaping: Alum., Cim., *Elat.,* Lyc., *Nux.*
with a sound resembling the neighing of a horse: **Elat.**

Goose flesh: Æsc., *Ang.,* Bar., Bell., Bry., Calc., Camph., Canth., Carbo an., Chin. s., Crot., *Hell.,* Lach., Laur., **Lyc.,** *Mercurialis,* **Natr.,** Nat. s., **Nux,** Par., Phos., Plant., Sab., Sabad., Staph., Thuja.
when warm: Puls.

Hair, bristling of: **Bar.,** Dul., Grat., **Meny.**

Hands, blueness of: Gels., Natr., **Nux,** *Stram.*
clenched: Cimex.
cold: Acon., Agar., Ang., Apis, Arg. n., *Arn., Cac.,* **Camph., Canth., Carbo v.,** Ced., *Chel.,* Cinch., Cof., Con., Dig., Dory., *Dros.,* Eup., Eup. p., *Fer.,* Gels., *Hep.,* Hipp., *Hyos.,* Indigo, Iod., *Ipec.,* Jatr., Kali b., Kreos., *Led., Lyc.,* Manc., **Meny.,** Mang., Med., *Mer.,* Mer. c., Mer. s., *Mez.,* Nat. c., *Natr.,* Nit. s. d., *Nit. ac., Nux,* Oleand., *Op.,* Phel., Petr., Phos. ac., **Phos.,** Plumb., Polyp., *Puls., Rhus, Samb.,* Sabad., Sarr., **Sec.,** *Sep., Stan.,* Staph., Stram., Sul., *Tarax., Thuja,* **Ver.**
heat of: *Apis,* Cad. s., Ced., Cina, Ipec., Kali c., Med., Mez., Nit. ac., Nat. s., Sabad., Sep.

Hands, cold and moist: Brom., Sep.
livid: Ced., Stram., Ver.
numbness of: Cim., Fer., Lyc., **Nux m.**, **Puls.**, **Sep.**
paleness of: Ced., Cinch.
one cold, the other warm: Cinch., Dig., Lyc.
one cold and red, the other hot and pale: Mosch., *Puls.*
palms moist: Nic., **Sticta.**
palms rigid: Kali m.
stiffness of: Kali c.
sweat, cold, on: Cina.
veins, disappearance of: Eup.
veins distended: *Chel.*, *Meny.*, *Phos.*
wet, feeling as though: Ipec.

Head hot: Acon., Alum., **Arn.**, Asar., *Bell.*, Berb., Bry., Ced., Cina, Cinch., Eup., Gels., Lachn., Mang., Nat. s., Nux, Op., Rhod., *Stram.*, Ver.
hot, hands and feet cold: Nat. c.
only hot: **Arn.**, **Op.**
heat in, rest of the body cold: **Arn.**
pain in: Bell., Glon., Natr., Sep.
painful, externally: Hell.
pressure and dullness of: Berb.
screwed up, as if: Glon.
stitches in: Asaf., Crot.
stinging in: Aran.
sweat, profuse about the: **Op.**
trembling of: Coc.
vertex constricted, feeling as though: Kali b.

Headache: Acon., Anac., Ant. t., Anth., *Aran.*, *Bell.*, Berb., Bov., Calc. ars., Caps., Carbo v., Chin. s., Cim., Cina, Cinch., Coca, Cor. r., Dros., Elat., Eup., *Eup. p.*, Fer., Graph., Ind., Ign., Kreos., Kob., Mag. s., Mez., **Natr.**, Nux, Petr., *Puls.*, Sang., **Sep.**, *Sul.*
ceases entirely in open air: *Aran.*
forehead: Eup. p., **Natr.**

Headache, forehead, extending through: **Lac. ac.**
one-sided: Ign.
vertex: Hydr.

Heat to back, craves: *Caps.,* Eup. p.
to back, craves, but does not relieve: Eup. p.

Heart, palpitation of: Gels., Lil., Phos.
icy coldness about: Arn., Camph., Helod., Kali c., **Natr.,** Oleand., Petr.
spasms and pains in region of: *Calc.*

Heat: Bar. m.
shivering with flushes of: Guarea.
desire for: Gym.
sensation of: Benz. ac.

Held, desire to be: Gels., **Lach.**
desire to be, firmly: **Lach.**

Hoarseness: Hep.

Horripilation: Æth., Agar., **Bar.,** Cad. s., Guarea, *Meny.,* Psor., Sarr.

Hunger: Ailant., **Cina,** Nux, Phos., **Sil.,** Staph.
at beginning of: Phyt.

Hysteria: *Eup. p.*

Hot drinks, craving for: Ars., *Casc., Ced.,* Eup.

Ill-humor: Ign.

Ice, lying on, feeling as though: **Lyc.**
lying on, feeling as though back between scapulæ: Lachn.

Internal, with external heat: Astac., Calc., Col., Plumb.
with external heat, with yawning and stretching: Nat. s.

Incisors, sensation as if elongated: Gamb.

Irritability: Anac., Caps., *Cina,* Gels., Hyos., **Ign.,** Kali b., Kreos *Nit. ac.,* Plat.

Jerkings: Stram.

Joints, pains in: Cim., Hell., *Pod.,* Polyp.
sticking in: Hell.
pains in large: Polyp., **Pod.**

Kidneys, pain in left: Mill.

Knees, cold: **Apis, Carbo v.,** *Ign.,* **Phos.,** *Sil.,* Stan.
pain in: Ang., *Cim., Pod.*
stitches in: Aran.

Lachrymation: Elat.

Lassitude: Amb., Aran., Carbo v., Caust., Kob., Mercurialis, Natr.

Leg, coldness of right: *Bry.,* Chel., Elaps, Sab., Sep.
coldness of left: Carbo v., Caust., Ol. an., Thuja.

Legs, coldness of, excessive: **Meny.,** Sec., Stram.
cramps in: Cup., Elat., *Nux.*
drawing sensation in left tibia: Brom.
goose flesh of: Chin. ars.
heaviness of: Ther.
jerking of: Ign.
lameness of: Ign.
involuntary movements of: Tar.
numbness of: *Eup. p., Nux.*
numbness of and coldness of: Lept.
pains, aching in bones: Eup., Eup. p., Polyp.
position of, must change: Cim., Pyr., Rhus.
stretch out, inability to: Cim.
soreness of: Bell.
tired feeling of: Gels., Rhus.
weakness of: Senega.

Lie down, desire to: Bry., Ced., Dros., Fer., *Lach.,* Mer., Nux, Puls., *Sep., Sil.,* Ther.
desire to be near the fire and: **Lach.**

Light, dread of: Bell., Psor.

Limbs, coldness of: Acon., Æth., Amb., Ant. t., Arg. n., Ars., *Bell.,* Berb., Calad., Calc., Camph., Canth., Carbo an., Carbo v., Caust., Cham., Chel., Cic., Cinch., Col., Con.,

Dig., Graph., Hell., Hyos., Ipec., Kali c., **Laur.**, Led., Lept., Lyc., Lys., **Meny.**, Mer., *Mez.*, Natr., **Nit. ac.**, *Nux, Op.*, Phos., Plant., *Puls.*, Plumb., *Rhus*, **Sec.**, Sep., **Stram.**, Sul., Tar., Thuja, Ver., Verb.
contraction of: Caps., **Cim.**
involuntary movements of: Tar.
heaviness of: Ant. t.
pain in: Acon., Anth., Ars., Bell., Bry., Dios., Dulc., Elat., *Eup.*, Eup. p., Graph., Hell., Lach., Led., Lyc., Mercurialis, *Mez.*, Natr., *Nux*, Op., *Puls.*, Pyr., *Rhus, Sabad.*, Sep., Sul., Tub.
paralysis of: Stram.
paralysis of upper: Phos. ac.
stretching and bending of: Alum.
trembling of: Bell., *Chin. s.*, Con., *Sabad.*
twitchings in: *Nux*, Stram., Tar.

Lips, blue: *Chin. s., Eup. p.*, Ipec., **Natr.**, *Nux, Sec.*

Liver, pain in the region of: Ars., Bry., *Cinch., Nux*, **Pod.**, Ver.

Loins, pains in: Ars., Kreos., Lach., Nux, Ver.

Loquacity: **Pod.**, Mar.

Lungs, pains in: Dios.

Malaise, with: Anth.

Mental exertion, aversion to: Kob.

Mind and disposition symptoms, alternating with: Plat.

Moaning: *Eup.*

Mottled and corrugated: Kali b.
and blue: Arn., Crot., Nux.

Mouth, dryness of: *Mez., Petr.*, Thuja.
dryness of, without thirst: Berb.
dryness of, posteriorly, saliva anteriorly: **Mez.**
foam at: Cina, (?) Ther.

Muscular pains intense, must walk about for relief: Pyr., Rhus.

Mucus, vomiting of: *Puls.*

Muscles, pain in: **Arn.,** Bap.

Muscles, involuntary movement of: **Tar.**

Nails blue: Apis, Arn., Ars., *Asaf.,* Aur., *Carbo v.,* Chin. s., *Cinch.,* Coc., Con., *Dros., Eup. p.,* Ipec., Jatr., Mer. s., Mez., **Natr., Nux,** *Petr.,* Phos. ac., Sul., *Thuja.*
finger, white: Sil.

Nausea: Alumen, Arg. n., *Ars.,* Aur., Bell., Bry., Chel., Cina, Cinch., Eup. p., Hydr., Ign., Ib., Ipec., Kali b., Kali c., Kob., Lach., *Lyc.,* Lob., Mer., Mer. s., *Natr.,* Petr., Puls., Rhus, Rum., *Sabad.,* Sang., Sep., Ver., Ver. v., Zinc.
drinking, after: *Ars.,* Arn., *Eup.*
and involuntary urine: Dul.
relieved by swallow of water: *Lob.*

Neck, nape of, aching in: Gels., Nat. s., Ver. v.

Nervousness: Coc., Eup. p.

Noise, dread of: *Bell.,* **Caps.,** *Hyos.*

Neighing like horses: Elat.

Nose cold: Apis, Ant. c., Ced., Chel., Colch., Iod., Meny., *Polyp.,* Sil., Sul., *Tarax.*
cold, tip of: **Ced.**
red: Bell.
sweat on, cold: Cina.

Numbness: Cinch., Fer., Lyc., Puls., *Sep.*
sensation of, in face: Plat.

Numb ache, in arms and legs: Carb. ac.

Pain, in parts rested on: *Bap.,* Pyr.
paroxysm of: Ars., Cinch., Eup., Puls., Rhus.

Parietal bone, sudden pain in: Calc.

Parts, single, get icy cold: Asar.

Photophobia: Hep., *Psor.*

Prostration great: Anth., Astacus, Cup., Phos. ac.

Ptyalism: Caps.

Pulled sensation in whole body: Calad.

Pulse, full: Ant. t., Chin. s.
hard: Cinch.
intermittent: Acon., Dig., Mer.
irregular: Ant. c., Cinch.
perceptible, scarcely: Kalm.
quick: Cinch., Nat. s.
slow: Meny.
thread-like: Acon., Apis, Chel.
weak: Ced., Gels.

Pupils, contracted: Acon., Gels.
dilated: Acon., *Bell.,* Ipec.

Recollect, inability to: Ars., Caps., Stram.

Respiration difficult: **Apis,** Ars., Bry., Gels., Kali c., Mez., Natr. Puls., Senega, *Thuja,* Zinc.

Restlessness: Anth., *Ars.,* Bell., Eup. p., Kreos., Plant., Rhus, Ter.

Rheumatic pains, severe over whole body: Pyr., Rhus, Tub.

Ribs ache: Calend.

Rigor and stiffness of limbs: Agar., Sul. ac.
followed by heat through whole body: Ter.
and cold to touch, but patient feels burning: Acon

Sacrum, pain in: Ars., Gamb., Hyos., **Nux,** Ver.

Saliva, spitting of: Alum., Caps., Rhus.

Scapula, pain under: Elat.
pain under left: Cim.
pain from right side to right: Aran.

Sensation, loss of: Lach.

Shivering, with: Clem., Kali br., Mur. ac., Sul. ac., Sab., Zinc.
with hot cheeks and cold hands: Mur. ac.
in paroxysms: Sul. ac.

Shuddering with goose flesh: Sab., Zinc.

Shoulders and elbows, sticking in: Hell.

Sight, obstruction of: Bell., Cic., Hydr. ac., Sabad.

Skin, blue: Arn., Cad. s., Cinch., Mer., Natr., Nux m., *Nux*.
blue and mottled: Arn., Crot., **Nux.**
cold, damp, clammy: Anth., Corn., Fer., Lach., Lachn., Mer. c., Pyr., Tub., **Ver.**, Ver. v.
cold and pale, covered and dripping with sweat: Mer. c.
cold and burning alternately: Dory.
coldness, icy, of: Nat. s., **Sec.**, *Stram.*, **Ver.**
contracted sensation of: Par.
dry: Anth., Ars., Asaf., Iod
dry and cold: Crot.
hot: **Coll.**
itching of: *Hep.*, *Petr.*
moist: Bufo.
painful: Camph., *Nux*.
sore to touch: Camph., Cinch.
stinging: *Hep.*, Samb.
warm to touch: Ars., Calend., Cor., Elaps, Gamb.

Sleep: Amb., Ant. c., Ant. t., **Apis**, Bor., Cim., Gels., Grat., *Kali i.*, Lyc., Mer., *Mez.*, *Natr.*, **Nux m.**, Nux, **Op.**, Pod., Psor., Sil.
deep snoring: Laur., **Op.**

Sleepiness: Æth., Amb., Asp., Aster, Hell., Iris, Kali b., *Kali i.*, Mez., *Natr.*, *Nux m.*, Nux, **Op.**, Phos., Tar.

Sneezing: Psor.

Snow, feet and ankles, as if in: Fer., Petr.

Soreness, feeling of: Arn., Bap., Camph., Pyr.

Spasms: *Calc.*, Camph., Tar., Ver.
clonic: Camph.

Speak, unable to: Tar.

Spine, painful to pressure: **Chin. s.**
coldness of the: Canth., **Meny.**
pain in: Lys.
shooting pain in, and arms from occiput: Crot.

Spleen, pain in the region of: *Bry.*, **Chin. s.**, *Eup.*, **Pod.**
stitches in: Bry.
swelling of: Caps., Cean., (?) Cinch., Petr.

Staggering: Caps.

Staring: Cic.

Stiffness, and rigidity of the body: **Op.**
of limbs with rigors: Agar.

Stretching: Alum., Ars., Brom., Bry., Caps., Cim., Cof., Elat., *Eup.*, Ipec., Kreos., Laur., Mar. v., Mez., Mur. ac., Nat. s., Nit. ac., Nux, Prun., Petr., Polyp., *Rhus.*

Stomach, heat in: Aran., Lob.
movements in, as if would faint: Calend.
pain in: Ars., Eup., Lyc., Mercurialis, Sil., Sul.
weight in, sensation of: *Bell.*

Stomach, sensation as of hot water in: Phos.

Stool, shiny: Dios.

Sun, desire for the heat of: *Con.*

Sweat, cold, from beginning of chill: Tar.
cold and clammy: Cup.
cold all over, so that a drop is on every hair: Hell.
with: *Acon.*, Alum., Anac., Ant. t., Apis, Ars., Bell., Bry., *Cad. s.*, *Calc.*, Caps., Carbo v., **Cham.**, *Cinch.*, Cina, **Eup.**, Fer., Graph., Hep., Ign., Kali c., Kali b., **Led.**, Lyc., Mez., Natr., Nit. ac., Nux, *Op.*, Phos., **Puls.**, **Rhus,** Sabad., Sep., Sul., Tar., Ter., Thuja, **Ver.**, Ver. v., Zinc.

Sweat of face: Alum.
without: Graph., Mal., Nat. s.

Taste, bitter: Alum., Ars., Dios., Eup. p., **Hep.**
insipid: Aur.
metallic: Alumen.

Teeth, incisors, sensation of elongation of: Gamb.
chattering of: Stan.

Tendons, feeling as though too short: Cimex.

Tenesmus: Canth., Caps., Col., Mer.

Thighs, heat of: Thuja.
weakness of: Ver.

Thirst: Acon., *Alum.,* Amm. m., **Apis,** Aran., **Arn.,** *Ars.,* Bar. m., Bell., *Bry.,* Calad., *Calc.,* Camph., **Caps.,** *Carbo v., Chin. s.,* Cinch., Coral., Croc., Cur., Dul., Elat., Elaps, **Eup.,** *Eup. p., Fer.,* Gamb., Graph., **Ign.,** Kali c., Kali i., **Lach.,** Lachn., Laur., *Led.,* Lob., Mag. s., Med., Mer., Mez., Mur. ac., Nat. c., *Natr.,* Nat. s., Nit. ac., Nux, Plant., *Plumb.,* Psor., Puls., *Rhus, Sec., Sep.,* Thuja, **Ver.**
much: *Alum., Apis, Arn.,* **Bry., Caps., Eup.,** Gamb., Graph., **Ign.,** Led., Mez., **Natr.,** Puls., Rhus.
for large quantity of water which relieves: **Bry., Natr.**
for small quantity, frequent drinking: *Ars.,* Cinch., *Eup.*
without: Agar., *Ang.,* Amm. m., Anac., *Ant. c., Ant. t., Aran.,* Ars., Asar., Bar., *Bell.,* Bov., *Cac.,* Calad., *Camph., Canth., Carbo an.,* Caust., *Ced., Cham.,* Chel., *Cim., Cina, Cinch., Coc.,* Cof., Col., Cur., Cyc., *Dros.,* Dul., Elaps, Euph., *Gels.,* Graph., Guaj., Hell., Hep., Hyos., *Ipec.,* Kali b., Lach., Lyc., Meny., Mer., Mur. ac., Nit. ac., Natr., Nat. c., Natr. s., Nux m., Nux, Oleand., Petr., Phos. ac., Phos., Pod., *Puls.,* Rhus, Sabad., Samb., Sil., Spig., *Staph.,* Stram., Sul., Ther.

Throat, rattling in: Camph.
swelling of glands in and below ear: Cist.

Throbbing through the body: Zinc.

Toes, coldness of: **Fer.**, **Meny.**
pain in: Ang.

Toothache: **Carbo v.**, Kali c., Graph., Rhus.

Torpor of affected side: Puls.
of affected parts: Caust.

Trembling: *Agn.*, Anac., Ant. t., Ars., *Cina*, Coc., Croc., Con., *Eup.*, Fer., Gels., Mer. i., *Par.*, *Petr.*, Plat., Sul. ac., Sabad., *Zinc.*

Trismus: Lach.

Unconsciousness: *Bell.*, Camph., *Hep.*, **Natr.**, Nux, Op., Puls., Rob.

Uncovering, pains from: **Stram**
chill from, yet smothers if covered: Arg. n.

Uneasiness: Calc., Caps., Hyos., Sil.

Urethra, pains in: *Canth.*, **Petros.**, Sars.

Urinating, frequent: Canth., Dul., Gels., Hyper., Mer., *Petros.*
urging to: Card. m.
desire to: Hyper., Indigo.

Urine, acid: Sep.
brown: Sep.
dark: Ver.
diminished: Mer. s.
incontinence of and nausea: Dul.

Uterus, pains in: Calc. p.

Urticaria: Apis, **Hep.**
over whole body, when chills were suppressed: Elat.

Veins distended: Ars., Bry., Calad., Caps., Caust., Cim., Cina, Elat., Eup., Gamb., Kob., Laur., Lyc., Mar., **Meny.**, Mer., Mez., Murex, Natr., Nat. s., Oleand., Par., Phos., Polyp., Sil., Thuja.

Vertebræ, pain in dorsal: **Chin. s.**
coldness in, sensation of: *Canth.*

Vertigo: Alum., Anth., Calc., Caps., Cinch., *Eucal.*, Glon., Kali b., Laur., Lyssin, Natr., Nux, Phos., Puls., Rhus, Sul.

Vomiting, in all stages: **Eucal.**, Ver.

Alum., Arn., *Ars.*, Asaf., Bar. m., **Eup.**, Fer., Gamb., Ign., *Ipec.*, Glon., Hydr., Lach., Lyc., Natr., Nux, Puls., Rhus, *Ver.*, Zinc.

of bile: Ars., Cina, Cinch., **Eup.**, Ign., Ipec.

drinking, after: *Arn.*, **Ars.**, **Eup.**, Nux.

of ingesta: **Fer.**, Ign., Eup.

of mucus: Caps., Ign., **Puls.**

of mucus, white not transparent: Kali m.

sour: **Lyc.**, *Rob.*, Sul. ac.

Warmth, desire for, but does not relieve: Alum., Aran., Camph., *Cic.*, Cina, Coc., *Con.*, Hep., **Lach.**, Lyc., Meny., Nat. ars., Nux, Phos., Pod., Ptel., Sil., Ver.

desire for, especially heat of sun: **Con.**

desire for, without, or dread of open air: **Mez.**

external, unbearable: *Apis*, *Ipec.*, **Puls.** **Sep.**

Waves, chill comes in: Chin. ars., Gels.

Weakness: Amb., Anth., Aran., Calc., Carbo v., Caust., Dros., Hep., Ipec., Kob., Lach., Laur., Mercurialis, *Natr.*, Op., Phos., Psor.

Wrists, tearing in: Phos. ac., **Pod.**

Yawning: Ars., *Bry.*, Brom., Calad., Caps., Caust., Cim., *Cina*, **Elat.**, **Eup.**, *Gamb.*, Kob., Laur., Lyc., Mar. v., *Meny.*, Mer., Mer. s., Mez., *Mur. ac.*, Murex, **Natr.**, Nat. s., *Oleand.*, Par., Phos., *Polyp.*, Sil., Thuja, Zinc.

CHILL FOLLOWED BY:

Anxiety, internal, with short breath: Berb., Kali c.

Bloating of hands and face: Lyc.

Breathing, oppressed: Berb., Cimex.

Chest, spasmodic pain in: Kali c.

Colic: Anth.

Collapse, deadly: Anth.

Cough, dry, uninterrupted, from tickling in larynx: Cimex.

Cyanosis: Anth.

Ears, roaring and tingling in: Cahinca.

Eructations, foul: Dig.

Eyes, redness of: Ced.

Eyelids, itching of: Ced.
bluish: Dig.

Face, heat of: Cahinca, Dros., Guarea.
yellow: Dig.

Feet, coldness of: Petr.

Fever, low, with bronchial or pulmonary complications: Stan.

Fingers, drawings in: Lyc.

Forehead, dull pain in: Mer. s.

Hands, icy coldness of: Ced.
and arms mottled blue: Arn., Crot., Kali b., Nux.

Head, heaviness of: Dros.
weight in: Cahinca.

Headache, frontal: Ant. t., Ced., Chin. s., Mer. sul., **Natr.**
throbbing, occipital: Dros.
severe, with soreness of lungs: Ailant.

Heart, icy coldness about the: Helod., **Natr.**

Heat flushes: Nat. p.
with trembling and rapid swelling of glands below ears and in throat: Cist.
with sweat and thirst: Ant. c., Ant. t., *Caps.*
with sweat: Guarea.
with sleep: Nat. c.
and perspiration: Polyp.
and perspiration, cold: Lyssin.

Hunger: Ars.

Itching, violent, of the skin: **Petr.**

Languor: Med.

Lips, dryness of: Kali b.
bluish: Dig.

Lungs, soreness of: Ailant.

Mouth, dryness of: Kali b.

Nausea: Acon., Anth., **Eup.,** Kali c., Zinc.

Nose, coldness of the tip of, rest of the face burning hot: Ced.

Occiput, throbbing pain in: Dros.

Pains: Cof., Kali c.

Prostration: Ars., Natr.

Restlessness: Apis, Camph.

Retching, after drinking: Ant. t.

Saliva, much sour: Zinc.

Shivering: Lyc., Sep.
after drinking and while eating: Caps., Lyc.
after every drink: Caps.

Shuddering: **Caps.,** Cup. s.

Skin, itching of: **Petr.**
hot and dry: Nat. ars.

Sleep: **Apis,** Ars., Camph., Lyc., Mez., Nux m., Nux, Sab.

Sweat: Amm. m., Apis, **Ars.,** Bell., *Bry.,* Cac., **Caps.,** Carbo v., Carbo an., **Caust.,** Ced., Cham., Coc., Dig., Dros., **Eup.,** Eup. p., Gels., Graph., Hyos., *Ign.,* **Ipec.,** Kali c., Kali m., Lach., **Lyc., Mez., Nux, Petr., Puls.,** Rhus, Sabad., Sep., Spig., Thuja, *Ver.*
cold: Anth., Ars., Mal., Pyr., Ver.
without heat or thirst: Amm. m., Bry., Caust., Pyr.
then heat: Bell., Mal.
sour: **Lyc.**

Swelling of glands below ears and in neck: Cist.

Taste bitter: Dig.

Thirst: **Ars.**, Bar., *Cim.*, **Cinch.**, **Dros.**, Hep., Kali b., Kreos., Mag. s., Puls., **Sabad.**, Thuja.
without heat: Canth.
yet cannot drink, makes headache unbearable: Cimex.

Urticaria: **Apis.**

Vomiting: Ant. t., Anth., **Eup.**, Kali c., *Lyc.*, **Natr.**
and spasmodic pain in chest: Kali c.
of bile: **Eup.**, Kali c., **Natr.**
sour: Lyc.
sour masses: Nat. p.
after every draught: **Eup.**

Weakness: **Ars.**, Lyc.

Weariness: Cimex, Lyc.
of the feet: Lyc.

Weep, desire to: Cof.

Wrists, drawing in: **Lyc.**

HEAT AGGRAVATED BY:

Air, in open: Cur., **Nux.**

Bed, in: *Mer.*

Carriage, when riding in a: Graph., **Psor.**

Drinking, by: Calc., Coc.

Eating, after: Amm. c., Brom., **Caust.**, Coc., Cof., Fluor. ac., Sep.

Evening, towards: Fer.

Exercising, when: Ant. c., Ant. t., **Camph.**, **Cinch.**, Cur., Nux, Stram., **Sep.**
light: Con.

Midnight, after: *Dros.*

Motion, by: Alum., Ant. t., *Camph.,* **Cinch.,** Cur., **Nux,** *Sep.,* Stram.

Night, at: *Cina,* Cur., **Sil.**

Noise: Con., Nux?

Sitting, while: Phos., Sep.

Sleep, in: Dul., Petr., Samb., Viol. t.
after: Calad., Cina, *Lach.*

Smoking, by: Cic., Cof., Ign.?

Stooping, when: Mer., Mer. c.
when, but cold when rising: Mer. c.

Vexation, after: Petr., Sep.

Walking, when: *Camph.,* Cinch.

Warmth, by: **Apis,** Bry., **Ign., Puls.**
of room, by: Amm. m., **Apis,** Ipec., Natr.

Weather, by damp: Cur., Dul., Mer., Rhus.

HEAT AMELIORATED BY:

Air, in open: Canch., Natr.

Carriage, by riding in a: Nit ac.

Eating, after: Anac., Cinch., Cur., Fer.

Heat, by artificial: Ars., **Ign.**

Motion, by: **Caps.,** Fer.

Sitting, when: **Bry.,** Nux.

Speaking, when: Fer.

Uncovering, by: Acon., Ars., Bor., Bov., Ign., Puls., Sul.

Walking, when: *Caps.*

HEAT ABSENT:

Amm. m., Agar., Aran., Benz., Bov., Cac., Camph., Caps., Caust., Cimex, Coc., Dios., Hep., Lyc., Mag. c., Mez., Phos. ac., Rhus, Sabad., Staph., Sul., Thuja, Ver.

HEAT IN GENERAL:

Acon., Æsc., Æth., Alst., Alum., Amb., Amm. m., Ang., Ant. c., **Ant. t.**, *Apis,* Aran., **Arn.**, **Ars.**, Asaf., Asar., *Bap.,* Bar., **Bell.**, *Bry.,* **Cac.**, Calad., Calc., Canch., Canth., Carbo an., Carbo v., *Casc.,* Ced., Cham., *Chel.,* **Chin. s.**, Cic., Cina, **Cinch.**, Cof., Con., Corn., Croc., Cup., *Cur.,* Cyc., Daph., Dig., Dros., Dul., Elat., *Elaps,* Eucal., **Eup.**, Eup. p., Euphor., *Fer.,* Gamb., **Gels.**, Glon., *Graph.,* Ham., *Hell.,* Hep., Hyos., *Ign.,* Iod., **Ipec.**, Iris v., Kali b., Kali c., **Kali i.**, *Lach.,* Lachn., Laur., Led., Lob., **Lyc.**, Mal., Mar., Mag. c., Mag. s., Meny., *Mercurialis, Mer.,* **Mez.**, Mosch., Mur. ac., *Natr.,* Nat. s., *Nit. ac.,* **Nux m.**, **Nux**, *Op.,* Par., Petr., Phos., Plant., Pod., Polyp., Psor., **Puls.**, Pyr., **Rhus**, Rob., Sabad., Sab., *Samb.,* Sarr., **Sec.**, *Sep., Sil.,* Stan., Spig., Staph., Stram., Sul., Tarax., Thuja, Tub., Val., Ver.

HEAT, SYMPTOMS DURING:

Abdomen, coldness in: Zinc.
coldness in, after midnight with hot feet: Calad.
burning in: Coca.
distended: Ars.
rumbling in: Lachn.
heat in: Apis, *Cac.,* Calad., Canth., *Cic.,* Cinch., Fer., Lach., Selen., Spig., Stan.
pain in: Ars., Caps., Carbo v., Cina, Elat., Ign., Lept., Nux, Pyr., *Rhus.*
puffed up, sensation as if: Calc. ars.

Abdomen, pulsations in: **Kali c.**
weak: Anac.

Air, cold, sensitiveness to: *Bar.,* Camph., *Coc.*
as if there was none in the room (breathing difficult): Plant.
of room intolerable: **Apis.**
of room seems hot and close: Plant.
warm, sensitiveness to: *Coc.*

Anguish: Hyper.
and oppression excessive: **Acon.**

Anxiety, with: Asaf., Berb., Casc., Guarea, Mer. c., Nicc., Plumb

Appetite, loss of: Cinch., Lach.

Apples, desire for: Ant. t.

Arms, cold: Kali b.
veins of, distended: *Chin. s.,* Cinch. (See Blood-vessels, Veins).

Aversion to dressing, clothes too heavy: Euphor.

Back, heat in, lumbar region of: Sarr., Spig., Stan.
heat in, and neck: Par.
heat in, with coldness of nape of neck: Zinc.
and loins, burning in: Kalm.
pain in: Alst., Arn., Ars., Caps., Carbo v., Chin. s., *Eup.,* Hyos., Ign., Kali c., Lach., Laur., Lyc., Natr., **Nux,** Puls., Rhus, Ver.
pressure in, and forehead: Lyssin.

Backache: Ind. m.

Beer, desire for: *Nux,* Spig.

Besotted: Gels.

Bladder, pain in: Cac.

Blood, feeling as though hot: *Ars., Bell.,* Cham., Med., **Rhus.**

Bloodvessels, distention of: *Bell.,* Camph., Cham., *Chin. s.,* **Cinch.,** *Croc.,* Puls.

Body, red: Canth.
purple: Curara.
was too heavy, clothes seemed burdensome: Euphor.
upper part chiefly, heat of: Agar., Lac. ac.

Bones, pains in: Ars., *Eup.*, *Eup. p.*, Ign., Mag. c., Natr., Puls.

Brandy, longing for: Ailant., Asar., Psor.

Breath, hot: Calc. p.

Breathing, anxious and rapid: Acon., Puls.
deep: Lach.
difficult, as if no air in the room: Plant., Sul.
oppressed: **Apis,** Ars., Bov., Cac., Carbo v., *Cim.*, Elaps, *Ipec.*, **Kali c.,** Myg., Plant.
short: Cac., Cina, Con., *Sil.*

Bruised, feeling as though: Arn., Bap., Bellis, Pyr.

Burning pain over whole body, except feet: Mer. s.
intense: **Gels.**

Calves, cramp in: Mag. p.

Carotids, throbbing: Hyper.

Cheek, heat and redness of one: Cof., *Ign.*, *Ipec.*, Puls.
red spot on the left: Lyc.
red spot on the right: Lachn.
redness of one, the other pale: Acon., Bar., **Cham.,** *Ipec.*, *Puls.*

Cheeks, burning and dark red: Chel., Eup., Lachn., Mercurialis.
red and hot: Carbo an., Chel., *Cina*, *Coc.*, Cof., Dig., **Eup.,** Fer., Kreos., Kali c., Lach., Lyc., *Meny.*, Mer., Nux, Rhus, Rob., *Ver.*
red and hot subjectively, although objectively are not warm: **Cinch.**
chilly on motion: Ind. m.
glowing: Daphne.
swollen: Guaj.

Chest, burning in: Amm. m., *Apis,* Cham., Puls., Senega, Stan., Sul.
faint feeling in: Calend.
oppression of: Acon., **Apis,** Ars., Berb., Bov., Carbo v., Hyper., Ipec., Kali c., *Lach.,* Mer., Plant., Puls.
pain in: Ars., Ant., Caps., Carbo v., Cinch., Guarea, Kali c., Nux.
sensation as of pressing together: Mer. i.
stitches in: Acon., **Bry.,** *Kali c.,* Nux.

Coldness: Arundo.
of lower part of body, heat of upper: Guarea.

Cold in one part, heat in another: Mag. s.

Coma: **Arn.,** Cac., Ign., Laur., Op., Tar.

Comatose, with eyes closed: Tar.

Consciousness, almost loses: Phos. ac.

Constipation: Chin. s., Lyc., Natr., Nux.

Convulsions: Cur., *Hyos.,* **Nux,** Op., **Stram.**
epileptiform: Hyos., *Stram.*

Cough: **Acon.,** *Bry.,* Dros., Cinch., Eup., **Ipec.,** Lob., Sul.
with pleuritic stitches: *Acon.,* **Bry.**
short, hacking, from tickling in throat-pit: Lob.
exciting nausea and vomiting: **Ipec.**
tearing: Hyos.
tight, dry: Guarea.

Conjunctiva, jaundiced hue of: Chin. s.

Cover, desire for: Mancinella.

Cramps: Cur., Cup., Mag. p., Rob.

Deafness: Cinch., Lachn., Sul.

Debilitating: Cup., Cup. s.

Debility: Lob., Nicc.

Delirium: Ailant., Ant. t., **Arn.**, Ars., Bell., Carbo v., **Chin. s.**, Cina, Cinch., Cof., Dul., Doryph., Gels., Hep., Hyper., Iris, Ign., Lach., Lachn., Mal., Myg., **Natr.**, Nit. ac., Nux, Op., **Pod.**, *Psor.*, Pyr., Sabad., Sang., Sarr., Sec., Spong., Stram., Sul. ac., *Ver.*

Despondency: Myg.

Diarrhea: Anth., **Cina**, Con., Elat., Puls., *Rhus*, Thuja, Ver. v.
bilious: Iris.
black: Lept.?, Ver. v.
constant on the days free from fever: **Iod.**

Dressing, aversion to: Euphor.

Drinking, repugnance to: Con., Hell., Nux.

Drinks, feel too cold: *Bell.*
cold, nausea after: Lyc.
little at time: **Ars.**, **Cinch.**, Lyc.
warm, desire for: **Casc.**, Ced., **Eup. p.**

Drowsiness: Aran., Bis.

Dyspnea: Acon., Anac., **Apis**, *Arn.*, Ars., Bov., Cac., Camph., Carbo v., Cimex, Crot., Elaps, Ign., *Kali c.*, Lob., Lyc., Phos., Plant., Puls., Sep.

Ear, heat and burning of one: **Ign.**

Ears, coldness of: Ipec.
heat of: *Caps.*, Cinch., Dig., Elaps, Lach., Lyc., *Meny.*
heat of, and face: Mer. sul.
humming in: Benz. ac., Nux.
pain in: Calad.
redness of: *Camph.*, Caps., Cist., Elaps, **Ign.**
ringing in: Chin. s.
roaring in: *Nux.*

Eating, after: Cyc., Val.

Epigastrium, fullness in: Aran., *Ars.*

Epistaxis: Crot.

29

Epilepsy: **Hyos.**, Stram.

Eructations: Rob.

Esophagus, pressure in: *Cimex*.

Excitability, nervous: *Acon.*, Con.
mental: Mar. v.

Exhausting: Cup., Cup. s.

Extremities, pains in: Elat., **Eup.**, Eup. p., *Rob*.
twitchings in: Gels., Ign., Rob.
clammy and cold: Mer. c.
weakness, great, of: Ver. v.

Eyelids, cannot open: **Gels.**
heat of: Chel.
burning in, on opening: Ham.
swelling of upper: Apis, **Kali c.**

Eyes, pupils contracted: Gels., Laur., Op., Phys., Ter., Ver.
pupils dilated: *Bell.*, Calc., Cic., Cina, *Hell.*, Ipec., Stram., Ver.
dim before: Chlor.
rubbing of: Cina.
weakness of: Carbo v., **Natr.**, Sep.
burning: Anth., Cinch.
brilliant: Gels.
swollen: Guarea.
pain in: Guarea.

Face, burning but not red: Plat.
burning and redness of the: Croc., Phel., Zinc.
burning as if sweat would break out: Bap.
burning with cool body: Zinc.
bloated: Hyper.
bathe, wants to: Fl. ac.
coldness of: Ang., *Ipec.*, Puls., Rheum.
flushed: Glon.
flushes of heat on, and neck: Med.

Face, flushes of heat over: Æsc., Asaf., Bap., Cac., Carbo v., Croc., Cup., Glon., Hydr., Ib., Kali i., Mar. v., Ver. v.

flushes of heat in, rest of body chilly: Calc. p., Sab.

and hands, heat on, with chill in the back: Asar., Spig.

heat in, sensation of: Calad., Plant., Sep., Tarax., *Thuja.*

heat in, ascending from pit of stomach to head: Glon.

heat in, after eating: Asaf., Caust., Cham.

hot: Anac., Bell., Cac., Camph., Caps., Carbo v., Caust., Cham., Chel., Cic., *Cina,* Cinch., Coc., Cof., Cyc., Dig., *Eup.,* Gels., Fl. ac., Ind., Ipec., Kali b., Kali c., Lach., Laur., *Lyc., Mag. c.,* Meny., Mercurialis, Mer., Nit. ac., Par., Phos., Phos. ac., Plant., *Polyp.,* Rhus, Sabad., Sab., *Samb., Sarr.,* Sep., Sul., Tarax., *Ver.,* Ver. v.

jaundiced hue: Chin. s.

paleness of: Ars., Bry., Caps., Cina, Croc., *Ipec.,* Lyc., Rhus, Rob., Sep., Sul. ac.

paleness of, when rising up: *Acon.*

red: Acon., Alum., Amm. m., Asaf., Astacus, **Bell.,** Bry., *Cac.,* Calc., Camph., Caps., *Carbo v.,* Ced., Chel., *Chin. s.,* Cic., **Cinch.,** Cof., Con., *Croc.,* Crot., Cyc., Dul., Elaps, Euph., **Fer.,** Glon., Grat., Hep., Hyper., *Ign.,* Kali i., Kreos., *Lachn.,* Lyc., Mag. c., Mag. s., Meny., Mer., Myg., Natr., Nux m., Nux, Op., *Petr., Polyp., Puls.,* Plumb., Rhus, Sabad., Sarr., **Sep., Sil.,** Spig., Spong., *Stram., Sul.,* Tarax., Ter., Ver.

red and pale alternately: Acon., Bell., Bov., Caps., Croc., Ipec., Mag. s., Nux, Op., Phos., Puls.

red and flushed: Crot.

red when lying: *Acon.*

red and burning, one side of: Ign.

red and burning in the eyes: Zinc.

red, right side of: Lachn.

redness of, dark: **Lachn.,** Rob., **Sil.**

redness of, and distention of bloodvessels: Cham., Cinch., Croc., Glon.

Face, redness of, mahogany: Crot., **Eup.**
sweat on: Dig., Dul., Lob., Val.
sweat on, gushes of: Med.
sweat on, cold: Dig.
spotted: Guaj.
swollen: Amm. m., Ars., Bell., Cac., Chel., Cina, Lyc., Puls.
swollen and bloated, sensation of: Croc., Fer.
yellow: Ars., Cina, Eup., Natr.

Fainting: **Acon.**, Anac., **Arn.**, Bell., Calc., Eup., Mer., **Natr.**, Nux, Op., Phos.
when rising up: **Acon.**

Falling, fear of: **Gels.**
sensation of: **Gels.**

Fanned, desire to be: Bap., **Carbo v.**, Pyr., Zinc.

Fauces, dryness of: Chin. s.

Fear: Acon., Med., Myg.

Feet, coldness of: Anac., Ant. c., *Arn.*, Asaf., Bell., Calc., Calad., Caps., Cinch., Chin., Coc., Fer., Graph., Hydr. ac., Ib., Ign., Ipec., Iris, Kali c., Lach., Meny., Nux, Petr., Phos. ac., Ptel., Puls., Rheum, Sabad., Sab., *Samb.*, **Stram.**, **Sul.**, Tar.
coldness of, continued: Tar.
burn: Calend.
hot: *Led.*, Mercurialis, Nux, Plant., Polyp., Ran., Sarr., Staph.
pain in, from cold on uncovering: Nux, Stram.
soles burning: Æsc., Canth., Cup., Cup. s., *Fer.*, Graph., *Lach.*, **Sul.**
soles burning and palms, must be uncovered: Æsc., Fer., **Lach.**
sweat on: Staph.
and toes, heat in: Asaf.

Fingers, heat of: Lyc.
alternately hot and cold: Par.
nervous movement of: Led.
pain in: Elat.

Flatulence, with: Cinnab., Rob.

Flushes of heat: Amyl.
of heat with burning face: Arum.

Food, aversion to: Cinch.
cold, desire for: Phos., Ver.

Forehead, coldness of: Cina, Cinch., Puls.
hot: Chel., *Stram.*
pressure in, and back: Lyssin.
sweat on: Ant. t., Ipec., Lachn., Mag. s., Sars., Staph., **Ver.**

Formication rising in loins to face: Arundo.

Forgetfulness: Guarea.

Gagging: **Cimex,** Kali c.

Gaping: Calc. p.

Genitals, burning on: Prun.

Hair on head, moist: Hyper.

Hands, cold: *Arn.,* Asaf., Canth., Caps., Cyc., Euph., Ipec., Iris, Ib., Nit. ac., Puls., Sab., *Thuja.*
heat of: Agar., Asar., Bell., Calad., Ced., Chel., Cur., Cyc., Dig., Graph., Ham., Hydr., Kali b., Lach., *Led., Mag. c.,* Mercurialis, *Nit. ac.,* Nux m., *Nux,* Petr., Phos., Plant., **Puls.,** Sab., Stan., Staph., **Sul.**
heat of one, the other cold: Cinch., Coc., *Dig.,* Puls.
heat of one, and coldness of the other in alternation: Coc.
heavy: Aran.
hot and clammy: Plant.
pain in, from cold, when uncovered: Nux, Stram.
palms of, hot: Æsc., Anac., Asar., **Fer.,** *Lach.,* Lyc., Mer., *Polyp.,* **Sul.**

Hands, perspiration, cold, on: Nit. ac.
sweat of: Bar., Hep., Nit. ac., Plant.
veins of, distended: *Bell.*, *Cinch.*, *Hyos.*, **Led.**, Meny.

Hard, feeling as though bed were: **Arn.**, Bap., Bellis, Mur. ac., Pyr.

Head, cold: Bell.
cold, also face, back and hands: Nit. s. d.
congested (cerebral): Doryph.
hot: *Bell.*, Cac., *Calc.*, Camph., Carbo an., Caust., Chel., Croc., Cur., Dig., Eup., Fer., Gels., Hyper., Ib., Ipec., Kali i., Kali m., Lyc., *Mag. c.*, Mercurialis, *Petr.*, Phel., Phos. ac., Plant., Rob., Rhus, Sab., Sars., Sil., Staph., Stram., Ver.
hot and body cold: Hell., Mag. s.
pain in, lancinating: Cac.
pain in, shooting: Corn. cir., Berb.
sweat on: Mag. c.
fullness in: Chin. s., Ib.
heavy: Boliv., Ced., Coc.

Headache: Acon., Æsc., Agar., Alst., *Ang.*, **Arn.**, *Ars.*, Astacus, **Bell.**, Berb., Bor., Bry., Cac., Calc., Caps., Carbo v., Chin. s., Cina, **Cinch.**, Coc., Col., Corn., Crot., Dros., Dul., Elat., **Eup.**, Graph., *Hep.*, Hipp., Irid., *Ign.*, Kali b., Kali c., Lach., Lac. ac., Lob., Lyssin, Manc., **Natr.**, Nux, Op., Plant., *Pod.*, Psor., Ptel., Puls., Rob., *Rhus*, Ruta, Sabad., Sep., **Sil.**, Sul., Val.
one-sided: Spig., *Thuja.*
stitches in the temples: **Nux**, Puls.
stitches unbearable in the: Asaf.
as if it would burst: Æsc., Bell., Corn.

Heart, beats violently: Æsc., Kali m.
constriction about: Lil. t.
palpitation of: Acon., *Bar.*, Calc., Mer., Sars., Sep., Sul.

Hips, burning in: Cur.
pain in: *Rhus.*

Hoarseness: Hep.

Hunger: **Cina, Cinch.**, Cur., Eup. p., **Phos.**
canine, or aversion to food: **Cinch.**

Ice-cream, desire for: **Phos.**, Ver.

Irritability: *Anac.*, **Cham.**, Bry., Med., Plant., Ptel.
in nursing children: **Anac.**, Cham., Sil.

Knees hot, nose cold: Ign.
weak: Anac.

Lachrymation: Eup.

Lassitude: Lyssin.

Leg, pain in one: Gels.

Legs, coldness of: Carbo an., Meph., Sep., **Stram.**
aching in: Lyssin.
heat in: Camph., Cur., **Led.**, Sarr., Stan.
burning in prevents sleep: Bap., Bufo.
numbness of: Ced.
veins of, distended: **Chin. s.**

Lie down, feeling as though he must: Natr.
still, wants to: *Bry.*, Gels.

Light, sensitiveness to: Bell., Psor.

Limbs, cold: Carbo an., **Stram.**
hot, but feel cold: Bap.
heaviness of: Aran., Calc.
pain in: Ars., Bry., Calc., Caps., Carbo v., Cinch., Eucal., *Eup.*, Eup. p., Guaj., Lach., Lyc., Ptel., Puls., Rhus, Sec., Sep., Sul., Val.
twitching of the: Gels., Op.

Lips, burning of: Cinch.
blue, body purple: **Guarea.**
dryness of: Con., Rhus.
fever blisters on: Chin. s., *Hep.*, *Ign.*, **Natr.**, **Nux**, **Rhus.**
fever blisters on upper: **Rhus.**
licks them, but does not drink: **Puls.**

Liver, pain in the region of: Ars., Cinch., Elat., *Nux.*

Loins, pain in: Crot., Kali c.

Loquacity: *Carbo v.,* Gels., **Lach., Mar. v.,** Meny., **Pod.**

Lungs, engorged, feel as if: Æsc.

Milk, desire for: Mer.

Moaning: Acon., Cham., *Eup.,* Lach., **Puls.**
during sleep: Eup.

Mouth, burning in: Æsc., *Petr.*
dryness of: *Ars.,* Chin. s., Cinch., Cinnab., **Nux m.,** Tar.
fever blisters around: *Hep., Ign.,* **Natr., Nux, Rhus.**
frequent spitting of mucus: Æsc.
open: Op.
paleness around: *Cina.*
yellow inside: Plumb.

Muscles, twitching of: Gels., Ign., Iod., Op.

Nasal sinuses, shooting pains through: Gels.

Nausea: Alum., Anac., Ant. t., Aran., Ars., Bor., Bry., *Carbo v.,* Cham., Cimex, Coc., Dros., *Elat.,* Eup., Eup. p., *Ipec.,* Lyc., *Natr.,* Nit. ac., *Nux,* Op., Phos., Ptel., Rob., Sabad., Sep., **Thuja,** Ver. Ver. v.
after eating: Ind. m.
from slightest motion: Fl. ac.

Neck, pain in: Graph.
nape of, coldness in: Zinc.
heat and fullness in, and head: Ib.
as if water were running upward, from back: Glon.

Nervous moving of fingers: Led.

Noise, sensitive to: *Bell.,* **Caps.,** Gels., Ptel., **Ther.**

Nose, cold: Ign.
end of, hot: **Caps.,** Chel.
paleness around: Cina.
picking of the: *Cina.*

Numbness: **Ced.**, Par., *Sep.*, Thuja.

Occiput, heat in: Camph.

Oppression and anxiety: ***Acon.***

Pain, in parts rested upon: ***Bap.***, **Bellis**, **Pyr.**

Painful, side lain upon: Bap., Phos. ac., Pyr.

Painfulness, of body when touched: Puls., Spig., **Stram.**
of body when uncovered: Mer., **Nux**, ***Stram.***

Pains, on uncovering, violent: Nux, ***Stram.***

Palate, heat of: Dulc.

Palpitation, heat in chest and: Calc. ars.
at times: Coc.

Paralysis: Cur.

Photophobia: Hep., **Psor.**

Position, desire to change: Arn., Bap., *Rhus.*
desire to change because bed is hard: **Arn.**, Pyr.
desire to change to relieve the pain: Rhus.
desire to move to a cool part of the bed: Bap., Op.

Prostration, marked: Ver. v.

Pulse, full: Acon., Camph., Ced., Chin. s., Corn., Nit. ac.
hard: Corn.
irregular: *Cinch.*, Nit. ac.
quick: *Acon.*, Camph., *Cinch.*, Corn., Dig., Iod., Myg., Rhus.
slow: Fer., Hell.
weak: Ant. t., Iod.
beat felt through whole body: Coc.
frequent: Fl. ac.
rapid at night: Med.
violent: Kali m.
violent in head preventing sleep: Benz. ac.

Pupils, contracted: Gels., Laur., Op., Phys., Ter., Ver.
dilated: *Bell.*, Calc., Cic., Cina, *Hell.*, Ipec., Stram., Ver.

Recollect, inability to: Ars., Natr., Phos. ac., Sep.

Respiration, rapid: Lob., Plant.
snoring: Con., **Op.,** *Laur., Lob.*

Restlessness: *Acon.,* Amm. c., *Arn.,* **Ars.,** Bap., Bar., Bell., Caps., Carb. ac., *Cham.,* Cina, Cinch., *Gels.,* Ipec., Lachn., Mag. m., Mancin., Nicc., Plant., *Puls.,* **Rhus,** Sab., *Sec.,* Val.

Room seems hot and close: Apis, Plant., Sul.

Saliva, profuse discharge of watery: Æsc., *Dros.*
frothy: Rob.
stringy: Con., Kali, Mer.

Salivation: Arundo, Mer.

Scapula, pain under the right: **Chel.,** *Nux,* Pod.
pain under the left: Sang.

Scrobiculus cordis, pain in: Eup.

Sensation, as if a hot wave, like vapor, surged through the body: Lyss., Mag. c., Sarr.

Shiverings, from uncovering: Apis, Arn., Bar., Hell., **Nux,** Stram.

Shoulders, pain between: *Rhus.*
hot: Calend.

Sighing: Ign., Puls.

Sight, obscuration of: Natr., Puls.

Skin, damp: Fer., Op., Ver.
dry: Acet. ac., Æsc., Apis, Ars., Bar., Carb. ac., Hyos., Ign., Iod., Ipec., Polyp., Sec., Sul.
excoriations of: Sarr.
fissures of: Sarr., Natr.
hot: Acet. ac., Acon., Æsc., Apis, Ars., Bar., Bell., Carb. ac., Chin. m., Corn., Fer., *Hyos.,* Nat. ars., Polyp., Sul.
itching of: Amm. m., Apis, *Ign., Rhus.*
itching of, worse from rubbing: *Rhus.*
hot and dry: Acet. ac., Acon., Agar., Lept., Sul., Ter.
hot and dry, and mucous membranes: Bry., Sul., Ter.
burning and pricking of: Mer. c.

Skin, pricking in: Croc., *Gels.,* Nit. ac., Polyp.
red: Ars., Tar.
scarlet: Tar.
stinging of: Amm. m., Cinch.
tingling of: Manc.
yellow: Mer. c.

Sleep: Abs., **Ant. t.,** Apis, Calad., Caps., Ced., *Cinch.,* **Eup.,** *Gels.,* Ign., **Lach.,** Lachn., Laur., Lyc., Med., **Mez., Natr.,** *Nux m.,* **Op., Pod., Rob.,** Rhus, **Samb.,** Stram.
disappears during: Calad.
at climax of heat: **Pod.**
deep snoring: Con., **Ign.,** *Laur.,* **Op., Rob.**
soporous: **Op., Rob.**
dreams during: Elaps.
inability to, after 3 A. M.: Ang.
starting in: *Cham., Chin. s.,* Con., Gels., Lyc.
starting when beginning to: Ign., Puls.

Sleepiness: Apis, Asaf., Ced., Cinch., *Gels.,* Hep., Ign., Lyc., Lyss., Nat. c., Nux m., Op., Phos., Plumb., Puls., Rhus, Stram., Ver., **Ver. v.**

Sleeplessness: Acon., Ang., Arn., Ars., Asaf., Bar., Cof., Con., Graph., Hyos., Nat. c., Puls., Staph.

Smothering, sensation of: **Apis,** Carbo v., Cimex, Natr., Sep.

Sneezing: *Chin. s.,* Cinch. b.

Somnolency: Ant. t., Arn., Ars., Cac., Dul., Gels., Ign., Lachn., *Natr.,* Nux m., Op., Phos. ac., Sep., Ter.

Speech, incoherent: Arn., Bap., Cur., Gels., Natr., Op., Ver.

Spine, painful to pressure: **Chin. s.**
heat from, to occiput: Nit. s. d.

Spleen, pain in region of: Ars., Carbo v., Eucal., *Nux,* Pod., Rob.

Staring, wild look: Hyper.

Stomach, heat in the pit of: Chin. s., Lach., Sarr.
heat in the, as if flames were spreading from: Manc.
pain in: Ars., Carbo v., Cina, Kali c., Rhus, Sec., Sep.
puffed up, with vomiting: Fer. p.

Stool, frequent: Lach.
urgency to: Caps.

Stretching: Æsc., Calc., Chin. s., Cina, Rhus, Sab.

Stupor and muttering delirium: Arn., Bap., Bry., Hyos., Rhus, Op., Ter.
state of apparent: Coc., Phos. ac.

Subsultus tendinum: Psor., Rhus, Ter., Ver. v., Zinc.

Swallow, constant inclination to: *Æsc.*

Swallowing, difficulty in: Cic., Cimex.
painful: Manc.

Sweat: Alum., Amm. m., Ant. c., Anth., Calend., Camph., Caps., Colch., Con., Hell., Mag. c., Nicc., Stan., Staph.
profuse: **Colch.**, Psor.
on forehead: Mag. s.
on head: Bell.

Teeth, chattering of: Ced.

Temperature, sensitive to change of: *Bar.,* Calc., Hep., Psor.
subnormal: Anth., Arg. n., Carbo v., **Pyr.**

Temples, throbbing pain in: Corn. c.
shooting pressive pains through: Gels.

Thirst: *Acon.,* Ailant., Alston., Amm. c., Amm. m., Ang., Anth., Ant. c., Apis, *Arn.,* **Ars.,** Arund., Bar., *Bell.,* Berb., Bov., *Bry.,* Cac., Calad., Calc., Canth., Caps., *Ced., Cham., Chin. m.,* Chin. s., *Cina, Cinch., Cof.,* Con., Croc., Cur., Elat., Elaps, Eup., *Eup. p., Hep.,* Hyos., Ind., Ipec., Kali bi., Lach., Lyc., Lyss., *Mag. c.,* Manc., Med., **Natr.,** Nicc., *Nux,* Phos., Plant., Plumb., Pod., *Psor., Puls.,* Rob., *Rhus,* Sab., Sarr., *Sec.,* Sep., *Sil.,* Staph., Stram., Sul., *Thuja,* Val., Ver.

Thirst, hot drinks, desire for: Ars., *Ced.,* **Casc., Eup. p.,** Sabad.
large quantities of water, desire for: *Acon., Alston.,* Bar., Bell., Bry., Myg., **Natr.**
large quantities of water, desire for, which relieve: **Natr.**
desire for, but unable to drink: **Cimex.**
much: Acon., Alston., *Arn., Ars.,* Bell., *Bry.,* Casc., Cham., Chin. s., Cinch., Elat., *Hep.,* Hyos., **Natr.,** Myg.
slight: Cac., Sabad.
uncovering, aggravated by: Bar.
vomiting after drinking, with: Alston., *Ars.,* Phos.
wanting: **Æth.,** Agar., *Alum., Ant. t., Apis,* Asaf., Bar., Bov., *Calc., Camph., Caps.,* Carbo an., *Carbo v., Caust., Cimex, Cinch.,* Coc., Coral., Cyc., Dig., *Dros., Fer.,* Gels., Hell., *Ign.,* Ipec., Kali c., *Led.,* Med., Meny., Mur. ac., **Nux m.,** Op., Phos. ac., **Puls.,** Rhus, Sabad., *Samb.,* **Sep.,** Spig., **Tar.**

Throat, pain in: Phos., Phos. ac., Sep.
burning dryness, constriction of: Æsc.
sore when swallowing: Berb., Phos. ac.
sore: Ind. m.

Throbbing, violent, through whole body: Lil., Zinc.
of left temporal artery: Arg. n.

Tongue, dry, without thirst: Cal. p., Nux m.
dry and brown: Myg.
coated: Guarea.

Toothache: Carbo v.

Trachea, dryness of: *Petr.*

Trembling: Ars., Calc., Cist., Eup., Kali i., Mag. c., Myg., Sep.

Tympanitis, excessive: Ter.

Unconsciousness: Laur., Manc., Natr.

Uncovered, desire to be: *Acon.,* Apis, Arn., *Ars.,* Bar., Bor., Calc., *Cinch., Eup.,* Fer., Fer. m., Fl. ac., *Hep.,* Hipp., **Iod.,** *Lach.,* Lyc., Mur. ac., **Natr.,** Nit. ac., *Op., Petr.,* **Puls.,** Spig., Staph., Ver.

Uncovered, aversion to being: *Apis,* **Arg. n.,** Ars., *Bell.,* Clem., Cof., Col., Con., *Hell., Hep.,* Ign., *Mag. c.,* Manc., Mer., Nux m., **Nux,** Phos. ac., Puls., Rhus, *Samb.,* **Stram.,** Stront.
chilliness when: Arg. n., *Cinch.,* **Nux,** Puls.

Urinate, after drinking, desire to: Cimex, Eup. p.

Urination, frequent: Arg., Bell., Ind., Kreos., Lyc., Mer., Phos., Rhus, Staph., Stram.
involuntary: Sul. ac.

Urine, brick dust sediment, with: Lyc., Phos., Sars.
whitish sediment: Phos., Sep.
pale: **Ced.,** Cham.
pale, frequent, large quantities of water: Phos. ac.
profuse: Ant. t., Arg., Ced., *Cham.,* Dul., *Eup. p.,* Ind., *Manc.,* Med., Mur. ac., *Phos.,* Phos. ac., Scill., Stram.
red: Nux.
suppressed: Cac.
turbid: Berb., Phos.

Urticaria: Apis, **Ign.,** *Rhus.*
during heat, disappearing with sweat: **Ign.**

Uterus, pain in the region of: Cac.

Veins, blood burns in: *Ars., Hyos.,* Med.
blood runs cold in: Ver.
as from hot water running through: **Rhus,** Pyr.
distended: *Agar., Bell.,* **Camph.,** *Chin. s.,* **Cinch.,** Croc., Cyc., Dig., **Hyos., Led.,** *Mercurialis,* Nit. s. d., **Puls.**

Vertex, hot sensation on: Nat. s., Sul.
pain throbbing in: Corn. c.

Vertigo: Ars., Bell., Berb., Bis., *Carbo v.* Coc., Eucal., Gels., Hep., Ign., Ipec., Laur., Mer., *Natr.,* Nux, Phos., Puls., *Sep., Stram.,* Val., Ver.
and heat, with sweat on forehead on raising head: Mag. s.

Vision, dim: Chin. s.

Vomiting: Alston., Ant. c., Ars., Bis., Bry., Cac., *Cham.*, *Cina*, Con., Doryph., Elat., **Eup.**, Eup. p., Fer., Fer. p., Ign., *Ipec.*, Lach., *Lyc.*, **Natr.**, Nicc., Nux, Puls., Stram., Thuja, Ver. v.
of bile: *Cham.*, *Cina*, **Eup.**, *Natr.*, Thuja.
bitter: Eup.
black: Sul. ac.
after drinking: *Ars.*
after cold drinks: Lyc.
frothy: *Elat.*
desire to: Guarea.
of ingesta: Cina, *Eup.*, **Fer.**, **Ign.**, **Nux.**
sour: **Lyc.**, Rob.
of water: Alston., Ars.

Voice, weak: Hep.

Wanting: (See absent).

Warmth, of bed, intolerable: Lach., **Led.**, *Puls.*
external, intolerable: *Apis*, Ipec., **Puls.**, **Sep.**
external, pleasant: *Ign.*

Wash with cold water, desire to: **Fl. ac.**

Weakness: Anac., *Arn.*, *Ars.*, Aspar., Bry., Calc., Carbo v., Clem., Coca, Cur., Eup., Ign., Ind., Ipec., Lyc., Lyssin, Nat. c., **Natr.**, Nux m., Phos., **Rob.**, Sarr., Sul.

Weeping: Spong.

Yawning: Æsc., Calc., Calc. p., **Chin. s.**, Cina, Kali c., *Rhus*, Sabad.

HEAT, FOLLOWED BY:

Chill: Amm. m., Ang., Apis, Asar., *Bell.*, *Bry.*, *Calad.*, **Cal.**, Caps., *Caust.*, Cinch., Col., Dul., Elaps, Eup. p., *Hell.*, Ign., Iris, Kali c., Lyc., **Mal.**, Meny., Mer., Natr., Nicc., Nit. ac., **Nux**, Petr., Phos., **Puls.**, Pyr., **Sep.**, **Stan.**, Staph., Sul., Thuja, **Tub.**
and gentle heat: Myr.

Chilliness: Aster., Hell., Mal., Meny., Mer., Tub.

Colic: Hell.

Debility: Aran., Hyd.

Drowsiness: Casc.

Exhaustion: Ars., Mal., Pyr., Tub.

Eyes, stinging in: Aran.

Face, paleness of: Scill.
paleness of and fainting when rising up: Acon.
redness of, worse on the right side: Lachn.

Headache: Ars., Cal., *Carbo v.,* **Eup., Natr.**

Hunger: **Cimex,** Dul., **Eup.,** Ign.
ravenous: **Cimex.**

Languor: Med.

Sleep: Apis, *Eup.,* Lob., Op.
with snoring: **Op.**

Thirst: Anac., Amm. m., Cac., *Cinch.,* Cof., Cyc., Mal., Nux, Op., Puls., Pyr., Stan., Stram., Tub.
absence of: Kali n., Op.

Vomiting: Aran., Cal., *Eup.*
bilious: *Eup.*

Weakness: *Ars.,* Dig., Natr., Pyr., Tub.

HEAT; CHARACTERISTICS OF:

Abdomen, of: Stan.
to head, in flushes: Ind.

Anxious, of whole body: Acon., Casc.
as if sweat would break out: Stan.

Anticipating: **Nux.**

Afternoon, without chill: Anac.

Ascends: Alum., Ang., *Cina,* Crot., Hyos., *Phos., Natr.,* **Sep.,** *Ver.*

Aversion to uncovering: Apis, Ars., Aur., Bell., Cal., *Eup.,* **Hep.,** Ign., Mag. c., **Nux, Psor.,** Pyr., Rhus, Samb., **Stram., Tub.**

Back, over the: Bap., Cur., Dul., Hyos., Phos., Stan.
from small of, in all directions: **Bap.**
descends: Laur.

Bed, in: Hell., Kali c., Mag. m., Mag. s., Sul., ac.
in, chilly when not: Mer.

Body, left side of: **Mez.,** Rhus.
left side of, coldness of right: *Rhus.*
right side of: **Alum.,** Meny., Mosc., **Puls.,** Ran., **Tub.**
of one side only: Asaf., Clem.
upper part of: Anac., Puls.
whole of: Æsc., Bap., Camph., Ipec., Ign., Kali bi., Led., Mal., Meny., Nit. ac., Nux, Op., Petr., Samb., Tub.
seems too heavy: Euphor.

Burning: *Acon., Arn.,* Ant. t., **Apis, Ars.,** Bar., *Bell.,* Bry., Cac., Canth., Caps., Cham., Chel., Cur., Dul., *Elaps,* Eup. p., Hell., *Hep., Hyos.,* Lach., Laur., Led., Lyc., Lyss., Mag. c., Mercurialis, Mer., Mer. s., Manc., Mosch., **Nux, Op.,** Phos., **Puls.,** Sabad., Sarr., Sec., Staph., Stan., **Tub.**
with internal chilliness: Hell.
with inclination to cover: Manc.
over all the body, with flushes to the head and face: Med.
in the face, with pimples: Mosc.
in the face, but not on the feet: Mer. s.
of palms and soles: Lach., Mur. ac., Sang., Sul.
on parts on which lain: Lyss.
intense, at first onset: Crot.
of whole body: Sab.
in throat and pharynx: Æsc.
in the mouth: Æsc.
which is not felt: Canth.

Burning, even when bathed in sweat: **Op.**
without external redness: Hyos.
interrupted by shaking chill: Sec.

Chest, in or on: **Apis,** Cic., Stan.

Chills, with shaking: Sec.

Chilliness, with: **Apis,** *Arn., Caust., Cur., Elaps,* Hell., Iris, **Kali bi.,** Kali c., Kali i., Lach., Lachn., *Mer., Nux,* Petr., Phos., *Pod.,* Plat., **Puls.,** *Rhus,* Sabad., Sab., Sec., *Sil.,* Sul.
with flushes of heat: Plat.
alternating with, not perceptible to the touch: Mer., Myr.
alternating with coldness here and there, over entire body: Arn.
during the day: **Dros.**
from putting hands outside bed covering: Arn., Bar., **Nux,** *Stram.,* **Tub.**

Clothing, and body too heavy: Euphor.

Coldness, with, except the face and head: Bell., *Op.,* Stram.
all over to the touch: Carbo v., Fer.

Day, during the, periodically: Sil.

Dry: *Acon., Æsc., Apis,* Arn., **Ars.,** Bar., *Bell.,* **Bry.,** Cac., Ced., Clem., Coc., Cof., Col., Con., Dul., Fer., Graph., Hell., *Hep., Hyos.,* Nat. s., Nit. ac., **Nux,** Op., Ol. an., *Phos.,* Phos. ac., Ptel., **Puls.,** Rhus, *Samb.,* Sarr., Sec., Sep., Stram.
on covered parts: Thuja.
at night: Clem.
as if blood boiling, cannot sweat: Chin. m.

Evening: Alum., Amb., Ang., Aran., *Berb.,* Carbo v., **Cinch.,** Dros., Fer., Hell., *Hep.,* Hyos., Lach., Lyc., Mag. c., Mer., Mur. ac., Phos., Phos. ac., *Psor.,* Sars., **Sil.,** *Sul.,* Sul. ac., Thuja.

Face, on: Acon., Æsc., Amb., Asar., Aur., Can. s., Cac., Cina, **Dros., Ind.,** Kali br., **Lyc.,** Mer. s., Stram.
of the, after eating: Asaf.
flushes in or over: Amb., Amm. m., Arn., *Bap.*, Bar., *Cac.*, Cal., Carbo an., Carbo v., Chel., Cinch., Graph., Hep., Ign., Iod., *Kali bi.*, **Kali c., Kali i.,** Kali br., Lach., Lyc., Mag. c., Meny., Natr., Nat. c., **Nit. ac.,** Nux, Petr., Phos., Puls., Sabad., Sab., Sep., Sil., Spig., Stan., **Sul.,** Sul. ac., Thuja, Val.
flushes in, always ending in sweat: *Amm. m.*
flushes, rise up to: Calad.
flushes, only on the: Crot., Euphor.
flushes on, rest of body chilly: Sab.
flushes on, with icy cold hands and feet: Sab.
flushes on, and neck: Med.
flushes in, sudden toward evening: Nat. s., Sul. ac.
flushes in, with desire to be fanned: Zinc.
flushes in, also chest and over back: Mang.

Flushes, hot, then sweat: Act.
hot, as if in a furnace, with coldness and chills: Kali br.
hot, with cold body: Hell.
every afternoon: Nat. p., **Tub.**
as if flames rose out of region of stomach: Manc.

Forenoon, in: Eup., Kali c., *Natr., Nux,* Rhus, Sars., Thuja.

Hands, palms of: Asar.

Head, mostly on: Cina, Cur., Dros., Hell., Mer., Sabad.
heat runs from, to toes: Calc. p.
hot, hands cold: Hell.
hot, then over whole body: Aster.

Hips, burning in the: Cur.

Hot water, on arms, chest, ears and legs, sensation of: *Cic.*
as if dashed with: Puls., Rhus, Sep., Tub.

Intense: *Acon., Ant. t.,* Arn., **Ars.,** *Bell.,* Bry., Cac., Canth., Caps., Chin. s., Colch., Dig., Hep., Kali i., Lyc., Mag. c., Mer-

curialis, **Mez.**, **Natr.**, Nux m., *Nux*, *Op.*, Puls., **Rhus**, **Sec.**, **Sil.**, Staph., Stram., Sul., **Tar.**, *Ver. v.*
alternating with icy-coldness: Tar.
with brain irritation and tendency to spasms: Ver. v.

Internal: *Acon.*, *Arn.*, *Ars.*, **Bell.**, Bry., Caps., Cham., Chel., Cic., Cinch., Con., Fer., Hell., Iod., Kali c., Mag. c., Mur. ac., Nit. ac., Nux, Phos., Phos. ac., **Puls.**, **Rhus**, *Sabad.*, Sec., Sep., Spig., Stan., Ver.
wants to uncover: Mur. ac.
with cold sensation in abdomen: Zinc.
with external coldness: Bell., Iod., Phos.
burning, external chilliness: **Mez.**
burning, as if between flesh and skin: Brom.
burning, external heat: Rheum.
chill: Ran.

Limbs, of: Kobalt, Stan.

Long-lasting: *Acon.*, **Ant. t.**, Cac., Hep., *Sec.*, Sil., **Sul.**, *Tar.*

Midnight, at: Rhus, **Stram.**, *Sul.*
before: *Ant. c.*, Calad., Laur.
after: **Ars.**, Kali c., Thuja.
and noon: *Stram.*

Morning: **Arn.**, Kali c., Mag. c., *Nux*, Rhus, **Sul.**, Thuja.

Night: **Alum.**, Ant. c., Ars., Bar., Bry., *Cal.*, Carbo an., Carbo v., Caust., Kali bi., Lach., Laur., Mag. c., Mag. m., Mer., Natr., Nit. ac., Petr., **Phos.**, Phos. ac., Polyp., Psor., **Puls.**, Rhus, Sab., Sarr., **Sil.**, Staph., Stram., Sul., Thuja, Zinc.
at, with palpitation: Mur. ac.
may last all: Rhus.

Noon: Lach., **Stram.**, *Sul.*

Pain, of limbs: Guaj.

Parts, affected, of: Acon., Bry., Sul.
covered, of: Thuja.
single, of: Stan., Zinc.
heat of one with chill of another at the same time: **Cinch.**

Predominating: *Ant. t.,* Bell., Cac., **Ipec.,** Sec., Sil.

Rising into head, with thirst: Mang.

Shiverings, with: Acon., Anac., Ant. t., *Apis,* **Arn.,** Cal., Carbo v., Caust., Cham., Cinch., *Cur., Elaps,* Eup., *Gels.,* Hep., Ign., Lach., **Mal.,** Meny., **Nux,** Petr., Phos. ac., Pod., Rhus, Sabad., **Sul.**
alternating with: Caust., Cinch., Cyc., Elaps, Hep., Lach., Mer., Phos. ac., Sabad., Tar.
drinking, from: *Caps.,* Eup., **Nux.**
motion, from: Apis, *Arn.,* **Nux,** Pod., Stram.
mingled with: Acon., Anac., Ant. t., Apis, Cal., **Caust.,** Cham., Mal., Petr., Pod., Rhus.
uncovering, from: **Arn.,** Apis, *Bar.,* **Nux,** Psor., **Tub.**

Short: Ant. t., Aran., Nit. ac.

Single parts: Tub., Zinc.

Slight: Lob., Lyc., Nux m.

Soles: Zinc.

Spine, along the: Hyos.

Spot, in one, which is cold to the touch: *Arn.*

Sweat, with: **Alum.,** Amm. m., **Ant. c.,** Camph., Canch., Caps., Ced., **Con.,** Eup., Ipec., *Kali i.,* Mag. c., **Mez., Op.,** Paris, **Phos., Pod., Psor., Puls.,** *Rhus,* Sabad., Sep., Stram., **Tub., Ver.**
with, on the face: Val.
with, on upper part of body: Paris.
with, on the head: Bell.

Warmth, over whole body, except the head: Ang.

SWEAT AGGRAVATED:

Air, exercise in the: *Bry.,* Casc., *Caust., Cinch.*
in open: *Bry.,* Cal., *Carbo an., Caust., Cinch.,* Ipec., *Psor.,* Pyr., Ruta, Tub.

Bed, getting out of: Lach.
in: Nit. ac.
in, and chilliness as soon as he gets warm: Arg. n.

Covered, on being: *Bell.,* **Cinch.,** Nit. ac., Tub.

Drinking, by: Coc.

Eating, by: Bar., Benz. ac., Bor., Cal., *Carbo an., Carbo v.,* Card., Cain., Coc., Con., Graph., Ign., Laur., Lyc., Natr., Nit. ac., Nux, Nat. c., Ol. an., Phos., Sars., Sep., Sul. ac.

Exercise, by: Bell., Berb., Brom., Bry., Cain., *Cal.,* Canth., Carbo v., Caust., *Cinch., Coc.,* Corn., *Fer., Graph., Hep., Kali c.,* Kali n., Led., Lyc., Mer., *Nat. c., Natr.,* Op., *Phos., Psor., Stan.,* Rheum, Sul. ac., Tub., Zinc.

Exertion, mental: Hep., *Kali c., Psor., Sep., Sul.,* Tub.

Eyes, upon closing the: *Con.*

Lying down, after: Mag. s., Meny.

Midnight, after: Alum., Amb., Amm. m., Bar., Clem., Dros., Kali c., Mag. m., Nux, Phos., *Sil.*

Morning, in the: Amb., Puls.

Motion: Alum., Amm. m., Arundo, Bell., Bry., Cain., Cal., Camph., Canth., *Carbo an., Caust.,* Chin. s., *Cinch., Coc.,* Cur., Fl. ac., Gels., Graph., **Hep.,** Ipec., Kali bi., *Kali c.,* Mal., Mag. c., **Mer.,** *Natr., Phos.,* **Psor.,** Pyr., **Sep.,** *Sil., Sul.,* Tub., Val., *Ver.*

Room, in a: Fl. ac., Tub.

Side affected, on: Amb.

Sitting, during: Anac., *Kali bi.,* Rhus, Sep., Staph.

Sleep, during: Ars., Bell., Camph., Cham., Chel., Cinch., **Con.,** Hyos., *Mez., Phos.,* Plat., **Thuja.**
during morning: Bor.
commencing to, when: Agar., Amm. c., Ars., Cinch., Con., Mur. ac., Tab., Thuja, Tub., Ver.
in first: Cal.

Smoking, by: Coc.

Stool, after every: **Ver.**

Vomiting, after mucous: *Ver.*
of sour masses: Nat. p.

Waking, on: Benz. ac., Canth., **Samb., Sep.,** ***Sul.***

Warmth of room: Plant.
of bed: Arg. n.

Weather, in damp: Cur.

Wind, by cold: Cur.

Writing, by: *Hep., Kali c., Psor.,* **Sep.,** *Sul.,* Tub.

Weakness: Apis, Ars., Bar., Camph., Fer., Iod., *Mer., Phos.,* Psor., Pyr., Puls.

Yawning: Caust.

SWEAT AMELIORATED:

Air, in open: Alum., Graph.

Bed, on getting out of: Hell.

Covered, by being: Acon.

Drinking, after: Chin. s.

Eating, after: Cinch., Lach., Phos.
by: Anac., Cur.

Food, after warm: Kali c., Sul. ac., Phos.

Morning, in the: Bor., **Lachn.**

Motion, by: **Caps.**

Sleep, in: Nux, Rum., *Samb.*
after: Hell.

Walking, on: Cham., Chel., *Puls.*, *Thuja.*

Wine, drinking: Sul. ac.

SWEAT, FOLLOWED BY:

Checked, if grave symptoms appear from: Cad. s.

Chill: **Carbo v.**, Corn., Corn. c., Hep., *Mal.*, **Nux**, Tub.
then sweat: Nux.
then sweat with heat: **Nux.**

Cough: Eup., Sil.

Debility and prostration: Tar.

Diarrhea: Puls.

Heat and thirst: Ant. c.

Hunger: **Cina**, Staph.
canine: **Cina.**

Madness, paroxysm of: Cup.

Prostration: Ars., Kali br., Tar., Ter.

Relief, of all complaints: Calad., **Psor.**, *Natr.*, Val.

Sleep: Nux m.

Stiffness of hands and fingers: Lyss.

Thirst: Bell., Bor., **Lyc.**, Nux, Sabad.
much: Lyc.

Vomiting: *Cina.*

Weakness: Ars., Mal., Pyr.

AGGRAVATION WHILE SWEATING:

Acon., Ant., Arn., **Ars.**, **Bry.**, Cal., **Caust.**, **Cham.**, Cinch., Cimex, Croc., Eup., *Fer.*, Ign., *Ipec.*, Lyc., **Mer.**, Mur. ac., *Nux*, **Op.**, Phos., Puls., Psor., **Rhus**, **Sep.**, Spong., **Stram.**, **Sul.**, **Ver.**, Tub.

AMELIORATION WHILE SWEATING:

Acon., Æsc., Æth., Ars., Apis, Bap., Bell., Bov., *Bry.*, Cal., Camph., Canth., Cham., Cimex, **Cup.**, Elat., Eup., **Gels.**, Graph., *Hep.*, *Lach.*, Lyc., **Natr.**, **Psor.**, **Rhus**, Samb., Sec., Stront., *Thuja*, *Ver.*

Except, the headache: **Natr.**
the headache which is made worse: *Ars.*, Chin. s., **Eup.**

SWEAT ABSENT:

Acon., Alum., Amm. c., Apis, *Aran.*, Arn., *Ars.*, Aspar., Asaf., *Bell.*, Bis., *Bov.*, Bry., Cal., Cham., Chin. m., Chin. ars., Cinch., Cof., Colch., Corn., Dul., *Eup.*, Gels., *Graph.*, Hyos., Ign., Iod., Ipec., Kali bi., Kali c., Lach., Led., *Lyc.*, Mag. c., Mer., Nat. c., Nit. ac., Nux m., Nux, Oleand., Op., Phel., Phos., Phos. ac., Plat., Psor., Puls., Rhus, Sabad., Sec., Seneg., Sil., Spong., Staph., Sul., Ver.

SWEAT IN GENERAL:

Acon., Æsc., Æth., *Agar.*, Alston., Alum., *Amb.*, Amm. m., Anac., Ang., Ant. c., **Ant. t.**, Apis, Arg. n., Arn., Ars., Asaf., Bap., **Bar.**, *Bell.*, **Benz.**, *Bov.*, **Bry.**, Cac., Calad., **Cal.**, *Camph.*, Canch., *Canth.*, *Caps.*, **Carbo an.**, *Carbo v.*,

Cain., **Caust.**, **Ced.**, Cham., Chel., **Chin. s.**, Chlor., Cic., Cim., Cina, **Cinch.**, Coc., Cof., Con., Corn., Cupr., Cur., Cyc., **Dig.**, Dros., Dul., *Elat.*, *Elaps*, Eup., *Eup. p.*, Euphor., **Fer.**, Gamb., *Gels.*, *Graph.*, Hell., **Hep.**, *Hyos.*, Ign., *Iod.*, **Ipec.**, **Kali bi.**, *Kali c.*, Kali i., **Lach.**, Lachn., Laur., Led., Lob., **Lyc.**, Mar., **Mag. c.**, Meny., Mercurialis, **Mer.**, *Mez.*, Nat. c., **Natr.**, Nit. ac., Nux m., **Nux**, **Op.**, Par., *Petr.*, **Phos. ac.**, **Phos.**, Plant., *Pod.*, *Polyp.*, **Psor.**, Puls., *Rhus*, *Rob.*, Sabad., Sab., **Samb.**, *Sarr.*, **Sec.**, **Sep.**, **Sil.**, Spong., Stan., *Staph.*

SWEAT PREDOMINATES:

Benz., **Carbo an.**, *Cinch.*, Fer., Hep., Kali bi., **Mer.**, *Nit. ac.*, Nux, Phos. ac., **Psor.**, **Samb.**, **Tar.**, *Thuja.*

Day, during the: Carbo an., Cinch., Con., **Fer.**, Lyc., Mal., Natr., Pyr., Sep., Stram.

Evening, in the: Bar., Samb., Sul., Tub.

Morning, in the: Alum., Amm. c., Fer., **Mag. c.**, Mer., Natr., *Nit. ac.*, **Psor.**, *Rhus*, *Sep.*, Stan.

Night, at: Alum., Ars., Asaf., **Carbo an.**, *Carbo v.*, Caust., *Cinch.*, **Kali c.**, **Mer.**, Mer. s., Myr., *Nit. ac.*, Phos., **Psor.**, *Pyr.*, Sep., **Sil.** Stram., **Sul.**, **Tarax.**, **Thuja**, **Tub.**, *Val.*, *Ver.*

SWEAT, PRODUCED BY:

Awakening, on: Ptel.

Covering, on slightest: **Cinch.**, *Spig.*

Cramps: Ced.

Eating: Benz. ac., Carbo v., Card., Guar.

Exertion, least: Æth., Agar., Brom., Bry., Corn., Dros., Fl. ac., Psor., *Tub.,* Val., Zinc.

Headache: *Fer.*

Hunger: Staph.

Produced easily: Æth., Agar., Colch., Tub.

Sleep, on going to: Æth., Agar., Cad. s., *Cinch.,* **Con.**
after 3 A. M.: Mercurialis.
only, ceases on waking: Plat.

Thirst: Cof., Thuja.

SWEAT, CHARACTER OF:

Acrid: All. s., Cad. s., *Caps.,* Cham., Con., Carb. ac., Fl. ac., Graph., Iod., Nat. p., Rhus, Tarax.

Ascends: Arn., Bell.

Awake, profuse while: **Samb.,** Sep.
profuse while, on going to sleep dry heat returns: **Samb.**

Bed, in: **Alum.,** Ang., Arg. n.
when getting out of: Lach.

Bloody: Cal., Clem., *Crot.,* **Cur., Lach., Lyc.,** *Nux m.,* Nux.
staining red: **Lach.**

Chill, after the: *Ant. c.,* Caust.
after, without previous heat: *Caps.*
alternating with: Ant. c., Cal., Glon., *Nux.*
simultaneously: Ant. c.

Chilliness, with: Ant. c., Bry., **Eup.,** Eup. p., *Natr.,* **Nux,** Petr., **Nux,** Psor., Tub.
from bathing: Arn.
from motion, or allowing the air to strike him: Eup., Hep., **Nux,** Psor., Tub.
changes to dryness and: Guaj.

Clammy: Acon., Anac., Ant. t., Anth., Arn., **Ars.**, Cal., Camph., Carb. ac., Cham., Coc., Corn. c., Cup. ars., Dig., Dios., Elat., *Fer.*, Fl. ac., Jatr., Hell., Hep., Iod., Lach., Lachn., Lyc., Mer., Mer. c., Nux, Op., Phos. ac., *Phos.*, Plumb., Spig., Ter., Tub., Ver., Ver. v.

Cold: Agar., Anac., **Ant. t.**, **Anth.**, Arn., **Ars.**, Asaf., Bar., Bar. m., Bry., Bufo, Benz. ac., Calad., **Camph.**, Canth., Caps., Chlorum, *Cina*, Cinch., Carb. ac., Crot., Coc., Cup., *Cur.*, Dig., Dul., Dros., Elaps, Fer., Fl. ac., Gels., Hell., **Hep.**, Hyos., Iod., *Ipec.*, Jatr., Kalm., Lach., Lachn., Lob., **Lyc.**, Mal., Mer., Mer. c., Mez., Nat. c., Natr., Nux, Op., Plant., Plumb., Pod., Puls., Rheum, Ruta, Sec., **Sep.**, Sil., Spig., Stan., Staph., **Stram.**, Sul., Sul. ac., Ter., Thuja, Tub., **Ver.**, Ver. v.
- all over the body: Crot., Hell., Mer. c., Spig., Ver.
- on forehead: Acet. ac., Acon., Asaf., Benz. ac., Gels., Graph., Lach., Lachn., Nux, Puls., Rheum, **Ver.**
- on forehead and limbs: Asaf.
- in sudden attacks: Crot.
- eating warm food, soon after: Sul. ac.

Coldness, with, on motion: Eup., **Nux.**
- with, on uncovering: Eup., **Nux**, Tub.

Debilitating, from least movement: Anth., Coc., Kalm., **Stan.**, Tarax.
- from least movement, on one side: Puls.
- when first appears: Ver.

Debility, not causing: Agar., Casc., Nat. s., **Rhus**, **Samb.**, Val.
- with great: Carbo v., Cinch., Sul. ac., Ter.

Discoloring: Bar. m.
- in old cases: Rhus, Sul. ac.

Dryness, alternating with: Apis, Nat. c.

Exhausting: **Benz.**, Carb. ac., **Cinch.**, Kali bi., Kali br., Kali p., Mil., Stan.

Easy: Ant. t., Bry., Calad., *Cal.*, Fer., Graph., *Lyc.*, **Natr.**, **Sep.**, **Sul.**, *Sul. ac.*, Zinc.

Face, cold on the: Coc., Nux, Tab.

Feet, beginning at the: Arn., **Bell.**

Flies, which attracts the: **Calad.**, Puls., *Sumbul*, Thuja.

Heat, with: Æsc., Ant. c., Apis, Bell., Hell., Hep., Kali bi., Laur., Lob., Nat. c., Op., Phel., Samb., Staph., Val.

Heat, dry, remaining sweat soon disappears: *Ant. c.*
internal and prostration, with: Calad.
with, during sleep: **Samb.**
with, in flushes: Ant. c., Bell., **Hep.**, Kali bi., Op.

Hot: **Æsc.**, **Op.**

Linen, making it stiff: Mer., Selen.
staining it bloody: **Lach.**, *Nux m.*
staining it red: Arn., Dul., *Lach.*, Nux.
staining it yellow: Ars., Bell., Bry., Cad. s., **Carbo an.**, Cinch., *Fer.*, *Graph.*, Ipec., Lach., Mag. c., **Mer.**, **Thuja**, *Ver.*

Lying down, after: Mag. s., Meny.

Long-lasting: Kali br., Zinc.

Oily: Agar., Arg., **Bry.**, *Cinch.*, *Mag. c.*, **Mer.**, Mer. s., Nux, Rob., **Stram.**, **Thuja.**

Oil, as if mixed with: **Cinch.**, Tub.

Partial: Cham., *Cinch.*, Mer., Nux, **Petr.**, Pyr., Stram., **Thuja**, Tub.

Profuse: Acet. ac., Acon., Æsc., Agar., Amb., Amyl, *Ant. t.*, Arg., Anth., *Bar.*, Bell., *Benz.*, **Bry.**, Cad. s., *Cal.*, Camph., Canth., Caps., **Carbo an.**, Carbo v., Carb. ac., *Casc.*, *Caust.*, *Ced.*, Chin. m., **Chin. s.**, **Cinch.**, Clem., Coca, Colch., *Dig.*, Elaps, Elat., Eup., Eup. p., *Fer.*, Gels., Graph., **Hep.**, Hyos., Iod., *Ipec.*, *Kali bi.*, Kali br., Kali p., Kali c., *Lach.*, Lact., Lith., **Lyc.**, Lob., *Mag. c.*, **Mal.**, Mang., **Mer.**, Mer. s., Mez., **Natr.**, *Nit. ac.*, *Nux*, *Op.*,

Par., **Phos. ac.,** *Phos.,* Pod., *Polyp.,* Petr., **Psor., Pyr.,** Rob., Rhus, Sabad., **Samb.,** Sarr., *Sec., Sep.,* **Sil.,** Stan., Staph., Stram., *Sul.,* Sul. ac., **Tarax.,** Tar., Ter., *Thuja,* **Tub.,** Val., **Ver.,** Ver. v., Zinc.

stinking at night: Carbo an., **Psor.,** Pyr.

after congestive chill: *Nux.*

on feet: Sab.

on covered parts: Cham., **Cinch.**

after light chill: **Eup.**

on uncovered parts, except head: **Thuja.**

Quinine, after abuse of: *Ipec.*

after 4 A. M. every day: **Stan.**

Room, in a: Ipec.

Shivering, with: Ced., Cof., Eup., *Nux.*

Slight: Ant. c., Apis, Calad., Cimex, *Cina,* Casc., Croc., Cyc., Elaps, *Eup.,* Eup. p., Ign., *Ipec.,* Kali i., Lach., Led., Mal., Nux m., Nux, Phel., Sep., Sil.

Smelling, aromatic: Benz. ac., Cop., Rhod.

bitter: Ver.

blood, like: Lyc.

camphor, like: Camph.

elder blossoms, like: Sep.

fetid: Æsc., **Psor.,** Pyr., Rob., Zinc.

mouldy: Psor., Puls., Rhus, **Stan.**

musk-like: Mosc., Puls., *Sul.*

musty: Cim., Rhus, **Stan.**

offensive: All. s., **Arn.,** Ars., *Bar.,* Bell., **Carbo an.,** *Carbo v., Carb. ac.,* Cimex, Con., Coc., Crot., Cyc., *Dul.,* Euph., Fer., Fl. ac., **Graph.,** Guaj., Kali c., Kali p., *Lach.,* Led., **Lyc.,** Mag. c., *Mercurialis,* **Mer.,** Mer. c., *Nit. ac., Nux,* Petr., **Psor.,** Puls., **Pyr.,** *Rhus,* Rhod., Rob., **Sep., Sil.,** Spig., Stan., Staph., Sul., Ver., Zinc.

on genitals: Aloe, Petr.

onions, like: *Bov., Lach., Lyc.*

onions, like, in axilla: **Bov.**

Smelling, pungent: Caps.
putrid: Daph., **Carbo v.,** Led., **Psor.,** Pyr., Rhus, Spig., **Staph.,** Stram., Ver.
rhubarb, like: Rheum.
sewer gas, like: Bov., Psor., *Pyr.*
strong: Fer.
sour: Acon., **Arn.,** Ars., Asar., **Bry.,** Cal., Carbo v., *Caust., Cham.,* Cimex, *Colch.,* Fl. ac., Graph., *Hep.,* Hyos., Iod., *Ipec.,* Led., **Lyc.,** *Mag. c.,* Mer., Natr., Nat. p., *Nit. ac., Nux,* **Psor.,** Rhus, *Sep., Sil., Sul.,* Sul. ac., Thuja, Ver.
sour, as in measles: Fer.
with fine sticking, itching: Zinc.
sulphur, like: *Phos.*
sweet: Calad.
urine, like: Berb., **Canth.,** Col., **Nit. ac.**
urine, like horses: **Nit. ac.**

Staining: (See Linen).

Sticky: Ant. t., Anth., Hell., Kali br., Lachn.
on forehead: Can. I.
about genitals: Gels., Petr.

Stool, before: Mer.

Strong: Aloe.

Sudden: Amyl, Ipec.
attacks, cold: Crot.
ceasing frequent: Val.

Suppressed or wanting: Colch.
grave symptoms appear: Cad. s.

Sweet, which attracts the flies: Calad., Sumb., Thuja.

Talking, when: Graph., Iod.

Viscid, profuse all over the body: Anth., Daphne, Kali br., Plumb.

Walking, after: Cad. s., Sul.
when: Agar., Amb., Benz. ac., Casc., Caust., Coc., Kali c., Led., Natr., Sil.

Warm: Acon., Ant. c., Benz., Camph., Cham., Coc., Dros., Ign., Kali c., Lach., Led., Natr., Nux, Op., Phos., Sep., Staph., Stram.
and very exhausting: Benz.

Warmth, easy sweating on exposure to: Carbo v.

Wash off, difficult to: *Mag. c.,* **Mer.,** Pyr.

SWEAT, TIME OF:

Afternoon: Berb., Mag. m., Mag. s., Natr., Nux, Sil., Staph.

Day, during the: Agar., Amb., Amm. m., Anac., *Ant. t.,* Bell., Bry., *Cal.,* **Carbo an., Cinch., Con.,** *Dul.,* **Fer.,** *Graph., Hep.,* Kali c., Lach., Laur., Led., *Lyc.,* Nat. c., **Natr.,** Nit. ac., Phos. ac., Puls., **Sep.,** Sil., *Staph.,* **Stram.,** Sul., Sul. ac., *Ver.,* Zinc.

Daily, same hour: Ant. c., Bov., Cina, Ign., Sabad., Spig.

Evening, during the: Bar., Calad., Mur. ac., **Samb.,** *Sul.*
every other: Bar.
toward: Calad.

Forenoon, during the: **Fer.,** Samb.

Long-lasting: **Fer.,** Kali br., Led., Zinc.

Midnight, after: Alum., Amb., Amm. m., Bar., Clem., Dros., Lachn., Mag. m., *Mercurialis,* Nux, Par., Phos., *Polyp.,* Stan.
before: Mur. ac.

Morning: *Alum.,* Amm. c., Ang., Ant. c., Arg. n., *Aur.,* Benz., Bov., Bry., *Cal.,* Carbo an., Carbo v., Caust., Chel., Chin. s., Cic., Clem., Coc., Cof., Dul., Dros., *Euphor.,* Eup., *Fer.,* Graph., Hell., Iod., Kreos., Lachn., Lyc., **Mag. c.,** Mag. m., Mag. s., Mercurialis, **Mer.,** Mosch., Mur. ac., Natr., Nat. c., Nat. s., Nicc., **Nit. ac.,** Nux, Par., **Phos., Phos. ac.,** Puls., **Rhus,** Sabad., *Sep.,* Sil., Spong., **Stan.,** Sul., Sul. ac.
every other, at precisely the same hour: **Ant. c.**

Night, at: Acet. ac., Acon., Agar., *Alum.*, *Amb.*, Amm. c., **Amm. m.**, *Anac.*, Ang., Ant. t., Arg., Arn., *Ars.*, Aur., Bar., Bell., Benz., Bry., *Cal.*, Camph., Casc., Carb. ac., **Carbo an.**, **Carbo v.**, **Caust.**, Cham., Cic., Cinch., Cist., Coc., *Col.*, *Con.*, Crot., Cup., Cur., Cyc., Dig., *Dros.*, *Dul.*, Eup., Euph., Fer., Fer. p., *Graph.*, Gamb., Ham., Hell., **Hep.**, Iod., Ipec., **Kali c.**, Lach., Laur., Led., Lob., Lyc., *Mag. c.*, Mag. m., Mag. s., Meny., Mercurialis, **Mer.**, *Mur. ac.*, *Natr.*, Nat. c., Nat. s., **Nit. ac.**, Nux, Petr., Phos. ac., **Phos.**, Polyp., Puls., Rhus, Sabad., Sab., Samb., Sarr., **Sep.**, **Sil.**, Spong., *Staph.*, Stram., *Stront.*, **Sul.**, Tab., *Tarax.*, Thuja, Val., Ver., Zinc.

at, relieving the headache: Psor.
at, relieved by drinking wine: Sul. ac.
at, profuse, every other: **Nit. ac.**
at, profuse, after 4 A. M.: Stan.
at, putrid-smelling: **Psor.**, *Pyr.*, Spig.
at, on chest and abdomen: Anac., Benz., Thuja.
at, only, cold and debilitating: Croc.
at 3 A. M., profuse: **Psor.**, Stan.
at, slight, over whole body, on waking from sleep: Cyc.
at, with itching: Mang.

Noon, at: Cinn.

Several hours after the heat: Ant. t., Ars.

Sleep, during: Æth., Agar., Ars., Bell., Bufo, Cad. s., Camph., Cham., Chel., **Cinch.**, **Con.**, Crot., Euph., Hyos., Phos., **Puls.**, *Plat.*, Prun., Sabad., Thuja.

after restless: Lachn.
in morning: Bor.
the first, until 12 P. M.: Mur. ac.

Walking, while: Cain.

SWEAT, LOCATION OF:

Abdomen: Act., **Anac.**, Arg., Cic., **Dros.**, *Staph.*

Arms: Ipec., **Mercurialis.**

Axilla: Asar., *Benz.*, *Bov.*, Cad. s., Caps., Casc., Card., Chin. s., Crot., Dul., **Kali c.**, Lach., Nit. ac., Petr., Rhod.

Back: Cain., Casc., Chin. s., *Cinch.*, Dul., Gym., Hyos., Ipec., Lach., Petr., Plant., Pod., Puls., **Sep.**, **Sul.**
lumbar and sacral region: Plant.

Body, all over the: *Ant. t.*, *Benz.*, *Caust.*, Coc., Cof., Col., Dul., Elaps, Gamb., Hyos., Iod., Led., *Lyc.*, Mang., *Mercurialis,* **Natr.**, *Nit. ac.*, Op., *Phos.*, Puls., Sec., Sep., **Sil.**, **Stram.**, Sul., *Tarax.*, Ter., *Thuja.*
all over except the head: *Thuja.*
all over except the right foot: Ars. hyd.
but not the face: **Rhus,** *Sec.*
front of: Agar., Arg.; *Cal.*, Graph., Mer., Phos., *Sel.*
lower part of: Croc., Cyc., Euph.
not on the limbs: Lyc.
upper part of: Arg., Asar., *Cham.*, Cina, Dul., Eup. p., Ipec., Kali c., Laur., Nux, Op., *Rheum,* Sep., Spig., *Sul. ac.*, Val., Ver.

Chest: *Agar.*, *Anac.*, Arg., Arund., *Benz.*, Bov., Cal., Cimex, Coc., Eup., Glon., Graph., Kali n., Sep.

Face: *Agar.*, Alum., Arg. n., Benz. ac., Cof., Cinch., **Dros.**, Glon., Lyss., Nat. s., Pod., Prun., **Psor.**, *Puls.*, Rhus, Rob., Sabad., *Samb.*, *Sil.*, *Stram.*
on, in beads: Arg. n.
with heat, on: Val.
all over excepting the: *Rhus,* Sec.
and head only: Æsc., Sil.
pale, cold sweat on the: Ver. v.
right side of: *Alum.*, Puls.

Feet: Bell., Cal., Calend., Camph., Canth., *Carbo an.*, Carbo v., Dros., Graph., Led., Med., Manc., *Petr.*, Phos., Puls., Sab., **Sil.**, Staph., Tub., Zinc.
profuse on the: Sab.
profuse, offensive: *Graph.*, **Psor.**, Pyr., San., **Sil.**, *Zinc.*
profuse, makes feet sore: Graph., San., Zinc.
soles of: **Nit. ac.**, Sabad.
from the, over the whole body: Euphor.
and hands: Hyper., Lac. ac.

Forehead: Ang., Can. I., Card., *Cina*, Crot. t., Elaps, Eup. p., Glon., Ipec., Kali bi., Led., Mer. c., Nat. c., Op., Ptel., Rheum, Stan., Stram., **Ver.**
and neck: Cann. s., Guaj.
and face, then spreads to body: Jab.
during stool, on: Ptel.
sticky, on: Gels.

Genitals: Aur., Canth., Con., Gels., Nat. s., **Petr.**, San., Staph.
male: Hydr., Petr., Psor., *Sep.*
profuse, offensive, of the: *Hydr.*, Petr.

Groin: Iris.

Hair, drop on every: Hell.

Hand, left: Anac.
right: Lyss.

Hands: Canth., *Cina*, Coc., Glon., *Kali bi.*, Led., Phos., Sec., **Sticta**, Zinc.
alternating on the: Coc.
palms of: Brom., Cal., Cof., Dig., Dul., Fl. ac., Guaj., Gym., Iod., Med., Petr., *Psor.*, Sep.
and feet: Hyper.
back of: Lith. c.

Head: Cal., Cimex, Cinch., Col., Eup. p., Mag. s., Mur. ac., *Op.*, Petr., Phos., Pod., Sabad., *Sil.*, Zinc.
occipital region: Sul.
profuse about the: Cal., Op., San., Sil.

Head, and extremities: Col.
only: *Sil.*
and face: Æsc.
and back: Mur. ac.

Inflamed surfaces: Graph.

Joints: Amm. c., Lyc.

Knees: Cal.
hollows of: Bufo, *Carbo an.*

Legs, on the: Euphor.

Limbs: Agar., Asaf., Cal., Col., Con., Euphor., Hyos., Kali n., Petr., Sarr.

Neck: Agar., Elaps, Euphor., Med., **Stan.**
nape of: San., Sil., Stan.

Nose: *Cina.*

Parts affected: **Ant. t.,** *Amb.,* Coc., Mer., Sep., Sil.
on affected side, worse: **Amb.**
covered: *Acon., Bell.,* Cham.
pressed by clothing: *Chin. s.*
single: *Acon.,* Bar., Bell., Bry., *Cal.,* Calc. p., Caps., Caust., Cham., Cinch., Graph., Hell., Hep., Ign., Ipec., Led., *Lyc.,* Mer., Nux, Nat. s., Petr., Phos., *Psor.,* **Pyr., Puls.,** Rhus, Sab., Samb., *Sel., Sep.,* Sil., Spig., Spong., *Stan., Sul., Thuja,* **Tub.,** Zinc.
upper: Fl. ac.
uncovered: **Thuja.**

Pelvis, region of: Canth.

Perineum: Chin. s., Con., *Hep., Kali c., Psor., Thuja.*

Scalp: Puls., Rheum, Rob.

Scrotum: Nat. s., Petr., *Thuja.*

Shoulders: Arundo.

Side, affected: **Amb.**, Nux.
left: *Bar.*, Fl. ac., Jab., *Puls.*, Phos.
not lain on: *Benz.*, San., Thuja.
on one: *Amb.*, Acon., *Bar.*, Benz., Bry., Cham., **Cinch.**, **Fl. ac.**, Lyc., Nux m., *Nux*, **Puls.**, Rhus, Sul.
on which he lies: *Acon.*, Bry., Cinch., *Nit. ac.*
right: Nux, *Puls.*

Sides: Mercurialis.

Thighs: Amb., *Carbo an.*, Euphor., *Hep.*, *Sep.*
inner surface of: *Thuja.*
only on the: Euphor.
sensation of cold sweat on: Caps.

SWEAT, SYMPTOMS DURING:

Abdomen, distention of: Stram.

Air, while walking in open: Zinc.

Appetite good: Stram.

Alternating with dryness: Act.

Anxiety: Arn., Benz. ac., Berb., Bry., Çal., Coc., Fer., **Mer. c.**, Nat. c., Nux, Phos., Plumb., Puls., Sep., Sul.
relieved: Acon., Bar., Natr.

Back, pain in: Carbo v.
chills up and down the: Amyl.

Body, lower part of, hot and dry: Op.
red, hot and dry: *Stram.*
hot and dry on going to sleep: Samb.

Bones, pains in: *Eup.*

Breathing, stertorous: Op.

Cheeks, heat and redness of: Kreos.

Chill: Amyl.
alternating with: Glon.

Chest, pain in: *Bry.*

Colic: Nux, Stram.

Cold and hot and hot and cold: Ced.

Convulsions: Nux.

Cramps: Fer.
from sides of waist: Corn.

Cough: **Arg. n.**, *Ars.*, Bry., **Dros.**, Ipec.
spasmodic: *Dros.*

Covered, desire to be: *Acon.*, Æth., Aur., Clem., Colch., Con., Nux m., **Nux**, *Samb.*, *Stram.*, *Stront.*

Debility: Amb., *Benz.*, Bry., Cal., Camph., Coc., *Carbo an.*, Chin. s., *Cinch.*, Croc., Dig., *Fer.*, Graph., Hyos., Ign., Iod., Lyc., *Mer.*, Natr., Phos., Psor., Sep., Sil., **Stan.**, Sul., Tarax.
at night, causing biting of the skin: Tarax.

Delirium: Thuja.
relieves: Æth., Agar.

Diarrhea: Acon., Chin. s., Stram., Sul.
nightly: Chin. s.

Dreams: Puls.

Drowsiness: Asaf.

Dyspnea: Anac., Cac., Mer.

Earache: Ign.

Ears, roaring in: Ars., Ign.

Epistaxis: Sul. ac.

Eruption: Con.

Excitability, nervous, relieved: Acon.

Exhaustion: *Benz.*, *Camph.*, **Carbo an.**, **Cinch.**, Ign.

Extremities, pains in: Ced.

Excoriation of parts lain on: Fl. ac., Pyr.

Eyes, burning in: Cinch., Stram.

Face, coldness of: Canch., Lach., Nux.
dry: *Kali bi.*
heat of: Bell., Nux, Sabad.
paleness, deathly, of: **Ver.**
red: Bell., Con., Sep.

Fainting: Anac., *Apis,* Ars., Cinch., Ign., Sul.

Feet, cold: Ced., Iod.
cramps in: Puls.
pains in: *Nit. ac.,* Staph.
soreness of: Graph., San., **Sil.**
soreness of the balls: **Nit. ac.**

Fingers, shriveling of, like a washer-woman's; *Ant. c.,* **Canch.,** *Mer.,* Phos. ac., **Ver.**

Forehead cool, with sensation of coolness inside: Cist.

Hands, cold: Canch., Ced., Kali bi., Nit. ac.
cramps in: Puls.
hot: Nux.

Head, congestion of blood to the: Thuja.
heaviness of the: Ars., Caust.
roaring in: Caust.

Headache: Ant. c., Arn., Eup., Fer., Natr., Rhus, Thuja.
commencing with: Fer.
relieved gradually: **Natr.,** Psor.
relieved by thirst: Chin. s.

Heart, palpitation of: Ced., Mer.

Hunger: *Cimex,* **Cina.**

Itching, with: Benz. ac.
with, and crawling in skin: Rhod.

Legs, pain in: Carbo v.
weakness in: Ars., Iod.

Limbs, cold: Lyss., *Sec.*
cold and livid: Lyss.

Lips, cold: Canch.

Loquacity: Puls.

Malaise, relieved by: Agar.

Mouth, dry: Ced.
open: *Op.*

Nails, blueness of: **Nit. ac.**

Nausea: *Dros., Ipec.,* Mer., Thuja.
relieves: Glon.

Nervousness: Cof.

Odor, smoky: Bell.
sulphur, of: Phos.

Pain, uncovering, on: Stram.

Pains, aggravated by coffee and tobacco: Ign.
continue: Eup., Kali c., Lach., Mer., Nat. c., Natr., Nux, Puls., Rhus, Tab.
relieved: *Arn.,* Bry., Calad., Chel., *Lach., Nat. m., Nux,* Sec.
relieved except headache, all: Eup.
relieved gradually: Bell., **Natr.,** Psor.

Periosteum, pain in: *Arn.*

Prostration, with: Ars., Cad. s., Calad., Mur. ac.

Pulse, intermittent: Sec.
weak: Chin. s., Pyr., Sec.

Respiration, hurried: Ced.
short, anxious: Mang.

Restlessness: Bry., Lachn.
if window is closed: Arg. n.

Rheumatic pains: Ant. t.

Sighing: Bry.

Side, stitches in: Mer.

Skin, biting of: Tarax.
biting itching that compels scratching: **Par.**
burning of: Mer., Op.
itching of: Apis, Col., Mang., Par., Rhod., Rhus.
parboiled: **Canch.**, *Cinch.*, Mer.
smarting of: Caps., Cham., Con.

Sleep: Agar., Arn., Ars., Bell., Calad., Carbo an., **Chel.**, **Cic.**, **Cina**, Cinch., Cyc., Euph., Fer., Hyos., Ign., **Kali c.**, **Lob.**, Mez., Mur. ac., Nit. ac., Nux m., **Op.**, Phos. ac., Plat., **Pod.**, Prun., Psor., *Puls.*, **Rhus**, Sabad., Sul.
deep snoring: **Op.**
restless: *Sul.*

Sleepy: Calad.

Sleepless, from profuse sweat: Corn.

Spleen, pain in: Tarax.

Spine, irritation of: Agar., Zinc.
painful to pressure: Chin. s.
irritation of: Agar., Zinc.
sensitive to touch: Agar.
weakness of: Agar., Sel.

Stretching: Caust.

Symptoms, aggravated while sweating: *Fer.*, **Ipec.**, *Mer.*, **Op.**
ameliorated while sweating: Fl. ac., Natr., Psor.
cessation of previous: *Æsc.*, Ars., Calad., Cimex, Elat., Gels., *Natr.*, **Psor.**, Samb., Sec.
cessation gradual: **Natr.**

Taciturn, during: Mur. ac.

Tenesmus: Sul.

Thirst: Acon., Anac., **Ars.**, Cac., *Ced.*, **Cinch.**, *Chin. s.*, Cof., Con., Gels., Hep., Iod., Mercurialis, **Natr.**, Phos. ac., Rhus, Sec., **Stram.**, Tarax., Thuja.
commencing with: Cof., Thuja.

Thirst, wanting: *Apis,* Bar., *Cal., Caps.,* Caust., *Cimex, Cina,* Eup., Euph., Hell., *Ign.,* Nat. s., *Nux, Samb.,* Staph., Stram., *Ver.*

Toes, soreness of: **Nit. ac.,** Petr., San.

Tongue and taste clammy and feverish: Gels.

Toothache: Carbo v., Cinch., *Cof.*
relieved by holding cold water in the mouth, returns when the water becomes warm: **Bry.,** *Cof.,* Caust., Nat. s., Puls., Sep.

Trembling: Apis, Ars., Nux, Rhus.

Uncovered, desire to be: *Acon.,* Cal., *Eup.,* Fer., Iod., Led., Mur. ac., *Natr., Op.,* Spig., Staph., Ver., Zinc.
cannot bear to be: Æth., Agar., Acon., Clem., **Nux.**

Uncovering, pain upon: Stram.
aversion to: Clem.

Urine, copious: Acon., Dul., Phos.
high-colored: Ced.
increased amount of: Ant. t., **Dul.**
milky: Phos.
scanty: Ced.
transparent: Dul.
turbid: *Ipec.,* Phos.

Urticaria: *Apis, Rhus.*

Veins, swelling of: *Agar.,* Cinch.

Vertigo: Arundo, Lachn.

Vision, dimness of: Stram.

Vomiting: *Ars.,* Camph., Cina, Cinch., *Dros., Eup.,* Ipec., Sul.
bitter: **Eup.**
drinks, after cold: *Ars.,* Cinch.
face cold when: Camph.
ingesta of: Cina, *Eup.*

Waking up, when: Anac., Natr., Nit. ac., Par.
up on, from a sound sleep: Rum.

Weakness: Apis, Ars., Bar., Camph., Fer., Iod., **Mer.,** *Phos.,* **Psor.,** Puls., Sel.

Walking, very copious when: **Psor.**

Yawning: Calad., Caust.

SWEAT SUPPRESSED:

Acon. Anth., Apis, Ars., **Bell., Bry., Cad. s., Cal.,** Carbo v., *Cham.,* **Chin. s.,** Clem., **Colch.,** Cup., **Dul.,** *Eup.,* **Graph.,** Hep., Kali c., Led., *Lyc.,* Mer., Nat. c., Natr., Nux m., **Nux,** *Op.,* Phos. ac., *Phos.,* Plumb., Puls., **Rhus,** Sabad., *Sec.,* **Sep., Sil., Sul.**

AGGRAVATION AFTER SWEAT:

Acon., Ant. t., Calad., Cal., Cham., **Cinch.,** Con., Ipec., Mer., Phos. ac., Phos., Puls., **Sep.,** Sil., Staph., *Sul.*

AMELIORATION AFTER SWEAT:

Eup., Gels., **Ipec.,** Lyss., **Natr., Psor.**
Limbs, pains in: Nux.

APPETITE, TASTE, TONGUE, ETC.

SYMPTOMS OF:

Appetite, good: Alum., Caps.
good as soon as paroxysm is over: Canch.
complete loss of: Apis, Lob., Op., Petr., Polyp., Sarr., Sil.
unimpaired: Caps.

Appetite, voracious: *Ver.*
want of: Apis, Dig., Lob., Tar.
between paroxysms of vomiting: *Ver.*

Aversion to, alcoholic liquors: Rhus.
bread: Natr., Nit. ac., *Nux.*
coffee: **Nux.**
fat: Hep., **Petr.,** Puls., Sec.
fat pork: **Puls.**
fat things: Carbo v., Hep., *Puls.*
fish: Graph.
fish, smell of cooking: Ars., *Colch.,* Sep.
food: Ars., Bry., Op., Sec.
food, cooked: Graph., Petr.
food and drink: Bry., Colch.
food, warm, boiled: Lyc., Petr., Sil.
food, warm things: Petr., **Ver.**
food, with loathing when looking at it, still more when smelling it: Colch.
milk, which causes flatulence: Carbo v., **Puls.**
meat: Alum., **Arn.,** Carbo v., Graph., Kali bi., Nit. ac., Petr., Rhus, Sec., Sep., Sil., Sul.
salt: Graph.
sweet things: Ars., Caust., Graph., Mer., Nit. ac., Phos., Sul.
sweet things, which disagree: **Caust.**
sour things: Coc.
tobacco: *Ign.,* Lyc., **Nux.**
water: **Nux.**

Breath, sour: **Arn.**
fetid: **Arn.,** Carb. ac., Crot., Gels., Mur. ac., Nit. ac.
fetid, if tongue coated thickly: Gels.
mouldy: Crot.
offensive: Plant., Pod., Psor.
offensive, objectively: Pod.
smells of onions: Sinapis.

Breath, putrid: Plant., Pyr.
cadaverous: Nit. ac.
urine, smells like: Graph.

Choke, when eating or drinking, apt to: *Anac.*, Kava.

Cough, caused by irritating things—salt, vinegar, pepper: **Alum.**

Cracking, in maxillary articulation, when chewing: Nit. ac.

Desire for, apples: **Ant. t.** (See Longing for.)
acids: Ant. c., Sec., Psor.
alcoholic drinks: Asar., **Sel.,** Spig., Tub.
beer: Caust., Kali bi., Puls., Rhus.
bitter food: Dig.
brandy: Ars., Nux.
coffee, but it nauseates: Caps.
cold drinks: *Dul.*, Phos., Puls., Sil., *Ver.*
cold food: *Phos.*, **Ver.,** Sil.
cold milk: **Rhus.**
cold water: Ars., Phos., Puls., Rhus, *Ver.*
cold fruits: **Ver.**
cold, everything: Phos., *Sil.*, **Ver.**
juicy fruit: Ant. t., Phos. ac., Ver.
juicy, refreshing, food: Phos. ac., Puls., **Ver.**
lemonade: Eup. p., Sec.
ice cream: *Eup.*, Phos.
ice water: *Phos.*, Puls., Rhus, **Ver.**
pickles: **Ant. c.,** Ars.
smoked meats: Caust.
sour things: Ant. c., Ant. t., Ars., Eup. p., Polyp., *Puls.*, Sec.
sour things, which always relieved: Polyp.
things, which are refused when offered: Bry., Staph.

Eating, better while, worse after: Caps.

Eats and drinks hastily: Anac., Bell., Cof., Hep.

Eructations, sour: **Lyc.**
sulphur, tasting of, lasting all day: Plant.

Faint, smell of fish, eggs, fat meat, makes him: **Colch.**
feels: Phos.

Food, cannot digest: Bap., Carbo **v.**
no desire for: Apis, Colch.
disgust for: Cyc.
disgust for, sudden, while at meals: Bar., Fer.
straw, tastes like: **Stram.**
dry, woody, tastes: Fer.
indifference to all, even when thinking of it: *Cinch.*
highly seasoned, can only digest: Nux m.
repugnance to: *Arn.*
regurgitation of, in mouthfuls, without nausea: Alum., Phos.
tasteless: *Ant. t.,* Dros., *Eup.,* **Ign.,** *Natr.,* Plant.
scarcely swallowed, comes up again: Phos.
sweet, wants: Sul.

Gums, loose and spongy: Dul., **Mer.,** Staph.
pale: Fer., Staph.
ulcerated, bleed when touched: San., **Staph.**
white: *Staph.*

Hemorrhage: Crot., Ham., Lach.

Hunger: Dig.
canine: Eup.
canine, after Quinine: *Nux,* Phos., Staph.
must eat before he can get up: Phos.
eating does not relieve: Ant. c.
and appetite between paroxysms of vomiting: Ver.
ravenous: Carbo an., **Meny.,** Petr., Ver.
ravenous, with nausea and thirst: Spig.
great, without appetite: **Psor.,** Rhus.

Hungry, but cannot eat: Bar.
head aches if he does not eat: *Lyc.*

Lips, dry and peeling off: Bry.
dry: Nit. ac., *Nux m.*
dry, without actual dryness or real thirst: Nux m.

Lips, cracked: Ars., Hep., Natr.
cracked, at commissures: **Cund.,** Eup., Natr.
cracked and sore as from cold: Graph.
pale: Eup., **Fer., Sec.**
pale, and bloodless: **Fer.**
sticky, dry: *Nux m.*

Longing for acids: Alum., Ant. t., Arn., Hep., Kali bi., Mag. c.
acid drinks: **Eup. p.,** *Mag. c.*
alcohol: *Arn.,* Ars., *Puls.,* Spig.
beer: Nux, *Sul.*
bitter things: Natr.
brandy: Nux, Sul.
chalk: Alum.
charcoal: Alum.
clean rags: Alum., Psor.
coffee: Caps., Cof.
coffee grounds: Alum.
dainties: Ipec.
fat: Nit. ac.
fat food: Nux.
food, refreshing, juicy: Phos. ac.
meat: **Canth.,** Mag. c., **Meny.**
milk, which agrees: Apis, Chel.
milk, which disagrees: Carbo v.
indigestible things: Alum.
oysters, which disagree: **Lyc.**
tea grounds: Alum.
salt: Cal., **Natr.**
strong tasting things: Hep.
sour things: Con., Dig.
spirituous liquors: Op., Puls.
stimulants: Asar., Puls.
sweets: Ipec., Lyc., Mag. m., Sul.

Milk, disagrees, causes sour taste, sour eructations: Sul.

Mouth, bitter when not eating: *Bry.*
covered with a grayish white fur: Mur. ac.
dry: Ars., Bap., Bell., Bry., Mur. ac., *Nux m.,* **Tar.**
rawness of: Carbo an.
rawness of, relieved by eating: Carbo an.
odor rotten from the: Graph.
offensive, objective odor from the: Hep., Psor., Stan.
offensive odor: Petr., Pod., **Psor.,** Stan.
sore and ulcerated, corners of: Natr., Nit. ac.
rinse the, must: **Nux,** Puls.
rinse the, must get up at night to: Thuja.

Nausea, with restlessness: Colch.
soon as he begins to move: Tab.

Nauseates, the smell of broth: Ars., *Colch.,* Sep.

Papillæ, red: *Ant. t., Bell.,* Mez., Nux m., Pyr., Stram.
red and elevated: Acon., *Ant. t.*
red, bright and raised: **Bell.**
red, large and elevated: *Mez.,* Pyr.
red, large and elevated, as in scarlatina: Ant. t., *Bell.,* Mez.

Potatoes, disagree, cause colic: Alum.

Salivation: Dig., Dul., *Iod.,* **Mer.,** Pod
constant: Dig., Mer.

Saliva, blood colored: Gels.
acrid: Nit. ac.
"cotton-like:" Nux m.
fetid: **Mer.,** *Nit. ac.,* Psor.
iron, tastes of: Cimex, **Mer.**
metallic: **Mer.**
on middle of tongue: Cimex.
profuse: Ipec., Mer., Nit. ac., Pod.
salty: Ant. c., Iod.
soapy: Dul.
sour: Ign.
stringy, ropy: Hydr., **Kali bi.,** Lyss.

Saliva, tastes bitter in the mouth: Chel.
tenacious: Dul., Hyd., **Kali bi.**
thready: Con.

Satiety: Carbo v., Lyc.
a few mouthfuls fill him up: Lyc.

Stomach, deranged: Cac., Hep.

Taste, acute, too: Cinch.
bad: Hyos., Kali c., Sarr.
bitter: Ant. c., Aran., Arn., Bap., Bov., **Bry.,** Cal., Carbo v. Cham., **Chin. s., Cinch.,** Con., Dul., Elat., ***Eup.,*** Eup. p. Gels., Graph., Hep., Ipec., Kali c., Lyc., Mag. c., Nat. Nat. s., **Nux,** Polyp., *Psor.,* **Puls.,** Staph., Sul., Thuja.
bitter, bread, after eating: Rhus.
bitter, goes off after eating or drinking: **Psor.**
bitter, after smoking: **Anac.,** Puls.
bitter, after eating: Nit. ac., Puls.
bitter, before and after eating: Carbo v., **Puls.**
bitter, in morning food tastes natural: Sul.
bitter, with clean tongue: Chin. s.
bitter, bread tastes: Dig., Dros.
bitter, sweetish: Meny.
bitter, everything tastes: **Bry.**
bitter, everything, but water: **Acon.,** Stan.
bitter, water: *Ars.*
bitter, all food tastes: Fer.
blood, of: Sil.
coppery: Asc., Kali bi., Polyp.
disgusting: Psor., **Puls.**
fatty: Lyc.
flat: Anac., Bap., Kali c., Cyc.
foul: Cal., Gels., Pod., **Psor., Puls.**
fruit, juicy, tastes dry: Stram.
herring brine, like: Anac.
ink, like: Cal.
insipid: Eup., Fer.

Taste, iron, like: Cal.
iron, like, with salivation: Æsc.
lost: Anth., Canth., Nat. s., Nux, **Pod.,** Sil.
metallic: Æsc., Coc., Hep., Mer.
nauseous, relieved by smoking: Aran.
oil, of: Sil.
offensive: Anac., *Bell.,* Cal., Cyc., Hyos., Plant., Puls., Stan.
offensive in throat when eating or drinking, although food tastes natural: **Bell.**
of rotten eggs: **Arn.,** Fer., Graph., **Pyr.,** Sil.
pappy: Eup., Petr., Pod.
pasty: Pod.
putrid: **Arn.,** *Bell.,* Bov., Cham., Cyc., Hep., Hyos., **Nux,** Petr., Plant.
qualmish: Cyc.
qualmish, water has a: Caps., Nat., Spig.
qualmish, food after eating: Rhus.
rancid oil, like: Ipec.
salt, too: Sep.
salty: Graph., Iod., **Nat.**
slimy: Petr., **Puls.**
soapy: Coc.
soapsuds: Sil.
sour: Caps., Cham., Graph., Ign., Iod., *Lach.,* **Lyc.,** Mag. c., Mag. m., Nat., **Nux,** Pod., Stan., Thuja.
sour, at night: Mag. m.
sour, everything turns: *Lach.*
sour, everything tastes: Pod.
sweetish: Anth., Ipec., Stan.
too fresh: Cal.

Thirst: Æsc., Eup., Cic., Cimex.
with inability to swallow: Æsc., Cic., Cimex.

Tip, burning on the: Carbo an., Ter.
burning on, relieved by eating: Carbo an.
bluish and sore: Sabad.

Tip, dry: Rhus, Thuja.
painful, sore to touch: **Thuja.**
red: Ars., Rhus, Ver.
red, brown in centre: Lach.
red, dry, triangular: **Rhus.**
sore: *Æsc.,* Kali c., Rhus, **Thuja,** Sabad.
sore, as if full of blisters: Sabad.
sore, as if ulcerated: Æsc., Kali c.
sore and painful: Hep., Thuja.
and edges red: Lach., Sec., Ter., **Ver.**

Tongue, adhering to roof of mouth: **Nux m.**
bleeding: Cur.
bluish: **Ars.,** Carbo v., Mur. ac.
broad, with indented edges: Chel., Hydr., *Kali bi.,* **Mer.,** Pod., Rhus.
broad too: Hydr., Mer., Puls.
burning tingling, as if needles were pricking it: Arum, Carb. ac.
burnt, tip feels, as far as middle: Psor.
clean: *Alum.,* Cac., Caust., **Cina,** Dig., Gels., Dros., Elaps, Ign., Ipec., Mag. c., Pyr., Sil., Stram., Sul.
clean, with dry, red tip: Sec.
clean, on left, coated on right: Lob.
clean, on one side: Rhus.
clean, but dry: Lyc.
clean, in old cases: Apis.
clean, never: **Arn.**
coated, back of, like dried clay: Cal. s., **Hep.**
coated, brown: Anth., Ars., Carb. ac., Hyos., Lyc.
coated, brown mucus: Sil.
coated, brownish white: Sarr.
coated, center, in: Sabad., Sec.
coated, dirty: Elat.
coated, dirty brown fur: Elat.
coated, greenish-gray or greenish-brown at base of: Nat. s.

Tongue, coated, white: Arn., Cinch., Pod.
coated, white or dirty yellow: Op.
coated, downy white: Colch.
coated, downy white, which **wears off during the day and becomes red and clean in the evening: Sul.**
coated, heavily: Bry., Canth., Nux.
coated, heavily, brown along the centre: Bap., Eup. p.
coated, middle, only in: Phos.
coated, middle, streak down the: Arn., Bap., Crot., Eup. p., Iod.
coated, slightly: Aran.
coated, thick: Anth., Bry., Canth., Polyp.
coated, thick fur: Phos.
coated, thick fur, grayish or white: Kali m.
coated, thick milky white: **Ant.,** Hydr.
coated, thick yellow: Kali bi., Carb. ac., Pod., Polyp., Spig., Stan.
coated, thick yellow with red tip: Polyp.
coated, white: *Acon., Æsc.,* Anac., Bar., Cal., Carbo v., Carb. ac., Chin. s., Cinch., Coc., Cyc., Dig., *Eup.,* Fer., Graph., Hydr., Ipec., Kali c., Lob., Mag. c., Nux m., Plant., Pod., Polyp., Psor., *Puls.,* Rhus, Sep., Spig., Staph., Sul., Ver.
coated, white, edges and papillæ red: Bap., Ter.
coated, white, dry: Coc.
coated, white, centre, in, dark streaks on the sides: Petr.
coated, white, edges, on, brown in centre: Iod., Phos.
coated, white, fuzzy: Bar.
coated, white, middle, in, edges red: Bap., Bell., Gels.
coated, white, morning, in, tip and edges clean: Mag. m.
coated, white, sides, on, red in middle: Caust., Cham.
coated, white, or brown, red edges, dark in centre: Crot., Phos.
coated, white, or grayish fur: Kali m.
coated, white, yellow: Æsc., Arn., *Nit. ac.,* Nux, Psor., *Puls.,* **Sul.**
coated, white, yellow in centre, pale on sides: Chin. s.
coated, white, yellow brown: Ver.

Tongue, coated, white, pasty fur: Ant. t., Cinch., Pod.
coated, white, thick: **Mez.,** Pod.
coated, yellow: Bov., Ced., Cham., Cinch., Eup., *Kali bi.,* **Pod.,** Polyp., Sec., Tar.
coated, yellow mucus: Stan.
coated, yellow mucus, tough: Camph.
coated, yellow brown, dry in centre: Crot.
coated, yellow, slimy: Kali s.
coated, yellow, white: Ars., Carb. ac., Cham., Gels., Ipec., Nat.
coating, peels off in patches, leaving bright red spot: Ter.
cracked: Cur., Lyc., Spig.
cracked and ulcerated: Bap.
dry: Anth., Arn., Carbo v., Caust., Dul., Lach., Lyc., Pod., Rhus, Stram.
dry, shiny, as if glazed: Carb. ac., Crot., **Mur. ac., Pyr.,** Ter.
dry and sticky: *Con.*
dry waking in the morning: Cal., Nit. ac.
blisters, burning pain on: Caps., Carbo an., Mur. ac.
blisters on sides, pain as if burnt: Carbo an.
blisters, on: Bor., Caps., Cham., Lyc., Med., Nat., Nit. ac., Sars., Sep.
fissured: Carbo v., Cur.
flabby: Camph., Chel., Chin. s., Hydr., **Mer.,** Pod., Pyr.
heavy, hinders talking: Mur. ac.
insensible: Colch.
itching: Ced.
large, too: Hydr., Mer., Puls.
mucus, slimy, covered with: Nat. s.
painful, raw: Apis.
mapped: Lach., Nat., Ran., Tarax., Ter.
pale: **Fer.,** *Ipec.,* **Sec.**
paralyzed, partially: Hyos.
pricking, in early morning, goes off after eating: Ced.
protrudes it with difficulty: *Crot.,* Hyos., **Lach.,** Stram.
protrudes it with difficulty, catches behind the teeth: Lach.
quivering: Op.

Tongue, red and white in alternate streaks: ***Ant. t.***
red papillæ here and there: Ant. t., Bell., **Carb. ac.**
red papillæ elevated: Ter.
red, dry: Bell., Crot., Lach., Ter.
red, dry and cracked: Ars., Crot., Ter.
red: Lyc., *Rhus,* Stram., Ter., **Thuja.**
red, bright: Colch., Lyc., **Pyr., Ter.**
red, deep: Crot., Cur., Elaps, Hyos.
red streaks down the middle: *Ars.,* Phos. ac.
red, smooth and polished: Crot., Mur. ac., *Pyr.,* Ter.
rough and white: Anac.
scalded, feels as if: *Æsc.,* Carb. ac., Cimex.
scalded, gums and palate feel as if: Cimex.
sensation as of a hair on fore part of: Sil.
sensitive: Graph.
sore: Apis, Hydr., Mur. ac., Sul., Sul. ac.
sore and cracked: Rhus.
sore, does not care to talk or protrude it: Apis.
spongy: Camph.
sticky, yellow: Sec.
stiff: Colch., Con., Lyc., **Ver.**
stiff and painful: Con.
strawberry: Acon., Bell., Ter.
swelling of: Apis, Cic., Dul., Thuja.
swollen and black: Elaps.
swollen: Stram., **Thuja,** Ver.
swollen, as if paralyzed with cold: Dul.
teeth, imprint of: Chel., Hydr., Kali b., **Mer.,** Pod., **Rhus.**
tender: Apis, Graph.
trembles: Camph., Canth., Lyc.
trembles when protruded: Lach.
very thick: Bar.

Tobacco, has no taste: **Ant. t.**
tastes bitter: Coc.

Toothache, when infant nurses: **Cinch.**

Throat dry: Æsc., Cimex, Bell.
dry causing drinking: Cimex.

Ulcers, flat: Caps.
deep, with black bases: Mur. ac.
irregular: **Mer.**
lardaceous: Caps., **Mer.**
lardaceous base, surrounded with dark halo: **Mer.**
apt to run together: *Mer.*
have a dirty look: Mer.
on gums, tongue, cheeks and throat: **Mer.**
spreading: Caps., **Mer.**
with undefined edges: **Mer.**

Vesicles, painful burning on sides and tip: Carbo v., Thuja.
on tip: Carbo an., Sep., Thuja.

Vomiting, on assuming the upright position: Colch., Stram.

Water, dread of: Canth., Hyos., *Lyss.*

APYREXIA; SYMPTOMS DURING:

Abdomen, bloated: *Ars.,* Cinch., Graph., Nat., Sil.
cramps in: Ver.
distended after eating: Carbo v., *Kali c.,* Lyc.
pain in: Ant. t., Led., Petros., Polyp., Ran., Sul.

Acids, longing for: *Ant. c.,* Arn., Ars., Dig., **Eup. p.,** Kali bi., Polyp., Puls., Sec.
longing for, especially pickles: **Ant. c.**

Air, sensitiveness to cold: Bar., *Hep.,* Nux m.

Alone, cannot bear to be left: **Ars.,** Bis., *Kali c.,* **Lyc.,** Ver.
wants to be: **Cinch.,** Ign., Nux.
dreads being, but avoids society: Con.

Anemia, with: **Ars.,** Carbo v., **Cinch., Fer.,** Eup.

Anasarca, after ague: Dul.

Anxiety, with: Acon., Camph.

Appetite, good: Alum., **Canch.,** Caps.
loss of: Acon., *Ant. c.,* Apis, *Arn.,* Ars., Bry., Caps., Carbo v., Coc., Cinch., *Corn.,* Cyc., Dig., Graph., Ign., Ipec., Kali c., Lob., Nat., **Nux,** Petr., **Pod.,** Polyp., Puls., Rhus, Sabad.

Backache: Æsc., Eup., Rhus.

Bed, must be in: Canth.

Beer, desire for: *Nux,* Puls.

Black, everything looks: *Nux.*

Bladder, pain in, from drinking: Canth., Lyss., Med.

Body, every spot of, painful to pressure: *Bap.,* Bellis, **Bry.,** *Pyr.*

Bones, pain in: **Arn.,** Bry., Caust., **Eup.,** Mer., Nux, *Rhus,* **Tub.**

Bowels, rumbling in: Carbo v., **Lyc.,** Pod.

Brain, symptoms, congestion of: Acon., **Arn.,** Bell., Cinch., Hell., Hyos., Lyc., **Nux, Op.,** Phos., Sep., Stram., Sul., Ver. v.

Brandy, desire for: Nux, Puls.

Bread, aversion to: Bell., Con., Cyc., Ign., Kali c., Lyc., **Nat.,** Nit. ac., Nux, Phos. ac., Phos., Puls., Rhus, Sep., Sul.

Breath, fetid: Gels., **Pod.,** Psor.
offensive: **Pod.,** Psor., Puls.
offensive, which he notices: Hep.
offensive, which he does not notice: Puls., Pod.
shortness of: *Cal.*
smelling like urine: Graph.
sour: *Arn.,* Nux, Rob., Sul. ac.

Bruised, feeling as though: *Arn.,* Bap., Bellis, Nux m., Pyr.

Burning, intense: Anth., Ars., Euphor.
from mouth to anus with bilious diarrhea: Iris.

Carried, desire to be: Ars., **Cham.,** Cina, Puls.

Cerebral congestion, symptoms of: Bell., Hell., Laur., *Op.*

Chest, constricted feeling of: Ars., Caps., Carbo v., Coc., Ign., Kali c., Nat., Puls., Sabad., Samb., Spig., Stan., Stram., Sul., Ver.
pain in: Sabad.
pressure on, cannot bear: Lach.
weakness of: Dig., **Stan.**

Chilly, constantly: Anac., **Ars.,** Bry., Caps., Coc., Dig., **Hep.,** Led., Nat., Puls., Sabad., Sil., Ver.

Clear: Caps., Dros., Ign., Sabad.
not: *Acon.,* Cal., Carbo an., Chel., *Cina, Colch.,* **Eup.,** *Gels.,* Ipec., **Nat.,** Rhus, Sep., Sil., Sul., Thuja.

Cold, easily takes: Bar., Cal., Caust., Dul., Hep., Psor., **Tub.**

Colic: Cham., Col., Nux, Petros., Pod.

Conjunctiva, jaundiced: Chel., **Eup.,** Fer., Lyc., **Mer.,** Pod., Sabad.

Convulsions: Alum., Ars., Bell., Cal., Camph., Caust., **Cham.,** Cina, Dig., Dros., Hyos., Ign., Mer., *Nux,* **Op.,** Phos. ac., Stan., Stram., Val., Ver., Ver. v., Zinc.

Constipation: Æsc., Alum., Anac., Ant. c., **Bry.,** Cal., *Canch.,* Carbo v., Cinch., Coc., Con., Fer., Graph., Ign., Led., *Lyc.,* Mag. m., **Nat., Nux, Op.,** *Phos.,* Polyp., Sabad., Sil., Staph., **Sul.,** *Ver.*

Cough: Ant. t., Apis, Arn., Ars., Bell., Bry., Cinch., **Cina,** Coc., Con., **Dros., Eup.,** Hep., Hyos., Ign., Ipec., Lyc., Mer., Nat., Nux m., Nux, Op., Phos., *Puls.,* Sep., Sil., Spong., Stan., Sul.

Countenance, sallow: Cinch., Eup., *Iod., Lyc., Nat.,* Sep., Sec.

Covered, must be: **Hep.,** Psor.

Covering, aversion to: Camph., *Sec.*

Debility: Ced., Cinch., Corn., *Eup.,* Eup. p., *Lob.,* **Nat.**

Diarrhea: Ant. c., Ant. t., *Ars., Cal.,* Caps., Carbo an., Cham., Cina, Cinch., Corn., Dig., Dros., Dul., Gels., Ign., **Iod.,** Mer., Mag. c., Nit. ac., Nux, Op., Phos. ac., *Phos.,* Puls., Rhus, Sab., Sil., **Sul.,** Val., Ver.
early morning: Aloe, Pod., Rum., **Sul.**
exhausting: **Carbo an.**
from taking cold in damp weather: Dul., Mer.
painful: Corn., Mer., Nux, Ver.

Drinks, cold, desire for: Dul., Pyr.

Dropsy: Ars., Apis, Cinch., Fer., Eup.
from suppressed sweat or eruptions: Dul., Mer.

Dyspepsia, intermittent, every other day: Ipec.

Ears, ringing in: **Cinch.,** Chin. s.

Edema: Apis, Ars., Cinch., Fer., Eup.

Emaciation: Ars., Carbo v., Cinch., Fer., Iod., Mer., **Nat.,** Nux, Op., Phos. ac., Tar.

Eructations: *Alum.,* Ant. c., Ant. t., *Arn.,* Cinch., Corn., Lyc., Petros., Puls., Sabad.

Eyeballs, sore to touch, as if drawn back into head: Hep., Oleand., Par.

Eyelids, agglutination of: Graph., Kali c.
half open: *Pod.,* Stram., *Sul.*
swelling of upper: Apis, **Kali c.**
swelling of lower: **Apis.**

Eyes, pupils dilated: Bell., Cal., Laur., Stram.

Face, bloated: *Ars.,* Eup., Fer.
clay colored: *Ars.*
emaciated: Tar.
flushed after exertion: Fer.
pale: Anac., *Ars., Camph.,* Carbo v., Cina, Cinch., **Fer.,** Ign., Lyc., Mez., Nux, Petr., Phos., Puls., *Sec.,* Spong., Stan., Sul., Ver.
sunken: *Ars., Camph., Sec.,* Ver.

Face, yellow: **Arn.**, **Ars.**, Caps., *Cinch.*, **Eup.**, Fer., **Nat.**, **Nux**, Petr., Rhus, *Sep.*
yellow spots on: Fer., **Sep.**

Faintness: Arn., **Ars.**, Bry., Cal., *Carbo v.*, Caust., Cina, Cinch., Coc., Con., Dig., Ign., Ipec., Lyc., Nat., Nit. ac., Nux, Op., Puls., Sabad., Sul., *Ver*

Fats, aversion to: Carbo v., *Cyc.*, Hell., Hep., Nat., Petr., **Puls.**, Sec.
longing for: Nit. ac., Nux.

Feet, coldness of: Carbo v., Graph., Hyos., Lyc., Rhus, Sep., Sil.
dampness about: **Cal.**, Graph., Sep.
heaviness of: Canth.
sensitive to touch, especially the soles: Kali c.
swelling of: Apis, Ars., Bry., Caps., Caust., Cinch., Fer., Lyc., Nux, Puls., Sep., Sil.

Flatulency: Carbo v., Cinch., **Kali c.**, Lyc., Petros., Polyp., Psor.

Food, aversion to: **Ant. c.**, Ars., Ipec., Kali c.
cold, desire for: Phos., Ver.
cold, aggravates: Lyc.
juicy, craves: *Phos. ac.*, Ver.
desire for, changeable: Bry.
fluid, desire for: Staph.
little satisfies: Cinch., Lyc.
tasteless: Ant. t., Canth., **Dros.**, Plant., Sil.
warm and cooked, aversion to: Colch., **Petr.**, Sec.

Fretting: Ant. c., Ant. t., *Cham.*, **Cina**, *Gels.*, Sil.

Fruit, longing for: Alum., **Ant. t.**, *Phos. ac.*, Ver.

Gastric symptoms: *Ant. c.*, Ant. t., Bry., **Carbo v.**, Colch., *Cyc.*, Dros., Ipec., Nux, **Puls.**, Psor., Sul.
symptoms predominate: Acon., **Ant. c.**, Ant. t., Bell., Bry., Cad. s., Carbo v., Cham., Cof., **Colch.**, Corn., *Cyc.*, Dig., Ign., **Ipec.**, **Nux**, Petros., **Puls.**, Rhus, Sul.

Glands, affections of: Apis, *Bar.*, *Bar. i.*, Bell., *Cal.*, Carbo an., Cina, Coc., Iod., **Psor.**, Spong., Staph., *Sul.*, Tub.

Grief, bad effects of: **Ign.**, Lach., Op., *Phos. ac.*, *Staph.*

Gums, bleed when touched: Carbo v., Staph.
feeling as though scalded: Cimex.
scorbutic condition of: Nat., *Nit. ac.*, San.
spongy: Staph.
white: Fer., Staph., Val.

Hemorrhage: Cac., **Cinch.**, Crot., Fer., Ham., *Ipec.*, Nit. ac., **Phos.**, *Psor.*, **Tub.**, Ter.
labor-pains cease from: Cinch.
from bowels: Crot., Ham., Ipec., Nit. ac., Rhus, Ter., Tub.

Hemorrhoids: **Æsc.**, *Aloe*, **Mur. ac.**, **Nux**, **Sul.**

Head, vertex, burning heat in: Cal., Graph., Lach., **Sul.**
vertex, coldness of: Sep., Val., Ver.
vertex, tightness over: Cinch.

Headache: Arn., Ars., Bell., Bry., Caps., Carbo v., Cinch., Coc., Dros., Fer., Gels., Ign., Mez., **Nat.**, **Nux**, *Op.*, Phos. ac., Polyp., Puls., Rhus, Sep., Spong., Stan.. Val.
menstrual: Glon., **Nat.**, *Puls.*

Heart, palpitation of: Acon., *Ant. t.*, Cinch., Ign., Lach., Lil., Mer., **Nat.**, Sep., Spig., Sul., Ver.
pulsations of, shake the body: **Nat.**
sensation as if would stop beating if she moved: Dig.
sensation as if would stop unless constantly on the move: Gels.

Heat, aversion to: Apis, Puls., Sec.
when asleep: *Samb.*

Hunger: Ant. c., Arn., Bar., *Carbo an.*, Carbo v., **Cina**, Cinch., Dig., Graph., Ign., **Iod.**, Lyc., *Meny.*, Nux, Petr., Rhus, San., Sep., **Staph.**, Stan., Sul., **Ver.**
but cannot eat: Bar., Elaps, Ign.
which eating does not relieve: Ant. c.

Hypochondrium, right, tender to the touch.: Bry., Chel., Card., *Eup., Kali c.,* Mer.

Hypochondria, painful, swollen: Card., **Cinch.,** Chin. s., Mer., Pod.

Ice-cream, desire for: Eup.

Irritability: Acon., *Anac.,* Bell., *Bry., Cham.,* Cina, Cinch., Cof., Gels., *Ign.,* Mer., **Nux,** Puls., Sil., Tub., Val.
excessive physical: Nit. ac.

Jaundice: Car., *Chel.,* **Crot., Mer.,** Pod.

Joints, pain in: Apis, Arn., Ars., **Bry.,** Caust., Cham., Cinch., Coc., Ign., Ipec., Phos. ac., *Pod.,* Puls., Rhus, Sab., Sul.
soreness of: Apis.

Labiæ, ulceration of commissures of: **Nat.,** Nit. ac., San.

Leucorrhea, staining the linen yellow: *Carbo an.*
exhausting: Alum., Carbo an.

Light, aversion to bright: Nux.

Limbs, cramps in: Cup., Sul., Ver.
pain in: Cal., Caps., Carbo v., Caust., Cinch., Dros., *Eup.,* Graph., Lyc., Nat., Nit. ac., Nux, Puls., Sab.
paralytic immobility of: Canth.
soreness of: Apis, Arn.
weakness of: Bar., Nux.

Lips, burning of: Apis, Ars.
cracked: Graph., Ign., Hep., Rhus.
dry: Ars., Bry., *Con.,* Ign., *Nux m.,* Rhus.
eruption on: Hep., Ign., **Nat., Nux,** *Rhus.*

Liver, pain in: Ars., Bell., *Bry.,* Card., Cham., *Chel.,* Cinch., Dul., **Kali c., Lyc.,** *Mer.,* **Nat., Nux,** Polyp., Pod., Puls.
sensation as if swollen: Cinch.

Love, disappointed, bad effects of: Cal. p., Hyos., **Ign.,** Nat., Staph.

Meat, aversion to: Alum., *Arn.,* Ars., Bell., Cal., Carbo v., Cham., Fer., Graph., Ign., Lyc., Mer., Nit. ac., Op., Petr., Puls., Rhus, Sabad., Sec., Sep., Sil., Sul.
desire for: **Canth.,** *Mag. c.,* **Meny., Tub.**

Menses, suppression of: Ars., Cal., Cham., Cinch., Con., Fer., Graph., Kali c., Lyc., Mer., Nux, Puls., Sep., Sil., Sul., Tub.
too early: Acon., Alum., Arn., Ars., Bar., Bell., Bry., **Cal.,** *Cal. p.,* Carbo v., Cham., Coc., Fer., Hyos., Ign., Iod., Kali c., Led., Mer., Nux, Petr., Phos., Rhus, Sab., Sep., Spong., Staph., Sul., Ver.
too late: Bell., Caust., Cinch., Con., Fer., Graph., Hyos., Ign., Ipec., Kali c., Lyc., Nat., **Puls.,** Sabad., Sil., Sul., **Tub.**
too profuse: Acon., Aran., Ars., Bar., Bell., *Cal.,* Cham., Cina, Cinch., Fer., Hyos., Ign., Ipec., Led., Lyc., Mer., Nat., Nux, Op., Phos., Sab., Sep., Sil., Spong., Stan., Stram., Sul.
too scanty: Alum., Con., Cyc., Graph., Lyc., Nat., Phos., Puls., Sabad., Sil., Sul., **Tub.,** Ver.
too exhausting: Alum., Carbo an., Coc.
flow intermits: Fer., Puls., Sul., Tub.
morning sickness during: Graph., Psor.

Metrorrhagia between the periods at every little accident: Amb.

Milk, aversion to: Puls., Sil.
desire for: Apis, Chel.
desire for, but causes flatulence: Carbo v.

Mouth, corners of, eruptions at: Hep., *Ign.,* **Nat., Nux,** *Rhus.*
corners, sore and ulcerated: Nat., Nit. ac.
desire to rinse the: **Nux,** *Thuja,* Puls.
mucous membrane of, pale: *Eup.,* **Fer.**
rawness of: Apis Carbo an.

Nausea: Ant. c., Ant. t., Arn., Ars., Caps., Dros., Eup., Graph., Hep., Hyos., Ipec., *Nux,* Petros., Rhus, Sabad., Sil.
relieved by drinking: **Lob.**

Neck, pain in back of: Fer.

Nervousness: Ced., *Cham.*, Cinch., Cof., *Gels.*, Ign., Nux, Puls., Rhus, Val.

Night-sweats: Cinch., Kali c., Nat., Stan., Tarax.

Pain, sensitive to: Cham., Cinch., Cof., Ign.
better while thinking of it: Camph.

Palpitation from mental emotion: Cal. ars.

Palate, scalded, feeling as though: Æsc., Cimex.

Perspiration: Ars., Cinch., Lach., Sul.

Prolapsus ani: **Ign.**, *Lach.*, *Lyc.*, Mer., Nit. ac., Plumb., **Pod.**, **Rat.**, *Sep.*, *Sul.*
from moderate straining: **Ign.**
from stooping: **Rat.**
from overlifting or straining, after parturition: Pod.

Pulse, accellerated by motion: Ant. t., *Dig.*, Gels.
full: Acon., Bell., Bry., Dig., Fer., Gels., Glon., Hyos., Lach., Op., Stram.
rapid, then slow: Ant. c.
suddenly increases, and then rapidly decreases to below normal: Tub., Ver. **v.**
slow: Chel., Cinch., **Dig.**, Sec., **Ver.**
slow, soft, weak: Ver. v.
third, fifth or seventh beat intermits: *Dig.*
thread-like: Acon., Gels., Lach.
weak: *Acon.*, Ars., *Carbo v.*, Cinch., Cup., Fer., Gels., Lach., Laur., *Op.*, Psor., *Sil.*, *Stram.*, *Ver.*, Ver. v.

Rectum, burning and dryness of: Æsc.

Remission, slight: Bap., **Eup.**, Gels.

Restless, continually moving from place to place: Pyr., Rhus.

Restlessness: Apis, Ars., Bap., Ced., Colch., Iod., Rhus.

Rheumatism: *Acon.*, Ant. t., Arn., *Bell.*, *Bry.*, Carbo v., *Caust.*, Cham., Colch., Nux, *Puls.*, *Rhus,* Thuja, Val., Ver.

Saliva, acrid: Nit. ac.
bitter, collection of, in the mouth: Chel.
bloody: *Bufo,* Crot., Gels., Mer., *Nat.,* **Nit. ac.,** *Phos.,* Sec.
bloody, before menses: Nat.
cotton-like: Nux m.
saltish: Ant. c., Iod.
secretion of, profuse: Ipec., Mer., Pod.
sticky: *Nux m.*
sour: Ign.
thready: Con., Crot., Hydr., *Kali bi.,* Lach.

Salivation: Æsc., Iod., Mer., **Pod.**

Scapula, pain under inferior angle of right: Chel.
pain under inferior angle of left: Sang.

Sick feeling all over, indescribable: Bap.

Side, better when lying on painful: *Bry.*
left, pain in: Apis.

Sighing: *Ign., Phos. ac., Ver.*

Sinking: *Camph., Carbo v.,* Ver.

Skin, blueness of: Carbo v., **Ver.**
itching of: Hep., Ign., Rhus.
yellow: Acon., Arn., Ars., Bell., Card., Cham., Cinch., Dig., *Eup.,* Fer., *Nat., Nux,* Pod., Polyp., Psor., Puls., Rhus, Sul., Tar.

Sleep, dreams with: Acon., Ign., Nat., Stram.
restless: Acon., Bap., Cina, Fer., Ign., Rhus, Stram.
snoring with: Ign., *Op.*

Sleepiness: Acon., **Ant. t.,** Bell., Bry., Cal., Carbo v., Cham., Coc., Hyos., Mer., **Op.,** Puls., Rhus, Sabad., Spig., Stan., Stram., Sul., Val.

Sleeplessness: Ars., Bell., Bry., Carbo v., Cinch., Cina, Cof., Hyos., Ipec., Led., Mer., Nat., Nit. ac., Op., Puls., Ran., Rhus, Sil., Spig.

Sour things, aversion to: Coc.
things, desire for: *Ant. c.,* Arn., Ars., Coc., Dig., Eup., Hep., Kali bi., Polyp., Puls., Sec.

Spine, irritation of: **Agar.,** Ang., Gels., Nux, *Sil.,* **Zinc.**

Spleen, enlarged: Aran., Ars., Bell., Carb. ac., *Cean., Cinch., Eup.,* Fer., **Iod.,** Mer., Mez., Nit. ac., Pod., Puls.
pain in region of: Apis, Ars., Chel., Cinch., Fer., **Nat., Nux,** Pod., Tarax.
region of, sensitive to pressure: Apis, Ars., *Chel.,* Cinch., Chin. s., Fer., **Iod.,** *Nux,* Pod., Puls.

"Spoiled cases" by Quinine and ague cures: Apis, **Ars.,** Chin. s., *Ign.,* **Ipec.,** *Lach.,* Lyc., **Psor., Puls., Sep.,** Sil., **Sul.**

Sputum, bloody: Nux m.

Stomach, cramps in: Cup., Ver.
distention of: Nux, Petros., Sabad.
fulness of, sense of: Carbo v., Lob., *Lyc.,* **Nat.,** Pod., Rhus.
oppression at pit of: Lob.
pain in: Acon., Arn., Ars., Cal., Caust., *Chel.,* Coc., Con., Fer., Ign., Lyc., Nat., Nux, Petros., Puls., Rhus, Sabad., Sep., Sil., Stan., Ver.
pressure in the region of: Ant. c., Rhus.
relaxed as if hanging down: Ipec., Staph.
spasms in: Ars., Bell., Bry., Carbo v., Cham., Coc., Fer., Ign., Nat., Nux, Puls., Sil., Stan., Sul., Val., Ver.
weak sensation in: Lob., Phos.

Stool, during, presence of others is unbearable: Amb.

Sweating: **Cinch.,** Nux, **Samb.,** Sil., *Ver.*

Sweat, debilitating: **Cinch.,** Eup., Tarax., **Tub.**
debilitating, not: **Samb.**
profuse, when awake: **Samb.**
profuse, of head: Cal., Mag. m., San., Sil.

Taste, acute: Cinch.
bitter: Ant. c., Aran., **Arn.**, Ars., *Bry.*, Cal., Carbo v., Cham., **Chel.**, *Chin. s.*, **Cinch.**, **Col.**, Con., Dros., Dul., Eup., Fer., Gels., Graph., Hep., Ipec., Lach., Lyc., Mag. c., Mer., Nat., **Nat. s.**, Nit. ac., **Nux**, Phos. ac., Polyp., Psor., Puls., Rhus, Sab., Staph., **Sul.**, Tarax., Thuja.
bitter, everything except water: **Acon.**, *Stan.*
sweet: *Meny.*
sweet, of tobacco: *Coc.*, Puls.
coppery: Kali bi., Mer., Ran.
herring brine, like: Anac.
ink, like: Arg. n., **Cal.**, Fluor. ac.
iron, like: Cal., Cimex.
lost: Canth., Nat., Pod., Psor., Sil.
metallic: **Coc.**, **Mer.**, Nux, Polyp., Rhus.
putrid: **Anac.**, **Arn.**, Bell., **Caps.**, **Carbo v.**, Cham., *Fer.*, *Graph.*, Hep., Hyos., Mer., Nat., Nit. ac., **Nux**, Petr., Plant., **Pod.**, **Psor.**, *Puls.*, **Pyr.**, Rhus, Sil., Staph.
putrid in morning: **Ars.**, Chin. s., Mer., *Rhus*, *Sul.*
salt: Ars., *Carbo v.*, Cinch., Mer., Nat., **Sep.**
soapy: Cac., Dul., Iod., Sil.
sour: **Arg. n.**, Cal., Caps., Cham., Graph., Ign., Iod., Lach., **Lyc.**, Mag. c., *Nux*, Petr., **Phos.**, Pod., Rob., Sep., Thuja.

Things, wants, which he repels when offered: Bry., **Cham.**, Cina, Iod., Staph.

Thirst: Canth., Cic., Cimex, **Cinch.**, Dul., Sul., Ver.
but disgust for all kinds of drink: **Canth.**
for cold drinks: Dul.

Thirstlessness, with nearly all complaints: Apis, Puls.

Throat, liability to sore: Bar., **Lac c.**, Psor.
dry, painfully sore: **Æsc.**
sore during menses: Lac c., Mag. c.

Tobacco, aversion to: Alum., Arn., Bell., Cal., Cinch., **Ign.**, Led., Nat., Nux, Phos., Rhus, Sep., Spig., Stan.
cannot bear: **Ign.**
has no taste: Ant. t.

Tongue, black: Elaps.
blistered: Caps., *Carbo an.*, Carbo v., Cham., Nat., Thuja.
broad, red, with indented edges: Kali bi., Mer., Pod., Rhus.
brown: Ars., Carbo v., Elat., Hyos., Iod., Lyc., Phos., Ver.
brown, edges white: *Iod.*
brown streak down the middle: *Arn.*, Eup. p., Iod., Lach., Phos.
burning: Carbo an., Carbo v., Cimex, Sang.
burnt, feeling as though: **Apis, Lyc.**, Psor., Mur. ac., Nit. ac., Sang., **Spig.**
catches behind the teeth: Lach.
clean: Alum., Apis, Cac., Caust., Chin. s., **Cina**, Dig., Dros., Elaps, Gels., Ign., Ipec., Lyc., Mag. c., Puls., Sec., Stram., Sul., *Thuja.*
coated thickly: **Ant. c.**, Arn., Bar., *Bry.*, Canth., Chel., Cinch., Iod., Kali bi., Mez., **Nux**, Phos., Polyp.
cold: **Camph.**, Carbo v., *Ver.*
contracted: Carbo v.
cracked: Cur., Lyc.
dry: Arn., **Bell.**, *Cal.*, *Carbo v.*, Caust., Dul., Lach., Lyc., *Nat.*, **Nux m.**, Pod., Puls., *Stram.*
dry at the back of: Hep.
dry at the edges: Coc.
edges red: **Ant. t.**, Bell., Canth., Gels., Phos., Sec., *Ver.*
edges red, white in the middle: Bell.
furred, with red streak down the middle: *Ars.*, Phos., Ver. v.
too large: Puls., Stram.
lead-colored: Camph., **Carbo v.**, Ver.
mapped: Lach., **Nat.**, *Ran.*, **Tarax.**, **Ter.**
mapped like herpes (ringworm), on the sides: **Nat.**
mucus, covered with: **Puls.**
mucus, yellowish, on: Camph.

Tongue, painful: Con., Graph., Hep.
pale: **Eup., Fer.**, Ipec., Kali c., *Sec.*
papillæ elevated: Acon., **Ant. t.**, *Bell.*, Mez., Nux m.
papillæ red: *Acon.*, **Apis**, *Bell.*, Mez., Nux, *Stram.*
protrude, cannot: Apis, *Lach.*, Stram.
red: *Ant. t.*, *Apis*, **Bell.**, Cur., Elaps, Hyos., Kali bi., Lyc., Sul., *Thuja.*
red and white in streaks: **Ant. t.**
red streak in centre: Phos. ac., Ver. v.
rough: Anac.
sore: *Apis*, Sul., Tarax.
spots on, dark, red and sensitive: **Tarax.**, Ter.
stiff: Con., Dul., Lyc.
strawberry: *Acon.*, Ant. t., **Apis**, **Bell.**, Ter.
swelling of: Dul., Cic., Elaps, Mer., *Thuja*, *Ver.*
tip blue: Sabad.
tip dry: Psor., *Rhus*, Sec.
tip dry and red: *Ars.*, Lach., Nux, Polyp., **Rhus**, Sec., *Ver.*
tip sore: Carbo v., *Hep.*, Kali c., Sabad., *Thuja*, Tarax.
tip red, triangular: **Rhus.**
shows imprint of teeth: Chel., **Mer.**, **Pod.**, Rhus.
trembling: Camph., Canth., Lach., *Lyc.*, **Op.**
ulcers on: Caps., Carbo an., **Mer.**, Mur. ac., Nit. ac.
vesicles on sides and tip: Carbo an., Caust., Lyc., Sep., Thuja.
white: Anac., *Ant. c.*, Arn., Ars., Bar., Cal., Carbo v., Chel., Cincn., Cina, Coc., Dig., Eup., Fer., Graph., Ipec., Kali c., Lach., Mag. c., Mez., Nat., Nit. ac., Nux m., Nux, Phos., Plant., Pod., Polyp., Psor., **Puls.**, Rhus, Sabad., Sarr., Sep., Staph., Stram., Sul., Ver.
white in centre, dark streak along the sides: Petr.
white, milky: **Ant. c.**
white at sides, middle red: Cham.
white or yellow in centre, margins pale: Chin. s.
white, or yellow with margins red: Chel., Gels.
yellow: Arn., Ars., Bov., *Bry.*, Canth., Carbo v., Ced., Cham.,

Chel., Cinch.; Eup., Fer., Gels., Ipec., Kali bi., *Mer.*, Nat., Nit. ac., *Nux,* Op., **Pod.**, Polyp., Psor., *Puls.*, Sec., Sul.

Tonsils, induration of: **Bar.**, Cal., Iod., Lac c., Lach., Mer., Psor.

Toothache, daily at same hour: Aran.

Touch, sensitive to: *Apis,* Bell., **Cinch.**, Kali c., *Lach.*

Urinary organs, irritation of: Canth., Clem., Dul., **Med.**, *Petr.*, Petros., Sars., Thuja.

Urination, difficult: *Canth.*, Sars.
frequent: Apis, Canth., Cham., *Eup.*, Med., Phos. ac., Plant.
frequent at night: *Phos. ac.*
frequent, flow intermits: **Con.**
painful: Canth., *Eup. p.*
profuse: Canth., **Eup. p.**, Phos. ac.
profuse but pale, clear as water at night: **Phos. ac.**
retarded, from stricture: Clem.

Urine, black: Canth.
brick-dust sediment: Chin. s., Cinch., **Lyc.**, **Nat.**, *Sars.*
brown: Camph., Cimex.
fatty: Chin. s.
green: Camph., *Plant.*
horses, smelling like: Absinth., **Nit. ac.**
hot: Cimex.
incontinence of: Caust., Dul., **Med.**, Nit. ac., Puls., Rhus, Sul.
milky, turning so, after standing: *Cina,* Dul., San.
odor, urinous, intensified: Benz. ac.
odor, offensive: **Nit. ac.**, Nux, Psor.
pale: Cham., **Eup.**, **Phos. ac.**, Thuja.
red: Bry., Camph., **Lyc.**, Nux.
red, yellow: Kali c.
retained, bladder full: **Op.**
retained from stricture, organic or inflammatory: *Clem.*, Med.

Urine, scanty: **Apis,** Bry., Cinch., Lyc., *Nat.*
scanty and painful: **Apis,** Canth.
suppressed: Stram., Tub.
turbid: Ant. t., Berb., Camph., Cina, Cinch., Dul., Graph., Ipec., **Lyc.,** Mer., *Nat., Nit. ac.*
white sediment, with: Berb., Graph.
yellowish: Camph.

Urticaria: **Apis,** Cop., Elat., **Hep.,** *Ign.,* **Rhus.**

Vegetables, longing for: Alum., Ver.

Veins, distended: Fer.

Vertigo: Acon., Arn., Ars., Bell., Cal., Caust., Cham., Coc., Con., **Eup.,** Fer., Hyos., Lyc., Nit. ac., Nux, Op., Petr., Phos., Polyp., Puls., Sep., Sil.
in occiput: Petr.
with sensation of falling to the left: Col., Eup., **Eup. p.**

Vomiting: Ant. c., Ant. t., Cina, Cinch., *Eup., Fer.,* Hyos., Ipec., Lyc., Mer., Nux, Petros., Sep., Sil., Ver.
bitter: Cinch., Eup.
bile, of: Ars., **Eup.,** Ipec., Mer., Nux, Stram., Ver.
ingesta, of: Ars., Cham., **Eup., Fer.,** *Ipec., Nux,* Puls.
mucus, of: Mer., Nux, *Puls.*
sour: **Lyc.,** *Rob.*

Walk, desire to slowly, which gives relief: *Fer.*

Weakness: Acon., *Alum.,* Apis, Arn., **Ars.,** Bap., Bar., Cal., Camph., **Carbo an., Carbo v., Ced.,** Chin. s., **Cinch.,** Corn., Dig., Eup. p., **Fer.,** *Gels.,* Ign., Iod., Ipec., Lyc., **Nat.,** Nit. ac., Nux, Polyp., Sul., Ver.
in stomach and abdomen: Chel., **Phos.,** *Sep.*
on going up stairs: Cal., Iod.

Weep, disposition to: *Cina,* Puls., Nux.

Worms, with symptoms of: *Cina,* Psor., Spig., Stan., Sul.

TYPHOID. TYPHUS, PRODROMIC STAGE.

In the early stages the following may be indicated:

Beginning sudden, flushed face, congestive headache: **Bap.**, *Bell.*
with frequent epistaxis: **Bry.**, Carbo v., *Rhus.*
with bleeding of gums: **Carbo v.**, Mer., *Pyr.*
with loss of appetite, belching, tongue coated white, frontal headache, heaviness of limbs and lassitude: Bry.
with heavily furred tongue, insidious, "walking typhoid:" Coc.
with tip of tongue and mouth dry: *Bell.*, Nux, *Rhus.*
with gastric symptoms, and acute shooting pains in various parts of body: **Bry.**, *Pyr.*
with acid or bitter belching and vertigo: Nux, Puls.
with loose, painless stool: *Bap.*, Rhus.
with excessive flatulence: **Phos.**
with gastric symptoms and delayed menses: *Puls.*, **Psor.**, Sul.
with vomiting and copious diarrhea: Ipec.
with copious, painful, watery stools, great prostration: Ver.
with chilliness on the slightest motion: **Bry.**, Nux, Sep., Sil.
with sleepiness, but unable to sleep: *Bell.*, **Op.**
with stiffness of joints: **Bry.**, Pyr.
with stiffness of joints and lameness of muscles: **Arn.**, *Bry.*, **Pyr.**
with wants to lie on one spot: **Bry.**, Rhus.
with trembling and weary limbs: Bell.
with heat unbearable, but uncovering makes chilly: Puls.
if the so-called nervous symptoms predominate: Gels.

SYMPTOMS OF THE MIND.

Anxiety: **Ars.**, Bry., Cham., Nux, Phos., *Psor.*
with nausea and cold sweat on forehead: Ver.
with frightful dreams and great weakness: Ars.

Anxiety, uncontrollable, even to suicide: Cinch.
does not know what to do with himself, < after midnight: **Ars.,** Psor., Kali c.

Apathy: Cinch., *Coc.,* **Op.,** Phos., **Phos. ac.,** Pyr., Ver.
with indifference: Cinch., *Phos. ac.*
and extreme dullness of the senses: Nit. sp. d.
makes no complaints: **Op.,** Hyos.
thinks he is well: Ars.
says he is well, nothing the matter with him: Arn.
unless questioned, does not speak of his condition, does not seem dangerous to him: Colch.
utters no desire, no will power: Hell.
does not ask for anything, has none of the usual wants: Nit. sp. d.

Indifference: Apis, *Arn.,* Carbo v., Cinch., Coc., **Op., Phos. ac.,** *Psor.*
even to the most loved child or dearest friend: **Phos.,** Sep.
to the most loved objects, wishes to die: Mer.
to everything: Nux, Sec.
and insensibility, with pale face: Cinch.
and insensibility, impelling to rub forehead: Ver.

Anxiety, faint-hearted, timid, inclined to weep, fears death: *Acon.,* **Ars.,** Coc., Rhus, Ver.
timid and fearful: Bell., Bry.
fear of being left alone: Ars., **Bis.,** Hyos., *Kali c.,* **Lyc.**
believes he is always alone: Stram.
dejected, debilitated, with aversion to thought: Bry.
either sorrowful, depressed or violent delirium: Bell.
depression of spirits, with timidity: Sec.
hopeless of recovery: Psor.
hopeless, thinks it useless to take medicine, is incurable: Ars.
hopeless and certain of death: Ars., Bap.
uneasiness of mind and body: Op.
wants to go from one bed into another: **Ars.,** Bell., *Col., Cina,* Cham., *Hyos.,* Mez., **Rhus,** Sep., Ver.

Anxiety, desire to escape: *Bell.,* **Hyos.,** Stram.
desire to get out of bed: Bry.
desire to escape from bed: **Bell.,** *Bry.,* **Hyos.,** Stram.
desire to go from one bed to another: Ars., Cal., **Rhus.**
desire to go home: **Bry.**
desire to jump out of bed: Bell., Hyos., Zinc.
desire to jump, calmed and restrained with difficulty: Zinc.
desire, springs from bed suddenly: **Bell.,** Nux.
frightful objects constantly before the mind; his expression is that of fear and terror; sees cats, dogs, etc.. approaching from all sides; sees ghosts: Stram.
fear of death: **Acon., Ars.,** *Bry.,* Coc., **Nit. ac.,** *Psor.,* **Rhus,** Ver.
fear, with, inclined to weep: Acon., Bry., Coc., **Ign.,** Rhus.

Loquacity: Apis, Bry., *Hyos.,* **Lach., Stram.**
afterwards stupid and irritable: Lachn.
talks all the time or not at all: Lach., **Stram.**
talks of the business of the day or the last few weeks: Bry.
talks to himself, continually: Rhus.
talks, constant muttering delirium: Hyos., Stram., Tarax.

Murmuring: Apis, Ars., Coc., Hyos., Lach., Lyc., Phos. ac., Phos., Tarax., Ver. v.
which cannot be understood: Hyos., Lyc., Phos. ac.
with picking bed clothes: Hyos., Op.
with apathy, hardness of hearing, and a pleasant, happy expression that looks strange: Apis.

Speaks, incoherently, no connection of ideas: *Alum.,* Bap., *Lach.,*
low and indistinctly: Hyos.
nonsense with eyes wide open: Hyos.
of dogs, wolves, cattle, soldiers, battles: Bell.
like a drunken man: Bap., Lyc., Op.

Sings, from time to time: Ars., Stram.
and laughs loud in delirium: Bell.
opera pieces, laughs, whistles, recites poetry: Stram.

Sings, whines, and don't know why: Hyos.
and moans loudly: Mur. ac.
and cries out suddenly: **Hyos.,** Lyc., **Stram.**

Picking the bed clothes: Arn., Ars., Bap., *Bell., Colch.,* **Hyos.,** Lyc., **Op.,** Psor., **Stram.,** Zinc.
the bed during sleep: Op.
with muttering delirium: Bell., **Hyos.,** Rhus.
with delirium while awake: Bell., Hyos.
or catching, grasping at flocks: Lyc., Phos. ac., Zinc.
or playing with his own hands: Hyos.
or motion with hands, as if grasping things: Phos. ac.
grasping about with hands: Op.
or waving hands as if getting things out of air: Psor., Stram., Sul.

Physical, does foolish things, behaves like a madman: Hyos.
beats and scratches others; the milder others talk to them the worse they get: Hyos.
abuses those about him: Hyos.
strikes, bites or spits at attendants: Bell.
strikes attendants, with fearful outcries; wants to bite and tear everything with his teeth, even his own limbs: Stram.
raving delirium, with pain in the head: Ars., Bell.
raving, motions never awkward, very dexterous: Stram.

Answers, quick, hasty: Bry., Coc., **Hell.,** *Hep., Hyos.,* Rhus.
if he talks at all it is quick and hasty: Ars., *Bry.*
refuses to: Camph., *Hyos.,* **Phos.,** Stram.
reluctantly and slowly, or short, unintelligible: Phos. ac.
slow: Ars. h., **Hell., Phos.,** Sul., Pyr.
wandering, as if semi-conscious: Bap., Lyc.
correctly, but in quick, violent manner, as if angry: Rhus.
correctly, but indignantly: Puls.
correctly, but slowly, as if cautious: Nux m.
correctly, but unconsciousness and delirium returns at once: Arn.
falls asleep in the midst of a sentence: Bap.
short with "yes" or "no:" Phos.

Taciturn, silent: Arn., Ars., Cinch., Bell., Bap., Bry., Coc., Hyos., Mer., Nux, Op., Phos., Phos. ac., Psor.
as if averse to everything: Nux.
with an unconquerable inclination to sleep: Coc., **Op.**
sits absorbed in silence: Op., *Phos. ac.,* **Psor.**
obstinate silence, will answer nothing: Cinch.
don't want to talk: **Phos. ac.**
averse to speaking, difficult to think: Rhus.
with confusion of mind: Mer.
reluctant to answer questions: Phos. ac., Rhus.
reluctant to speak: Bell.
short and incorrectly: Phos. ac.
declines to answer questions: Arn., Ars., Hyos.
scarcely answers, in spite of what is done to induce him to do so; appears to hear without comprehending what is said, or without it making any impression on him: Nit. sp. d.
permits no one to speak to him: Ver.
refuses things offered: Bell., **Bry.,** *Staph.,* Kreos.
refuses things, lies indolent, without sleeping or speaking; Nit. sp. d.

Indolence, sits in silence: Coc., Op., Psor.
of mind and body; in daytime averse to work or motion: in the evening averse to pleasure: extremely uncomfortable; does not know what is the matter: Sul.
aversion to all efforts of mind and body: Cinch., Coc.
does not know if he will take what is offered: Hyos. Sul.

Ill humor: Bell., *Bry.,* **Cham.,** Cinch., Lach., **Nux,** *Psor.,* Puls., *Rhus,* **Sul.**
quarrelsome: Bell.
vexed, irritated, wants to quarrel: Bry.
angry disposition: **Bry.,** Cinch.
chagrined: Nux, Staph

Irritable: **Bry.,** *Carbo v.,* **Caust., Cham.,** Cinch., Coc., **Gels., Lyc., Mer.,** Mur. ac., **Nux,** Phos., **Psor.**
too sensitive, easily offended, vexed from questions or gives curt answers: Bry.

Irritable, nervous, depressed, intolerant of noise and all external impressions: Cinch.
mutters, can endure neither noise nor contradiction, speaks hastily: Coc.
peevish, easily offended: Bry.

Unconscious: *Apis,* Arn., Ars., **Bell.,** Carb. ac., **Colch.,** Gels., **Hyos., Lach.,** Lyc., **Mur. ac.,** Nux m., **Op.,** *Phos. ac.,* Phos., **Psor.,** Rhus, *Stram.,* Sul., *Zinc.*
and insensible, muscles relaxed: Op.
with loss of functional sensation: Hyos.
like a deep sleep: Mer., **Op.,** Pyr.
with imbecility: Stram.
knows neither where he is nor what he does: Puls.
when spoken to, called, cannot be roused from lethargy: Hyos.
perceptions entirely lost, picking at the bed clothes: Colch.

Insensibility: Apis, Ars., Cinch., *Hell.,* Mer., **Op.,** Psor., Pyr., *Rhus,* **Sul.**
with stupor, feels neither pain nor pleasure: Op.
with indifference: Ver.
is compelled to rub the forehead: Ver.
and loss of consciousness; Apis, Hell., Rhus.
with loss of speech, pulseless, cadaverous, while natural heat of body is retained; is in a sleep-like state, from which he emerges with consciousness and speech: Mer.
stupid and embarrassed, avoids moving about: Sul.
to all external impressions: Stram.

Stupor: *Apis,* Arn., *Bap.,* Bell., *Bry.,* **Hyos.,** Kali c., Lach., *Nux m.,* **Op., Phos. ac.,** Psor., Rhus, Sul., Ver.
falls asleep in the midst of a sentence: Bap.
with profuse sweat: Kali c.
with apathy, unconsciousness, muttering delirium: Apis.
sinks into a state of apathy or stupefaction: Hyos.
takes no notice of what occurs; neither sees, hears, nor recognizes friends: Stram.

Stupor, with brown, parched tongue; teeth and gums covered with sordes: Rhus.

rush of blood to head, desire to lie down, as if drunk: Bry.

is conscious of no want except thirst: Hyos.

silly, stupid, sadness and weakened memory: Op.

momentary, does not know where he is: Mer.

sensibility entirely benumbed: Op.

giddiness and vanishing of thought: Nux m.

entire loss of speech: Hyos.

utter insensibility: Op., Psor., Pyr., Sul.

so profound cannot be brought to himself: Nit. sp. d.

when spoken to answers promptly, but unconsciousness immediately returns: Arn., Bell., Hyos., Pyr.

if aroused, soon returns: Hyos.

Memory lost: **Anac.**, Arn., Hyos., **Kali br.**, Kali p., **Lach.**, Mer., **Mur. ac.**, *Nux m.*, Natr., Op., Puls., *Rhus,* Sep., Sil., Ver., Zinc.

or weakened: Lach., Op.

forgets the word while speaking: Arn.

forgets time and place: Mer.

forgets what he has said: Mur. ac.

cannot remember the most recent events: Rhus.

almost entire loss of mind; remembers events only as dreams: Ver.

dulness, like a want of memory: Puls.

Memory weak: **Anac.**, Apis, *Bar.*, Bell., Bry., Carbo v., Carb. ac., Coc., **Colch.**, Crot., Dig., Graph., Hell., Ign., Kali p., **Lach.**, Lyc., **Mer.**, Mur. ac., Natr., **Nux m.**, **Nux**, *Phos.*, Psor., Puls., **Sep.**

mind occupied with things past and present: Mur. ac.

does not know those about, relatives or friends: Hyos.

knows neither relatives nor most familiar objects: Op.

knows his friends at one time and not at another: Bell.

Comprehension difficult: *Arn.*, Bry., Carbo v., Cham., *Coc.*, Con., Graph., *Hyos.*, **Lyc.**, Phos., Phos. ac., **Psor.**, Puls., Op., *Sul.*

when asked a question: Sul.

cannot find the right expression for his ideas, does not remember what has passed: Coc.

thinks right, but uses wrong words for the correct ideas he intends to express: Arn., Graph., *Hyos.*, **Lyc.**

in speaking great difficulty to use right expression: Puls.

talks slowly, answers do not correspond: Carbo v.

does not understand questions, does not answer: Sec.

does not understand questions or does understand and cannot speak: Hyos.

Comprehension difficult, makes irrelevant answers: **Hyos.**, Phos. ac., *Psor.*

when spoken to, appears silly, as if awakened from a dream, and can only comprehend and answer after a great effort: Sul.

recognizes what is said, but appears in a dream: Op.

sits as if in thought, yet thinks of nothing; like a waking dream: Arn.

Absent minded: Arn., **Agnus**, **Apis**, Bell., Caust., Cham., Colch., Hyos., Ign., *Kali br.*, Kali c., Natr., *Nux m.*, Phos., **Psor.**, Rhus.

with staggering or vertigo: Ars.

cannot fix his attention on business or manage his affairs: Sul.

as if absorbed in thoughts, yet a paucity of ideas: Rhus.

with insensibility, as if intoxicated: Nux m.

with absence of ideas: Sul.

with entire self-forgetfulness: Hyos.

Intellection: Arn., **Bap.**, *Bry.*, Carbo v., Cinch., *Colch.*, Hell., **Hyos.**, Mer., **Nit. sp. d.**, *Nux m.*, **Op.**, Petr., *Phos. ac.*, Phos., **Psor.**, Rhus, Sec., *Stram.*, Sul.

difficult thinking and speech: Sec.

Intellection, clouded, though he gives correct answers; unless questioned says nothing of his condition, it does not seem dangerous to him: Coch.

dull, stupid, as if sleepy or drunk: **Op.**, *Rhus.*

mentally obtuse, with great inclination to sleep: Mer.

sluggish, with inability to think: Carbo v.

slow movement of ideas: Cinch., Nux m., Phos., Rhus.

slow and difficult: Rhus.

ideas move slowly and constantly around one subject: Petr.

with confusion of head, as if bound: Carbo v.

dwells long on his answer, often does not answer: Nux m.

averse to thinking, debility of mind, vanishing of thought, like fainting: Bry.

difficulty of thinking, great forgetfulness: Bry.

weak, cannot bring two ideas into connection: Sul.

inability to think, cannot control or direct thought: Hyos.

slow comprehension of ideas: Op.

confusion of ideas: Bap.

stupefied, sits as if in thought, like a waking dream: Arn.

lethargy of the sensorium, a paresis of mentality: Nit. sp. d.

imbecility, dulness, stupidity: Op., Rhus, Stram.

stupid and disconcerted for many days: Phos.

stupidity with dilated pupils: Sec., Sul.

with constant heaviness in forehead, does not think: Arn.

cannot comprehend an idea; headache on waking in the morning: Phos.

Fixed ideas, when he has once grasped a thought it elevates him: Petr., Puls.

monomania, one idea haunting him: Stram.

the same disagreeable idea arouses him as soon as he falls into a light slumber: Cal.

great crowd of changing ideas: Lach., Puls.

Illusions: *Apis,* Arn., *Ars.,* Bapt., **Bell.,** *Bry.,* **Hyos., Lach., Op.,** *Plat.,* Phos., **Stram.**

Illusions, as if the body were cut in two in the middle; as if all the surrounding objects were very small, while he himself is very large: Plat.

that he is very large and tall: Pallad.

believes he sees a large company of people about him and grasps at them: Stram.

phantasies, in slumber and waking, as if she was on a distant island, had great occupation, was a lady of rank: Phos.

speaks to the absent as if they were present, calls inanimate objects by names of persons, while he takes no notice of his attendants: Stram.

does not believe to be in his own house: Op.

thinks he is in the wrong place: Hyos.

wants to go home: Bry.

believes he is always alone: Stram.

muttering stupor; thinks he is dead: Apis, Lach.

says there is nothing the matter with him: Arn.

thinks he is well: Ars.

of the senses and imagination: Hyos.

has visions of beauty or terror: Bell.

sees people standing at the foot of the bed: Bry.

imagines to be under strangers, wants to go home: Bry.

that head or body feels scattered about the bed: Bap.

thought she was three persons, could not keep them covered: Bap., Petr.

gets out of bed, does not feel as if he were at home: Op.

thinks he is elsewhere than at home: Ver.

talks continually of going home: Bell., Bry.

talks of starting on a journey, wants to be dressed, is ready to go: Op.

attempts to get out of bed: Bell., Hyos., Op., Stram., Zinc.

attempts to escape: Bell., Hyos., Op.

of sight, hearing and smell: Stram.

absent persons talk to him: Stram.

Visions, sees animals which he fears: Bell.
with fear and desire to hide or run away: Puls.
hides under bed covers: Stram.
frightful: Carbo v.
frightful phantasies, in the evening in bed, starts frightened on closing the eyes: Cinch.
sees things all the time: Bell., Cal., Stram.
vivid hallucinations: Mur. ac.
with frequent change of vision: Hyos.
when closing the eyes sees persons and events before him that are neither fearful nor anxious, mostly strange faces: Ars., Cal., Carbo v., Samb.

Delirium, mild: Arn., Ars., Bap., **Bell.,** Cal., *Cic.,* Con., Crot., **Gels., Hyos.,** *Ign.,* Lach., Laur., Lyc., *Mer.,* Mur. ac., **Nit. ac.,** *Nux, Nux m.,* **Petr.,** *Phos.,* **Psor.,** Puls., **Stram.,** *Sul.,* Ver.
mild, alternating with loud talking: Bell., Hyos., Stram.
in early stage, in sleep or on waking: Bell., Bry.
after two weeks: Cal., Hyos.
makes no complaint, with general heat: Hyos.
continued when awake, sees persons who are not and have not been present: Hyos.
constant, with congestion to head and face: Bap., Op.
constant, allowing no rest or sleep: Mur. ac.
after Cal. if the patient is harassed by muttering delirium, a tearing and stinging headache, lies in a quiet sopor, sometimes interrupted by screaming and scolding; with distended abdomen and borborygmus: Lyc.—Jahr.
talking, constant, thinks he is roaming over fields, swimming, lying in the water for hours: Rhus.
talking of old occurrences, with open eyes, and recognizes what is said to him only as if in a dream: Op.
talking of religious things, fulfilling vows, prayers: *Stram.,* Ver.
loquacity, mild or terrified: Stram.
talking constantly about his avocation: Bry.

Delirium, talking very loquaciously, with brilliant eyes and circumscribed redness of cheeks, afterwards stupid, irritable: Lachn.

talking loquacious, or loud and violent: Bell.

with singing, laughing, whistling; constant involuntary, odd motions; objects appear oblique: Stram.

talks of ghosts, devils, spirits, which surround his bed: Op.

changing images, past or present, keep him active and irritated: Mur. ac.

Delirium furious, at the height of the disease: Bell., Colch., Stram., Zinc.

amounting to madness: Hyos., Stram., Zinc.

raging, with loud talking, laughing and attempts to escape: Op.

raving, restless, obstinate, objects to sleep, redness and staring of eyes, with intolerance of light: Bell.

cries, strikes at all around: Canth.

cries, even to hoarseness, complete loss of voice: Stram.

with desire to escape from bed: Bell., Hyos., Stram.

maniacal, gets up, tries to run away, screams, roars, with sunken features, cold feet, quick pulse: Zinc.

violent, followed by vomiting and deep sleep: Sec.

stupid, with stupor: Bap., Nux m., Lyc.

stupid, with loss of consciousness: Puls.

stupid, as if intoxicated, with lassitude and weakness: Sec.

stupid, quiet, with great stupefaction and dullness of head: Phos. ac.

stupid, anxiety, headache, noise before the ears, restlessness, sleepless, trembling and anxious sweating: Ars.

stupid, with wide open eyes: Bell., Hyos., Stram.

stupid, on closing eyes, all sorts of frightful visions: Cal.

stupid, with sunken features: Zinc.

stupid, wild, alternating with stupor and stertorous breathing, with open mouth and depression of lower jaw: Mur. ac., Lach., Op., Pyr.

stupid, with hoarseness: Stram.

Delirium, stupid, with sleeplessness: Bell.
stupid, on going to sleep: Cinch., Ginseng.
stupid, as soon as he falls asleep: Gels., **Lach.**, Spong.
restlessness, jumps out of bed, attempts to run away: Hyos.
drunkenness, with indolence or staggering, frantic: Nux m.
prostration; with depression of spirits; weakness with inability to do any work; marked sinking of strength, with inability to move; want of tonicity: Op., Psor.
prostration of the mind, cannot bring two thoughts together, as if quite stupid: Rhus.
prostration and depression of spirits: Mer.
prostration, mentally restless, but too lifeless to move: Ars., Bell.

SENSORIUM.

Acute, increased, of all the senses: Bell., Coff., Gels., Ign., Mur. ac., Nux, Nux m., Op.
especially of hearing and smell: Op., Phos.
especially to noise: Cinch., Nux, Op., Ther.
sounds, talking, odors, lights are insupportable: Nux.
perceptions of the usual pains: Bry.
perceptions, followed by dulness: Rhus.

Dulness of all the senses: Stram., Sul.
slowness or not comprehended: Hell., Op.
with apathy: Nit. sp. d.
as if senses had ceased to act: Hell.
with heavy eyes and extreme weakness: Op.
sensorial action sunken: Carbo v.
is completely insensible, as if in a dream, neither sees or hears: Bell.
perception entirely lost: Colch.
loss of senses: Apis, Psor., Ver.
no complaints, has no pains when pinched or pricked: Phos.

Dulness, complete stupefaction: Stram.
with watery eyes: Op.
hallucinations of sight, smell and hearing: Stram.

Confusion of the head: *Arn.,* **Bap.,** Rhus.
unable to read or perform the least mental labor: Mer.
as if bound with slow ideas: Carbo v.
with vertigo: Puls.
and stupefaction of mind: Sec.
thinking difficult: Stram.
and heavy feeling: Bap., Gels., Puls.
like a want of memory: Puls.
with a rush of blood to head: Camph., Sul.
with bruised pain in forehead: Puls.
with cold sweat on forehead and hands: Coc., Ver.
and vertigo, when getting awake and sitting up, has to lie down: Op.
of the head, with dull vision: Stram.
beclouding of the head: Bap., Nux.
and stupefaction: Rhus.
as after a debauch: *Psor.,* Sul.
with indifference to all external impressions: Hell.
with rush of blood to head: Sul.
with lassitude and weakness: Lach., **Ter.**

Vertigo, like drunkenness: Hyos., Puls.
increasing after delirium: Sec.
as if he would fall after rising from the bed: Rhus.
with dulness in forehead, as if a board were before it: Coc.
with inability to stand erect: Sec.
the whole day whirling, while moving, especially the head: Carbo v.
increased by raising the head: Arn., Cinch.
when rising up in bed: Bap., **Bry.**
with nausea, compelling to lie down again: Coc.
as though swung to and fro in a cradle, or in a swing: Ign.

Vertigo, while lying on the back, like whirling, > when lying on the side: Mer.
- when standing: Lach., Sec., Sul.
- when sitting up: Bry., Phos. ac., Tarax.
- falls when trying to sit up: Phos. ac.
- while raising or moving the head: Arn., Bry.
- on rising from lying on the back, obscure vision: Coc., Nux.
- when moving, especially the head: Arn., **Bry.,** Carbo v., Puls.
- after motions: Bell.
- on rising: *Coc.,* **Bry.,** *Nux,* Rhus.
- compelling to lie down: *Bry.,* Coc.
- in morning on awaking, with weakness of limbs: Cinch.
- so that he cannot rightly comprehend an idea: Puls.
- with confusion and stupidity of the head, as if he would lose his senses: Phos.
- with anxiety and glimmering before the eyes: Bell.
- with headache and heaviness: *Bry.,* Cinch.
- on closing the eyes: Lach., **Ther.,** Thuja.
- on opening the eyes: **Tab.**
- on looking upwards: **Puls.,** *Sil.*
- on looking down: Kalmia, *Spig.*
- with nausea and subsequent heat: Cinch.
- with muscular restlessness: Nux m.
- and fainting while leaving the bed: Op.
- and sleepiness, as if drunk; does not know where he is and walks with eyes shut: Nux m.
- as if there was a whirling in a circle in the brain, with loss of consciousness: **Nux.**

HEAD: INTERNAL.

Congestion to the head: Apis, Arn., *Bap.,* **Bell., Gels.,** Op., *Stram.*
- with mild delirium: Apis.

Congestion in early stage, in violent cases, with great drowsiness, but inability to sleep, and frequent starting: Bell.
venous, with dark red face: *Bap.*, Gels., **Op.**, *Sul.*

Bruised pain, as if compressed: Nux.
pain in the forehead: *Bry.*, Puls.
pain in occiput, as if cerebellum was bruised: **Gels.**, Rhus.
pain, first in forehead, then in occiput: Nux m.

Headache, dull, stupefying, with confusion of ideas: Bap.
heaviness and confusion in the head: Bell., Bry.
in occiput, forehead, especially in membranes of brain: Hyos.
the brain seems to be the only organ affected: Hell.
with the delirium: Ars., Colch.
with violent pain in forehead: Bell., Bry.
< by moving eyes; eyes red, staring, prominent, brilliant: Bell.
< from opening and moving eyes: Bry., Rhus.
in the forehead and eyes: Bap.
does not allow opening of the eyes, with attacks of yawning and stretching: Ign.
when waking from sleep: Lach., Rhus.
in the evening with lassitude: Bry.

Heat, and burning in the brain: Cal., Phos., Sul.
and fulness: Bry., Rhus, Sul.
and chilliness in body: Coc.

Heaviness of the head: Bry., *Nux m.*, Op.
all things seem to whirl in a circle: Ver.
with empty confusion and severe pain: Hyos.
and dulness: Bap., *Gels.*, Puls.
and dulness as if muddled: Mer.
like lead in the forehead, severe pain: Carbo v.
with pressure in the brain and desire to lie down: Bry.

Heaviness, has difficulty in raising head: Puls.
of occiput, like lead, head constantly falls backwards: *Gels.*, Op., Petr.

Heaviness, with intolerance of light: Psor., Puls.
in morning, with drunken vertigo: Coc., Nux.
in vertex, with sensation of fulness: Sul.
with humming and buzzing almost the whole day: Phos.
cannot go to sleep, because she cannot get herself together; head feels scattered and she tosses about to get the pieces together: Bap.

Pressing outward in the temples: Mer., Rhus.
the sides together: Rhus.
in occiput outward; in the forehead, with pain in supraorbital bone, < when touched: Mer.
dull or stitching pains, < from motion and opening the eyes: Bry.
pain in forehead and temples: Ars., Bell., Bry., Glon., Hyos., Stram.

Stupefying pain: Ars., Bap., Bell., Bry., Hyos.
pressure in forehead, with rushing sounds in ears: Ars.
heavy pain in frontal region: Bry.
pressure in forehead, changing to shooting, tearing: Hyos.
pressing, contracting headache: Bell.

Tearing pain in the occiput: Tarax.
pain on the left side: Hyos., Lach.
as if the brain were torn: Rhus.
in the morning, on and after waking: Puls.

HEAD: EXTERNAL.

Throbbing of arteries: Bell., Op.
turns head from side to side: Ars.
often raises or jerks the head from the pillow: Stram.
movement of occiput, grasping it with hands: Carbo v., Gels., Op.
raises up the head, but it constantly falls backwards, and the mouth opens to its widest extent: Colch.

Throbbing of arteries, inability to hold up the head: Op.
can hardly hold head erect, and falls asleep: Cinch.

Forehead covered with cold sweat: Colch., Mer., Ver.

Head and extremities cold, body hot: Phos.

Scalp very sensitive to touch, like a boil: Rhus.

Impelled to rub the forehead, with a kind of insensibility: Ver.

EYES AND SIGHT.

Vision, intolerance of light: *Bell.,* **Psor.,** Puls.
sensibility to light: Lach.
shuns the light: Mur. ac., *Psor.*
shuns the light, lies with face buried in pillow: **Psor.**
hailucination of; objects appear oblique or double, or smaller and farther off: Stram.
obscured with vertigo: Nux.
and hearing diminished, or entire loss of these senses: Sec.
apparent loss of: Psor., Sul.
total blindness: Gels., Psor., Stram., Zinc.
total blindness with loss of, hearing and speech: Stram.

Pupils, much dilated, little sensitive to light: Carbo v.
dilated and immovable: Colch., Stram.
oftener large than small; no reaction to light; either contracted or greatly dilated and immovable: Bell.
immovable, but sees and talks: Stram.
immovable, but slightly dilated: Colch.
dilated, with restlessness: *Hell.,* Mer., Nux.
contracted, immovable; insensible to light: Op., Cinch.
first contracted and then dilated: Puls.
l. contracted, while r. is dilated: Colch.
contracted or dilated, with slow respiration: Coc., Hyos., Nux, Sec., Ver.
contracted: Ars., Op., Mur. ac., Stram., Sul.
contracted, with cloudiness of head: Arn.

Eyes, bright and injected: Bell., Glon., Hell., Hyos., Stram.
glistening: Ars., Bell., Tub.
glistening, with contracted pupils: Mur. ac.
brilliant, with delirium: Lach.
brilliant, unusually bright: Op.
red, sparkling, staring: Bell.
rolling about in their sockets: Hyos.
glassy: Bell., Op.
glassy and watery: Bry., Psor.
dull, lusterless: Ars., Gels., Hyos., Mer., Mur. ac.
dull, lusterless, pupils without reaction to light: Carbo v.
dull, without expression: Bap., Bell., Op.
dull, vacant look with dilated pupils: Hell.
heavy, hollow, sunken: Ars., Bap., Colch., Op., Pyr.
dim and sleepy: Phos. ac., Stram.
full and turned upwards: Ars., Op.
turned up when lying on back: Psor., Sul.
turned up, looking over forehead: Op.
rolling of the: Bell., Hell., Hyos., Sec.
distorted: Lach.
distorted and staring: Hyos.
squinting of: Bell., Hyos., Lyc., Stram.

Staring: *Bell.,* **Hyos.,** Op., Phos. ac., Sec., **Stram.,** Zinc.
with open eyes at one point: Bell.
at surrounding objects: Hyos.
with watery eyes, without comprehending what occurs or recognizing his relatives: Mur. ac., Op.
with slow comprehension and slow answers: Hell.

Eyelids, trembling and jerking: Coc.
open: Bell., Hyos., Lyc., Stram.
open, with sopor: Lyc.
open, and lies speechless: Op.
open, in delirium: Ars., *Bap.,* Op., *Stram.,* Ver.
half open: Colch., Psor.
half covering the dull eyes: Phos.

Eyelids, paralyzed, sunken, either cannot or will not open them: Coc., Colch., Lach., Zinc.

paralyzed, as if, heavy, drowsiness increases to coma: Coc.

droop: Ars., **Gels.,** Rhus, Zinc.

difficult raising of: Gels., Op.

on closing the, starts frightened: Cinch.

chronic soreness of: Psor., Sul.

pale, swelling like a bag over eyes: Kali c.

pale, swelling under the eyes: Apis.

sunken and heavy, with blue circles: Phos.

HEARING AND EARS.

Hearing, over-sensitive: Bell., Bry., Lyc., Mur. ac., Nux, Phos., Op.

over-sensitive to music: Bry.

noise is intolerable: Cinch., Coc., Nux.

every sound annoys him: Sul.

hardness of: Apis, Ars., Bry., Phos.

hardness, beginning with buzzing: Hyos.

hardness, in fevers: Bell., Carbo c., Hyos., Nit. sp. d., Phos. ac.

ringing in the head: Ars., Coc.

ringing and rushing sounds in the ear: Op.

buzzing, singing, rushing: Hyos.

rushing sound: Hyos., Mer.

rushing sound, like wind: Puls.

rushing sound, with humming: Sec.

rushing sound, with and thundering: Lach.

rushing sound, like rain or music: Mur. ac.

Deafness: Ars., Bap., Bell., Carbo v., Chlorum, Hyos., Lachn.. Lach., Mer., Nit. sp. d., Phos. ac., Psor., Stram., Sul.

as if ears were stopped: Ver.

with a rushing sound: Mer.

Great dryness in the ears, rapidly disappears after a dose of Sul. or Psor.

SMELL AND NOSE.

Bleeding: Arn., Bry., Carbo v., Gels., Hyos., Lach., Mel., Mer. s., Phos. ac., Phos., Psor., Rhus, Sec., Sul., Sul. ac.
- only from r. side, at night in sleep: Ver.
- nose, mouth and gums: Carbo v.
- mouth and gums: Sul.
- continued: Nux, Psor., Rhus.
- frequent and copious, mostly in the evening: Phos.
- profuse hemorrhage: Carbo v.
- profuse hemorrhage at night, in sleep: Bry., Mer., Rhus.
- profuse after midnight or in morning: Rhus.
- mostly at three A. M. or after rising, daily for many days: Bry.
- in the beginning of the fever: Rhus.
- with salivation: Hyos.*
- relieves: Mel., Rhus.
- does not relieve: Phos. ac.

Dryness, in the nose: Bry., Nux, Nux m., Phos.
- in the nostrils: Puls.
- of nose, lips, tongue: Mur. ac.
- of mouth and throat: Bell.
- of mucus, to hard crusts: Rhus.

Nostrils, widely distended: Op.
- widely distended and dry: Puls.
- dry and black: Colch.
- sooty, smoked: Ars., Chlor., Hell., Hyos.
- look smoked, with dry tongue and mouth: Chlorum.
- fan-like motion of: Lyc.

Nose, pointed: Coc., Phos., Ver.
- cold, and cold mouth: Camph., Carbo v.
- can endure no odors: Nux, Sul.
- smell and taste very acute: Mur. ac.

---

* Do not give Mercury in typhoid salivation.

Nose, smell frequent, bad: Ars., Psor.
smell, hallucinations of: Stram.
stopped up, must breathe through mouth: Am. c., Arum.
boring with fingers in: Arum.
constantly picking the, till it bleeds: Arum.
acrid, ichorous discharge, excoriating the alæ and upper lip, rendering them raw and sore: Ars., Arum.

FACE.

Cheeks, yellow, with deep flushes in centre: Bap.
reddened: Bap., Bell., Cal., Hyos., Mur. ac., Stram., Sul.
red and hot: Bell., Rhus.
red and hot, burning: Bry.
burning hot, with circumscribed redness: Ars., Mur. ac.
burning, in afternoon: Lyc.
burning, with delirium: Lach.
one red and the other pale: Cham.
alternately red and pale: Ver.
red or venous blue: Bell.
emaciation of: Tab.

Face, cold, covered with cold sweat: Carbo v., Ver. v.
covered with sweat: Colch.
sweats on the right side: Puls.
cold sweat on forehead; pale, cool, moist, death-like: Ver.
pale, with cold sweat: Sec., Ver. v.
pale, cold, sunken: Carbo v., Coc., Mur. ac.
pale, cold, sunken, cadaverous, blue circles around eyes: Ver.
hot, mostly in the evening: Bry.
wears a happy and strange expression: Apis.
wears a stupid expression: Colch., Stram.
wears a stupid expression, without collapse: Hell., Hyos.
wears a listless expression: Rhus.
besotted expression, apathetic and indifferent: Bap., Phos. ac.

Face, stupid aspect, relaxed and hanging facial muscles and lower lip: Op.
relaxation of the facial muscles: Op.
trembling and jerking: Coc., Nux.
trembling convulsion of lips and tongue: Op.
spasmodic motion of: Coc., Hyos., Stram.
sunken features: Ars., Carbo v., Coc., Zinc.
anxious, hippocratic: Ars.
expression of fear and terror: Stram.
expression wild, with fulness and redness of face: Bell.
dark red, bloated, with snoring: Op.
red with heat: Ver.
red and cracked: Zinc.
blue, venous congestion: Carbo v., Lach., Ver.
bluish-red, with feeble, intermitting pulse: Ver.
brown, black: Ars., Lach.
shining and puffed: Bell., Stram.
waxy, white or yellow: Sil., Zinc.
yellow and dirty color: Lyc., Mer.
yellowish, eyes sunken: Lyc.
yellowish and pale: Bry.
yellowish and pale suddenly, after the first week (often, in fact generally, fatal): Lyc.
pale, sickly features: Kali c., Sul.
pale, sickly, as after a long illness; great uneasiness, sunken eyes, with blue circles around them: Phos., Sul.
pale, dingy, earthy, sunken: Ars., Phos., Sec.
pale, with sharp nose, hollow eyes, with dark circles around them, insensibility and indifference: Cinch., Phos., Ver.
and eyes sunken: Cinch., Coc., Colch., Lach., Mer., Lyc., Phos. ac., Phos., Sec., Sul.
deathly appearance of: Ars., Mer.
hippocratic: Ars., Carbo v., Cinch., Colch., Phos., Sec., Zinc.
cadaverous and extreme prostration: Colch., Ver.
cadaverous, while heat of body is retained: Mer.
lower jaw, dropping of: Ars., Bap., Lach.

Face, lower jaw, hanging down of: Bap., Lach., Lyc., Mur. ac.
risus sardonicus: Colch.
distortion of muscles of: Bell., Coc., Hyos., Stram.

Lips, trembling: Stram., Sul.
trembling of lower lip: Arn.
and tongue pale: Phos.
bright red: Sul.
dark red and dry: Bell.
bluish red, black or brown: Ars.
bluish or pale: Carbo v., Cinch.
dry, with dry nose and tongue: Mur. ac.
dry and cracked: Ars., Bell., Pyr.
dry and bleeding: Lach., Pyr.
dry and brown: Bry., Nit. sp. d., Rhus.
dry and covered with brown crusts: Ars., Rhus.
dry and blackish: Ars., Bell., Bry., Lach., Phos. ac., Pyr., Rhus, Ver.
dry, covered with brown or black mucus: Ars., Cinch., Colch., Phos., Pyr.
dry, as if parched by thirst: Arn.
dry, with dryness of the palate: Phos.
dry, brown or black: Ars., Rhus.
dry crusts or sordes on: Ars., Rhus.
gums and teeth covered with brown or black mucus: Ars.
teeth and tongue covered with a thick brown coating: Colch.
cracked: Colch., Puls., Sul.
cracked, dry and black: Ver.
ulcerated and covered with vesicles: Apis.
and commissures sore and cracked: Ars., Arum, Mur. ac.
picking, until they bleed: Arum.
eruption on or around: Phos. ac.

Commissures, sore, bleeding: Ars., Arum.
pain in, as if cut; cracks, excoriation, ulceration: Mer.
and upper lip raw and sore; acrid, ichorous discharge: Arum.

Mouth, corner of, drawn down on left side: Ver. v.
distorted: Bell., Camph., Colch., Op.
open: Mer., Mur. ac., Phos. ac., Phos.
open to widest extent, falls back on lifting head: Colch.
frequent motions during sleep: Bry.
viscid, neither thirst nor appetite: Bap., Gels.
viscid, intolerably: Phos.
fetid breath from: Arn., Arum, Bap., Mer., Psor., Sul.
filled with slimy mucus: Mer.
frothy, soap-like saliva in, almost choking: Bry.
raw, ulcerated, sore: Arum, Mur. ac., Stram.
cadaverous, putrid odor from: Arum, Hyos., Nux, Psor.
hemorrhage from, and nose: Carbo v.
aphthæ: Bap., Sul. ac.
aphthæ, small and bluish, with putrid acid stench: Mur. ac.

Dryness, of mouth and tongue: Mur. ac., Nux m.
of mouth, food tastes like straw: Stram.
of mouth, forepart, and tip of tongue in early stage: Nux.
of mouth and fauces: Bell., Phos. ac.
from fauces into nose: Bell.
of mouth and throat: Nux, Nux m., Puls.
of mouth at night: Coc., Puls.
of mouth in morning, as from spirituous drinks night before: Nux.
or sense of, afternoon and after midnight: Rhus.
with or without thirst: Bry.
without thirst: Nux m., Puls.
severe, not > by drinking: Nux m., Phos., Rhus.
drinks large quantities at a time: Arn., Bry.
great, tongue sticks to roof of mouth: Nux m.

Gums, at the beginning, swollen and bleeding: Mer.
spongy, bleeding at the slightest touch: Carbo v., Mur. ac., Phos., Sul.
and teeth covered with brown or black mucus: Ars., Rhus.

Teeth, grinding of: Ars., Bell., Colch.
grating: Hyos.
champing: Ver. v.
sordes on: Bap., Pyr., Rhus, Stram.
brown or black mucus on: Ars., Hyos., Sul.
thick brown coating on: Colch.
covered with a dark mass: Hyos.

Speech, stammering: Ars., Bell., Carbo v., Lyc., Sec., Stram.
stammering, as if drunk: Bell., Lach., Op.
stammering, as if the tongue were too heavy, stuttering: Ver.
stammering, lisping, unintelligible: Ars., Bell., Op., Stram., Ver.
muttering, mumbling; it costs him great effort to speak the words plainly: Coc.
impeded, from a dry, hard, glazed tongue: Ars., Phos. ac., Pyr.
falters and hesitates, averse to the effort: Sul.
difficult, weak, indistinct: Hyos., Lach., Sec.
difficult, from dryness of mouth and throat: Bry.
slow and weak, as if to overcome an impediment: Sec.
slow, as if they could not move the tongue: Carbo v.
difficult, with heaviness of tongue: Lach., Phos. ac.
inability to speak loud: Nux, Pyr.
can only speak loud with great effort: Op.
from difficult respiration and debility: Bell.
loss of: Colch., Hyos., Pyr., Ver.
loss of, and consciousness: Mer.
loss of, with subsultus: Mur. ac., Sec.
loss of, as if paralyzed, lisping, stammering: Stram.
loss of, as if complete aphasia: Bell.
unable to talk, or protrude the tongue, which is cracked, sore, ulcerated: Apis, Arum.

Tongue, trembling: Ars., **Bell.,** *Gels.,* **Lach.,** Lyc., Sec., Stram.
hard to put out: Gels., Hyos., **Lach.,** Lyc.
trembles when put out: Bell., Gels., **Lach.,** Sec., Stram.
dry and cracked: Ars.

Tongue, spasmodically thrust to and fro between the teeth: **Lyc.**
comes out dry and black, with a snapping noise, and moves like a pendulum: Lyc.
trembling in the act of protruding: Sec.
tip remains under the teeth or lip, does not come out: Lach.
cannot protrude it, or if he does it trembles: *Gels.*, Hyos., **Lach.**, *Lyc.*
is put out with difficulty, can hardly withdraw it: Hyos.
protruded with difficulty: Colch., **Lach.**
cannot move it at will, even if conscious: Mur. ac.
stiff, numb, like a piece of wood: Ars., Colch.
stiff, motion difficult while swallowing: Lach.
immovable, from dry black crusts: Phos.
sensation as if too thick, while speaking: Nux.
with difficult speech, scarcely movable: Carbo v.
paralyzed: Bar., Bell., Hyos., Lach., **Mur. ac.**, Op., Stram.
paralyzed on right side (turns to the left): Bell.
as if burnt and insensible: Puls.
burning; looks like burnt leather: *Hyos.*
dry, rattles like leather: **Mur. ac.**
dry, red, hard: Bry., Hyos., Rhus.
dry, great thirst, drinks little at a time: Ars.
dry, great thirst, drinks large quantity: Bry.
not coated, with desire to drink: Rhus.
dry, as if burnt, yet no thirst: Mag. m., Op., **Puls.**
bright red: Bell., Colch., **Pyr.**
covered with raised papillæ: Ant. t., Ars., Bap., Bell., Crot., Lach., Lyc., Pyr., Rhus.
dry and dark red: Bap.
dry and cracked: Ars., Hyos., Lach., Rhus.
raw, painful, inflamed in middle: Gels.
clean, or slightly coated: Gels., Mur. ac., Pyr.
clean and dry: Stram.
clean, almost, with bright red edges and cracked lips: Op.
smooth, not very dry: Mur. ac., Phos. ac.
smooth, glossy, as if deprived of its papillæ: **Pyr.**, Ter.

Tongue, rough, dry, cracked, dark brown: Bap., Bry., Hyos., Stram.

covered with a thick, tenacious paste, like a layer of putty spread over it: Bry., Carbo v.

brown, black, dry, hard: Bap., Hyos., Sec., Rhus.

pale, bluish or lead color: Ars., Carbo v.

hard, thick mucus on: Rhus.

as if coated with a skin: Phos.

sticky, dirty, moist, yellow: Carbo v., Lyc., Puls.

thick, white or dirty white coating: Bry., Mer.

thick, white fur in the beginning: Coc.

white coating, with sore spots: Nit. ac., Tarax.

red margin and white centre: Bell., Gels., Sul.

coated in middle and back, not on edges: Bry.

dry, with a brown streak in middle: Arn., Bap.

with two white stripes on a red ground: Bell.

yellowish-brown, dry in centre: Stram.

white coating on sides: Caust.

white coating in centre: Bell., Bry., Gels., Phos., Sul.

mapped: Ars., *Lach.,* Mer., **Nat.**, Nit. ac., **Tarax.**

rough or dry, with whitish-yellow coating: Bap., Coc., Bry., Puls.

brown and dry, mostly in centre: Bap., Hyos., Puls.

grayish-white: Phos. ac.

thickly coated: Colch.

thickly coated and cracked: Bry.

brownish, thick crusts on: Phos. ac.

covered with dark brown sordes of an offensive odor; foul, with a thick layer of yellowish or brownish fur: Bry.

coating remaining after Bryonia: Nux.

cracked and parched: Apis, Carbo v.

as if scalded or burnt: Ars., Ver. v.

rough, dry, and dark brown: Bry.

thick: Chel., Mer., Nux, Nux m.

too red, dry, swollen: Stram., Ver.

atrophied, substance altered: Mur. ac.

Tongue, with imprint of teeth: Ant. t., Chel., Kali h., Mer., Pod., Rhus, Stram., Pyr.
coating, on removal leaves sore spots: Tarax.
coating whitish, on one side: Rhus.
tip red, undefined: Sul.
tip red, triangular: Rhus.
red and cracked, or cracked and bleeding: Lach.
fissures in the: Lach.
(For other symptoms of the tongue see page 515.)

Throat, fluids roll audibly into stomach: gurgling when drinking: *Ars.*, Coc., (?) **Hydro. ac.**
fluids roll audibly into, involuntary stool and urine: Mosch.
swallowing difficult: Apis.
swallowing difficult, chokes even with half a spoonful of water: Bap.
swallowing very slow: Hell.
swallowing, dryness hardly permits: Phos.
swallowing liquids, difficulty in: Bap., Bell., Hyos.
swallow, complete inability to: Stram.
choking sensation from stomach up into throat, > by belching: Ign.
intense burning in: Ver. v.
sore, with deafness: Bap., Lach.
sore, glands of, and neck swollen: Arum.
sore, swallowing very painful; tonsils enlarged; uvula enlarged: Bap.
sore, chewing or swallowing food, even drinking, causes pain in raw mouth: Arum.

Appetite, hunger in convalescence, begins to eat, does not enjoy it, everything is so bitter: Puls.
will not return: Psor., Sul.
loss of, with fulness of stomach: Nux m.
loss of, and prostration: Rhus.
loss of, would not eat or drink, no nausea: Iris.
they push back the food they wanted: Bell.

Appetite, asks for food, but refuses it when offered: Bry., Phos.
complete loss of: Bry., Nux, Nux m.

Thirst: Bell., Bry., Camph., Carbo v., Colch., Hyos., Mer., Mur. ac., Rhus, Stram.
unquenchable: Ars., Bry., Colch., Nat., Pyr.
excessive, with a red, dry tongue: Bell., Camph., Rhus.
with aversion to water: Nux.
not > by drinking: Ars., Rhus.
constant, for cold drinks, especially for water: Mer., Phos.
afternoon and evening, with cold sweat: Ver.
water disturbs the stomach: **Ars.,** *Phos.,* Pyr., Sul.
burning, but does not drink much: Bell.
liquids put into mouth are spit out: Bap.
constant, but only wets lips, every swallow becomes disgusting: Ars., Lyc.
for large quantities: Bry., Hyos.
does not ask for water, but when offered takes it hastily: Hep., Op.
but water does not taste well: Nat.
with heat, from 3 to 6 P. M.: Phos.
great, with trunk hot and extremities cold: Colch.
burning in head and coldness of trunk: Arn.

Desire, for refreshing acid things: Mer., Phos. ac., Ver.
for alcoholic drinks: Ars., Asar., Bry., Cof., **Psor.,** *Tub.*
for alcoholic drinks, which are readily borne: Agar.

Eating, after, chilliness: *Ars.,* Arum, **Bell.,** Cal., Carbo an., Carbo v., Coc., Ipec., **Kali c.,** Nux, Rhus, **Tarax.,** Zinc.
sour taste after: Nux.
diarrhea, immediately after: Phos.
or drinking, after, great chilliness: Tarax.

Drinking, hurts in the throat: Hydro. ac.
after, distention and pain in bowels: Nux.
after, hasty rumbling in bowels: Ars., Mer., Thuja.
after, cold fingers: Tarax.

GASTRIC.

Belching: **Bry.**, Carbo v., Coc.

Hiccough: Ars., **Carbo v.**, Hyos., Ign., ***Lach.***, ***Nux m.***, Sec., Stram., Ver., Zinc.

Nausea and retching: Ars., Bry., Coc.
and vomiting, stomach painfully sensitive: Bry.

Vomiting, and retching: Ars., Bry., Kali c.
> by swallowing water, but is returned when it gets warm in stomach: Phos.
water, sour taste: Phos.
water and green, slimy fluid, not what had been eaten: Ars.
watery, bilious, slimy masses, with great pain: Phos.
thick, black bile, mixed with sticky, bilious mucus, as if decomposed; a quart at a time: Sec.
after bile and mucus, black bile and blood: Ver.
when moving: Bry., Sul.
and watery diarrhea: Bry., Ver.
after delirium: Sec.
with burning heat: Cham.
with headache: Kali c.

Epigastrium, throbbing, pulsating: Puls.
sinking, weak feeling in: Ign.
great soreness to touch, pressure, motion: Arn., Colch., Carbo v., Lach., Mer., Nux.
pain and tenderness remaining after touch or pressure: Bry.
distention and painful sensitiveness to touch: Nux.
burning in, and sensitive to pressure: Ars.

Stomach, discomfort and sickness: Phos.
fulness in: Bap., Carbo v., Nux m.
to hip, sharp pain from: Bry.
sensitive to external pressure: Ars., Mer., Sec.
sensitive, even bed clothes cause pain: **Lach.**, Sul.
sensitive, least pressure is insupportable, excruciating pain from touch and cough: Bry.

Liver, region of, painful, sensitive: *Bell.,* Bry., *Chel.,* Lach., Lyc., **Mer.,** *Phos., Tarax.,* Sul.

region, enlarged, engorged: Mer., Psor.

region, hepatitis after: Bry., Lach., Lyc., *Mer.,* **Psor.**

Spleen, enlarged: Arn., Ars., Cal., **Cean.,** Carbo v., Chin. s., **Cinch.,** Coc., *Lach.,* Lyc., Phos. ac., Psor., Rhus.

rumbling in region of: Cal., Phos.

swollen, painful to pressure: Ars.

swollen, hardness of: Cean., Cinch.

Abdomen, distention of: **Apis,** Arn., Ars., Bap., Bry., *Carbo v.,* **Cinch.,** *Coc.,* **Colch.,** Lach., Mer., Lyc., **Phos.,** Phos. ac., Psor., **Ter.,** Tub., Ver. v.

distention as if from flatulence: Carbo v., Nux m.

distention as if diarrhea would set in: Bry., Cinch., Rhus, Ver.

distention as if raw; distended immediately after drinking: Nux.

heaviness in upper part of: Bry., Nat. c., Nux m.

pinching, grasping pains in: Puls.

colic pains, with looseness: Ver.

colic with frequent loose stool: Ars.

colic with violent gagging: Nit. s. d.

colic, < in the morning: Bry., Pod., Sul.

burning or heat in: Ars., Lach., Lachn., Sul.

soreness and bloating of: Apis.

very sensitive to touch: Bell., Ham., **Mer., Lach.,** *Nit. ac.,* **Phos.,** Psor., Pyr., Ter.

very sensitive in umbilical region: Mer., Phos.

very sensitive in ileo-cecal region: Ars., Bell., Bry., Gels.

very sensitive in left iliac region: Bap., Lach.

very sensitive, cecal and peritoneal inflammation: Bell.

hardness of: Arn., Bry., Coc., Colch., Ver.

hotter than rest of body: Colch., Lach.

as if inflated: Carbo v., Nux m., Sul.

sore during the crisis, with > from papescent stools: Ars., Carbo v., Mur. ac., Rhus.

as if raw and inflamed in hypogastrium, < by touch: Phos.

Abdomen, hemorrhage and intestinal ulceration: Crot., Nit. ac., Ter.
compressed, the whole: Rhus.
drawn in towards spine: Bell., Plb.
pain in, if pressed: Op., Sec.
soreness to touch: Apis, Arn., Cham., Ham., *Lach.,* **Nit. ac.,** Phos., Phos. ac., Pyr.

Flatulence: Ars., Bry., **Carbo v., Cinch.,** Coc., Colch., Gings., Hyos., *Lach., Lyc., Nux m.,* Phos., Puls.
rumbling in upper part of abdomen: Cinch.
rolling and gurgling: Ars., **Carbo v.,** Lyc., **Phos.**
rolling and grumbling: Nux m., Sul., Thuja.
fermentation, with diarrhea and offensive flatus: Carbo v.
loud gurgling in ileo-cecal tract: Gings.

Rumbling: Bry., *Carbo v.,* Coc., Colch., Hyos., Lach., Mer., *Nux,* Phos. ac., *Phos., Puls.,* Pyr., Ter., Ver.
after drinking or before every stool: Mer.
before stool: Lach., *Phos. ac.,* Phos., **Pyr.**
mostly in evening in bed, or at night: Bry.
painful; very offensive flatus: Phos., **Psor.**
diarrhea of decomposed blood, horribly offensive: Carbo v., Crot., **Psor.,** *Pyr.,* Ter.

Tympanitis: Cinch., **Colch.,** *Nux m., Op., Phos.,* **Pyr.,** Sec., *Ter.*
from accumulation of gas, though much is passed: Phos.
with pain in back: Colch.
very full and hard abdomen: Arn., Phos.
heaviness in upper part of abdomen, restless sleep: Nux m.
in the morning: Cinch.

Eruptions, roseola spots on abdomen: Apis, *Arn.,* Hyos., Mur. ac.
white, miliary: Apis, Ter.
petechiæ: **Apis,** Ars., Crot., *Mur. ac.,* Phos., Psor., *Rhus,* Sul., **Ter.**
petechiæ with hemorrhagic spots: *Sul. ac.,* **Ter.**

Diarrhea: Apis, Arn., **Ars.,** *Bap.,* Bell., Bry., Cal., Carbo v., Camph., *Cinch., Colch.,* Hyos., Lach., Lep., **Mer.,** *Mur. ac.,* Nit. ac., Op., *Pod.,* Phos., *Phos. ac., Psor., Puls.,* Pyr., **Rhus,** Sec., *Sul.,* Stram., Ter., **Ver.**

thin, watery: *Ars.,* Colch., Hyos., Mer., Mur. ac., *Phos.,* **Ver.**

worse at night: **Mer., Puls.,** *Rhus,* Ver.

in prodromic stage, < at night: Rhus.

with pinching, grasping pain: Puls.

painless: Cal., **Cinch.,** *Phos. ac.,* **Sul.**

painless, every half hour, after grumbling in the bowels each time: Sul.

painless, abdomen bloated, hemorrhages, slow convalescence: Cinch.

painless, with loud rumbling: Phos.

painless, in early morning: Pod., Sul., Tub.

profuse, blood-streaked, like meat washings; dry tongue: Phos.

frequent, frothy, with tenesmus: Sul.

excessive; stools sour: Cal., Sul. ac.

bilious, slimy: Bry., **Mer.**

yellow, watery, slimy: Phos. ac.

blackish, every hour: Stram.

blackish, from decomposed blood: Lach., Phos., Ter.

blackish, like coffee dregs: Ars.

blackish, only in the morning: Pod.

blackish, offensive, with severe pain: Colch.

blackish, or brownish: Arn., *Ars., Carbo v.,* Mer., Ver.

brownish, grayish: Carbo v.

greenish, grayish, watery: Phos.

greenish, acrid, offensive: Nit. ac.

greenish, slimy, great tenesmus: Mer., Nit. ac.

painful, frequent: Apis.

painful, with great sinking of the vital force: Cal., Tub.

at night, with pressure in the abdomen, as if from gas: Arn.

at night, after midnight: Ars., Kali c., Sul., Tub.

black, and epigastric oppression: Dul., Lep., Mer.

with headache, tearing pain down limbs during stool: Rhus.

Diarrhea, with bitter, sour belching: Bap., Puls., Phos.
with empty belching: Rhus.
bloody: Apis, *Arn., Ars.,* Carbo v., **Crot.,** *Ham.,* Lach., **Mer., Nit. ac.,** *Phos.,* Pyr., **Ter.,** Tub.
offensive, watery, with white flakes: Colch.
cadaverous, carrion-like: *Carbo v.,* **Pyr., Psor.,** Stram.
fetid: *Bap.,* Kreos., **Psor.**
fetid, whether formed or loose: *Lach.,* **Psor.**
thin and extremely offensive: Lach., Op., **Psor., Pyr.,** *Sec., Sul.*
putrid, colliquative: Nux m.
liquid, yellow, between 4 and 7 A. M.: Nuphar.
dark, watery, painful: Colch.
dark, tarry mixed with bloody mucus: Lep.
dark brown, odor like foul ulcers: Ars.
black, burning, acrid; colic and great restlessness: Ars.
thin, with glairy mucus, great urging: Mer.
thin, cutting, drawing pains, extending to thighs: Nux.
thin, foul: Apis, *Ars.,* **Psor.,** *Pyr.*
thin, very watery: Op.
followed by prostration: Ars., Kreos., Phos., Sul., Ver.
brownish, grayish or bloody: Carbo v., **Psor.,** *Rhus.*
gangrenous and bloody: *Ars.,* **Phos.,** *Pyr.*

Involuntary: *Apis,* Arn., *Ars.,* Bap., Bry., *Carbo v.,* Cinch., **Colch.,** *Hyos.,* Kali c., **Mur. ac.,** *Op., Phos.,* **Phos. ac., Psor.,** Pyr., *Rhus, Sec.,* **Sul., Ter., Tub.,** Zinc.
sudden, black-brown, every three hours: Bry.
after eating, with rolling and rumbling in bowels: Camph.
when passing flatus: **Aloe,** *Nat.,* **Nux m.**
painful, foul, bloody: Apis, Ars.
painful and frequent: Apis, Zinc.
painful, after hard stool: Nux m., Op.
stool and urine: Arn., Bell., **Mur. ac., Psor.,** *Pyr., Rhus,* Sul.
paralysis of sphincter ani: Apis, *Phos.*
paralysis of sphincter ani and vesicæ: Hyos.
at night in sleep: Puls., Rhus.
with stupefaction: Arn.

Hemorrhage: *Alumen, Arn.,* Ars., Carbo v., **Crot., Ham.,** *Mur. ac.,* **Nit. ac., Phos., Ter., Tub.**

fluid, dark, tar-like, large quantities: Ham., Ter.

bright, and does not clot: Arn., **Nit. ac.**

fluid, decomposed: Crot., Sec.

fluid, clotted, black, in the third week: Alumen.

after diarrhea, seventh day, from rectum *by the pound,* faints from slight motion, ileo-cecal region sensitive: **Nit. ac.**

from intestinal ulceration: Ars., **Crot., Mur. ac., Nit. ac.,** Phos. ac., **Ter.,** Tub.

pus, meteorism, somnolence, reduced to the verge of the grave: Carbo v.

black, clotted, like charred straw, more or less ground up, and epistaxis: Lach.

very sick, but no: Hell.

Constipation: Apis, Ars., Bap., **Bry.,** Hell., Hyos., *Lyc.,* **Nux, Nux m., Op.,** Phos. ac., Phos., **Psor.,** Puls., **Sul.**

alternating with looseness: Ars., Bap.

or watery, painless, offensive stools: Op.

no stool for a long time: Apis, Bry., Lyc.

no stool for six or ten days: Puls.

long, tough stools, with great straining: Phos.

little or no affection of mucous membranes, seldom any stool: Hell., Mur. ac.

if, still exists, intestinal ulceration has not begun; if sudamina and petechiæ have already appeared during inflammatory stage: Bry.

If not costive do not give Carbo v.—JAHR.*

It is always safe when the alimentary tract is diseased to keep it quiescent as long as necessary; danger lurks in diarrhea, especially in purgation. Cathartics in typhoid are often fatal.

---

*I have not yet lost a single patient, in whom, up to the time of the crisis, the bowels remained costive, inactive.—JAHR.

I said the same more than twenty years ago, and can repeat it now; even in the *third week* the non-appearance of a stool is to be regarded as significant. The same applies in child-bed.—HERING.

Urine, involuntary: **Apis,** Arn., Ars., *Bap.,* **Colch.,** Hell., **Hyos.,** Lyc., **Mosch., Op.,** *Phos., Rhus,* Stram., Ver., Ver. v.
involuntary, all night: *Arn.,* **Ars.,** Bell., *Hyos.,* Pyr., **Rhus.**
involuntary and copious: Stram., Ver.
involuntary and unconsciously in bed: Mer.
involuntary and stool involuntary, from paralysis of sphincter: Bell., Hyos., **Mur. ac.**
unconscious flow of: Apis.
unconscious, turbid, like horse's urine: Apis, **Nit. ac.**
retained: Ars., **Hyos., Op.,** Stram.
retained, as if from closing of bladder or loss of power: Op.
suppressed: Arum, **Canth., Colch.,** Psor., Sec., **Stram.,** *Sul.*
frequent, in small quantity: Coc.
frequent, copious: **Colch., Mur. ac.,** Stram.
frequent, copious and watery: **Mur. ac.**
frequent, scanty, with burning and urging: Ars., Canth., Sec.
difficult, constant desire: Sec.
bloody, thoroughly mixed: Ter.
dark: **Bry.,** Carbo v., Mer., Nux, Puls.
dark brown: Ars., *Bry.,* Puls., *Sul.,* **Ter.,** Ver.
dark, but clear: Bell., *Cal.*
clear and acrid: Apis, Mur. ac., Phos. ac.
clear, very high colored: Nux m.
offensive, alkaline: Ars., Bap., Psor., *Sul.*
first clear, then white or chalky: Mer.
brownish-red, brown, with burning, no sediment: **Puls.**
turbid: *Ars.,* Carbo v., **Ter.,** Ver. v.
turbid, like horse urine: *Apis,* Carbo v., **Nit. ac.**
turbid, after standing: Sul.
turbid, with white sediment: Mer., Phos.
turbid, with gray sediment: Puls.
turbid, reddish, dark colored: Carbo v.
turbid, greenish or dark brown when passed, and does not become clear on standing: Ars.
turbid, after depositing a sediment, not clear: Phos.
coagulates, like milk: Phos. ac.

Urine, odor like violets: Ter.
odor like violet roots: Phos.
odor ammoniacal, strong: *Nit. ac.,* Phos.
yellow, no sediment: Lyc.

Bladder, region of, painful and very sensitive to touch: Lyc.

Voice, weak and trembling, or hoarse, crowing: Ars.
nasal, indistinct: Lach.
the few words he speaks are whispered, but not irrelevant: Nit. s. d.
is lost, cries until it becomes hoarse: Stram.
hoarse and hollow: Hep., Sec., Spong., Tub.
unintelligible, stammering, as though the tongue were too heavy: Ars., Lach.
rough, hoarse: Hep., Kali h.

Sighing, frequent: Bry., Ign., Ipec., Sec., Op., Tub.

Breathing, audible, irregular, intermittent: Colch.
rapid, labored, interrupted: Mer., Mur. ac., Phos.
slow, intermittent, moaning: Hell., Op.
deep drawn, sighing: Nux m., Op.
deep sighing, groaning, and a sour odor of body, with or without sweat: Bry.
short, anxious, oppressed, rattling: Ars.
short, anxious, with vertigo: Phos.
short, cough, hands and feet cold, craves heat in room: Carbo v.
short, after each cough: Phos.
mucous râle during stupor or delirium: Hyos.
the more snoring the darker the face becomes: Op.
stertorous: Lach., **Op.**
breath very offensive: Arn., Bap.
breath cold: Carbo v.
loose, rattling, loud, difficult: Op.
oppressed, difficult, pleuritic stitches, harassing cough, thick yellow or reddish sputa: Phos.

Breathing, oppressed, from tension in stomach: Mer.
oppressed, anxious, with heaving of chest: Op.
oppressed, anguish in chest, as if pressed together: Phos., Sul.
oppressed, with sighing and hiccough: Sec.
oppressed, with extreme prostration: Ars.
oppressed, with pleuritic stitches: Arn., Bry., Ran. b.
gasping, could not draw a full breath: Bap.
suffocation, paroxysms of: Apis, Ars., Phos., Puls., Sul.
> from belching: Carbo v., Ign.
accelerated: Ars., Colch., Mur. ac.
oppressed: Ars., Lach., Phos., Sul.
rattling: Ant. t., Ars., Carbo v., Op., Phos.

Cough, dry: *Ars.,* Bell., **Bry.,** Mer., *Phos.,* Rhus, **Tub.**
short, hacking, from tickling under midsternum, < from talking or moving: Cal.
rattling and rattling breathing: **Ant. t.,** Nit. ac.
rattling, with tough, transparent, thick, yellow or reddish sputa: Phos.
hard, with stitching pains in right chest and liver: Bry., Kali c., Mer.
with tough, bloody sputa: Rhus.
with brownish, bloody sputa: Nit. ac.
with slimy, bloody sputa: Lach.
with tightness of the chest: **Phos.,** *Tub.*
< from evening until midnight: Phos., Puls.
with infiltration of lower lobes: Rhus.
gray hepatization, sputa falling to the bottom in water leaves a trail of tough mucus behind, like a meteor: Cal.
with dirty, gray, pus-like sputa; when falling on a hard surface will break and fly like thin batter: Phos.
with impending paralysis: **Ant. t.,** Carbo v., **Mosch., Nit. ac.**
ceases, mucus cannot be expectorated: Ant. t., Mosch.
ceases, mucus causes rattling in trachea: Ars., Phos.
ceases, the secretions cause loud rattling breathing: Carbo v.
mucus in throat, neither able to swallow nor expectorate: Bap.
mucus, tenacious, in throat: Apis, Stan.

Cough, mucus, tenacious, hangs on tongue and lips: Phos.
mucus hard to expectorate, in convalescence: Ars., Phos., Senega.
mucous râle, threatening edema: **Ant. t.,** Carbo v., **Phos.**
mucous râle, dyspnea and edema: *Ant. t.*
in pneumo-typhus or typhoid: *Apis,* Bell., Bry., Mer., **Phos.,** *Psor.,* Puls., *Rhus,* **Sul.,** Tub.
in tuberculous patients: Kali c., **Tub.**
pulmonary symptoms predominate: *Bry.,* Lach., Nit. ac., Psor., Rhus, Sul., Stan., Tub.
violent, racking, dry or thick, yellow, tenacious mucus: Lach.
lungs seemed filled with blood: Nit. ac., Tub.

Heart, action grows weaker: Ars., Mosch.
action rapid, frequent small beats: Coc.
action very slow: Hell., Dig.
action violent, when turning in bed, shaking left side: Ver. v.
impending paralysis of, blood stagnates in capillaries, cyanotic blueness of face, lips and tongue, body cold and covered with cold sweat: Carbo v.

Pulse, weak, feeble: Apis, **Ars., Carbo v.,** Hyos., **Lach.,** Mer., *Phos.,* Phos. ac., **Psor.,** Puls., Ver., Ver. v.
weak and irregular: Apis, Bap., Gels., Hyos., Nit. ac., Ver. v.
weak and small: *Ars.,* **Carbo v.,** Hyos., **Lach.,** Phos., Phos. ac., Pyr., *Rhus.*
weak, no energy: Carbo v.
weak, no energy, irritable, 120-130: Mur. ac.
weak, scarcely perceptible: Carbo v., Hyos., Zinc.
weak, imperceptible: *Ars.,* **Carbo v.,** Colch., Iod., Mer.
small, threadlike, wiry: Ars., Camph., *Carbo v., Colch.,* Hyos., **Lach.,** Phos., Psor., *Pyr., Rhus,* Zinc.
small, quick: **Ars.,** Colch., Psor., **Pyr., Rhus,** *Sul.,* Zinc.
frequent: **Ars.,** Bell., *Carbo v.,* Colch., Hyos., Iod., *Lach.,* **Mur. ac.,** Phos. ac., *Stram.*
frequent, by lifting or turning patient, but otherwise slow: Gels.
slow: **Bap.,** Gels., **Hell.,** Op., Sec.

Pulse, intermitting: Apis, **Ars.**, Hyos., *Kali c.*, Mur. ac., *Phos. ac.*, Sec., Ver., *Zinc.*
irregular: Apis, *Bap.*, **Gels.**, Hyos., Nit. ac., *Ver. v.*
irregular, omitting every third beat: Mur. ac.
tremulous: Ars., Cal., Phos.
full, with throbbing carotids: Bell., Glon., Hyos., Stram., Sul.
full, frequent: **Bap.**, Bell., Glon., Hyos., *Iod.*, Stram.
accelerated, full, 120 to 140: **Bap.**, **Bell.**, Gels., Kali c., Lach., *Phos.*, Pyr., Rhus, Sul.
accelerated and slow: Bap., Op.
accelerated and hard: Bap.
changing frequently: Apis, Bap., *Gels.*
increasing by least motion: Iod.

Back, pain in, typanitis: Colch.
pain in, and limbs: Bap., Gels., **Pyr.**
pain along spine from moving hands or feet: Fer.
sensitive when fever is coming on: Nux.
weak, must lie down after least exertion: Nux m.
great heat in, with cold sweat on head and limbs: Phos.

Hands, trembling, automatic motion of: Zinc.
trembling when trying to lift them: Gels.
trembling, with coldness of limbs: Zinc.
and feet cold: *Ars.*, **Colch.**, Gels., Lyc.
and feet cold, would not be covered: Sec.
one cold the other hot: *Cinch.*, Dig., Ipec., **Puls.**

Fingers cold after drinking: Tarax.
picking at tips of: Arum.

Lower Limbs: weak, weary, heavy: Ars., Phos., Puls., Tub.
fears will be paralyzed: Selen.
tremble when trying to walk: Cac., Gels.
unbearable, tearing pain in, when at rest, > by moving them: *Rhus*, **Tarax.**
pain in, < by moving: Bry., Pyr.
pain and convulsive motions of: Coc., Ign.
clonic spasms of, with paralytic weakness: **Laur.**

Lower Limbs, jerking of, and of whole body, awake or asleep: Lyc., Pyr.
muscles refuse to obey the will: Gels., Kali br.
bruised, sore feeling in: Bry., Pyr., Rhus.
weak from morning to evening: Sul., Tub.
cold and covered with cold sweat: Carbo v.
pain in, extending from elbows and knees: Lach.

Feet, great heaviness of: Bry., **Coc.**
soreness of soles: Cal.
one foot hot, the other cold: *Cinch.*, Ipec., **Lyc.**
sore and sweaty between toes: Bar., Graph., **Sil.**
intensely cold: Iod., **Lyc.**, *Zinc.*

Sleepy, drowsy: Arn., *Bap.*, Bell., Bry., *Cac.*, Cinch., Gels., Hyos., Lach., Mer., **Op.**, *Phos. ac.*, **Pyr.**, Puls., Rhus, Sec., Sul., Ver.
in daytime: Bry., Phos. ac., Rhus, Sul.
coma-like sleep: Coc., Gels., *Nux m.*, **Op.**, Phos., Puls., Sec.
with open eyes: *Colch.*, **Op.**
when left alone: Hell.
with falling eyelids: **Gels.**, Nux m.
but cannot sleep: *Bell.*, Mer., Mur. ac., **Op.**
but cannot sleep because she cannot get herself together; head feels as though scattered about: Bap.
while answering a question, falls into a deep sleep: *Arn.*, **Bap.**, Hyos.
can be roused to answer correctly, then falls asleep again: Phos. ac.
cannot be roused to full consciousness: Bap., **Hell.**, **Op.**, Phos., Ver.
with frightful visions on closing the eyes: Ars., **Bell.**, Cal., Ign., Mer., *Op.*
or deep sopor: Ars., *Lach.*, *Lyc.*, **Op.**, Rhus.

Sleep, during, groaning, moaning, muttering: **Hyos.**, *Mur. ac.*, Op.
during, chewing motions of the mouth: Bry., Carbo v., Op.
during, loud talking and laughing: **Lyc.**

Sleep, during, talking incoherently: Gels.
during, talking, loud blowing during expiration: Arn.
during, muttering delirium: Phos. ac.
during, starting frequently: Bell., Op.
during, pricking at bed clothes: Op.
during, pricking at bed clothes and murmuring: Rhus.
after, < of all the symptoms: Lach.
after, great exhaustion: Sec.
after, stammering, difficulty of moving the tongue: Op.
after, restless tossing about, throwing off bed covers: Lach.
after, awakens conscious, but apathetic, taciturn: Phos. ac.
after, weary, weak, sluggish lassitude: Bry.
after, weary as before: Bry., Nux, Puls., Tub.
after, exceedingly cross, irritable, scolding, screaming, disagreeable: Lyc.
after, dizzy, stupefied, as if drunk: Phos.
after, on sitting up, giddy, has to lie down again: Op.
after, cannot at once free himself from anxious, phantastic visions: Sul.
after, feels as if he had not slept: Puls.
after, feels as if he had too little sleep: Ver.
loss of, followed by great loss of strength: **Coc.,** Colch.

Sleepless, restless: Ars., Arum, Hyos., Phos., Sul.
restless during the night: Sul.
restless, tossing about the bed: Ars.
from over-mental activity, same idea rouses from sleep: Cal.
from nervous excitability: Hyos.
on account of visions as soon as he falls into a doze: Ign.
stupid, half sleeping, phantastic visions of ghosts, dragons, skeletons, spirits: Op.
frightful imaginations prevent sleep in the evening: Mer.
or constant sleep with muttering: Hyos.
from continuous delirium: Mur. ac.

Nervous, restless, anxious to go from one bed to another: Ars., Bell., Cal., Cham., Cina, Hyos., Mer., Sep., Rhus, Ver.
turns from one place to another: *Ars.,* Hyos., Pyr., *Rhus.*

Nervous, suddenly sits up, then lies down again: Hyos.
tossing about: Ars., Bell., Canth., Rhus.
continually changing position: *Ars.,* Cinch., Pyr., **Rhus.**
has no rest day or night: Sul.
constantly moving head and limbs, while the trunk lies still, on account of great weakness: Ars.
in the muscles, with vertigo: Nux m.
with dilated pupils: Bell., Hyos., **Nux.**
all night, put out his hands: Phos.
constant inclination to stretch limbs or change their position: Cinch.
cannot lie long anywhere: Bap., Pyr., Rhus.
great nervous restlessness: Bap.
great nervous restlessness of body and limbs: Camph.
every position feels too hard: Arn., Pyr.
feels > when lying down: Bry.
trembling of body and propulsion of tongue: Agar., **Lach.**
trembling of whole body: Stram.
trembling and jerking of limbs: Apis, Coc., **Zinc.**
trembling from weakness: Gels.

Restless, jerking and twitching: Bell., Hyos., Ign., Lyc., Op., Zinc.
jerking, especially in children: Bell., Cal.
automatic motion of muscles: Camph., Rhus.
automatic motion of hands and feet: Coc., Rhus.
involuntary motions: Bell., Colch., Hyos., Rhus.
involuntary odd motions of limbs and body: Stram.
involuntary twitchings the fourteenth day: Colch.
involuntary, raises or jerks the head from pillow: Stram.
involuntary thrusting out one leg and then drawing it up: Ver. v.

Convulsive motions: Hyos., Ign., *Nux.*
motions of mouth and face: Bell.
motions, intermittent, every two or three hours, at same hour: Mosch.

Convulsive motions, subsultus tendinum: **Hyos,** *Ign.,* Lyc., Psor., Pyr., Rhus, Sec., Sul., Ver., Ver. v., *Zinc.*
automatic: Camph., Coc., Rhus.

Paralytic symptoms: Carbo v., *Coc.,* Cup., *Nux,* **Psor.,** Sel.
muscles refuse to obey the will: **Gels.,** Kali br.

Weakness, muscular, but slight: Mur. ac.
general and pronounced: Ars., Camph., Coc., *Colch.,* **Phos. ac., Psor.,** *Rhus,* **Sec.,** Sel., Stram., Sul., *Ter.*
> from magnetizing: Phos., Sil.
and nervous prostration: Bap., Rhus.
and lassitude: *Arn.,* **Bap.,** Bry., *Phos.,* **Sul.**
as from physical exertion: Colch.
and bruised soreness, compelling to lie down: **Arn.,** *Pyr.*
in all the joints: **Bry.,** Coc., Phos.
joints too weak to carry the body: Carbo an., Carbo v.
muscular, from slightest exertion: **Lach.**
sinking of strength, great: Arn., *Bap.,* Hyos., *Phos.,* Phos. ac., **Psor.,** Tub.
sinking of strength rapid: **Ars.,** Carbo v., *Colch.,* Cinch., Nux, Phos., **Pyr.,** *Sec.,* **Ver.**
great prostration: Alumen, Arn., *Ars.,* Bap., Colch., *Gels.,* Mer., Phos. ac., Psor., **Pyr.,** *Rhus,* Stram., *Ver.*
great prostration in first stage: Gels.
great prostration, with cadaverous look: Colch.
great prostration, sliding down in bed: Apis, Ars., Bapt., Hell., **Mur. ac.,** *Pyr., Zinc.*
with fainting: Bry., *Camph.,* **Lach.,** Sec., Sul., **Tarax.**
from bodily movement, with facial distortion: Coc.

Position, lying on the back: **Ars.,** Bap., *Colch., Lach.,* Phos., *Pyr.,* Zinc.
lying on back, with limbs drawn up: *Ars.,* Hell., Puls.
lying on back, with thighs flexed on abdomen: Ver. v.
lying on back, with thighs flexed and forearm firmly flexed: Bell.
with head thrown back: Bap., Gels.

Position, any, bed feels too hard: Arn., Pyr.
constantly tosses hands about: Phos.
constant change of: Apis, *Ars.,* Bell., Cinch., Hyos., Ign., *Puls.,* **Pyr., Rhus.**
unable to lie long in any: *Bap.,* **Pyr.**
tossing about: **Apis, Bell.,** *Rhus.*
moves head and limbs, trunk lies still from weakness: Ars.

Skin, dry and hot: *Ars.,* Bap., **Mur. ac.**
dry or clammy and cold: Phos.
bluish, cold: Carbo v.
pale, relaxed, waxy: Phos. ac., Phos.
pale, wrinkled: Ver.
icteroid: Crot., Mer.
icteroid, with diarrhea: Lept.
surface very sensitive: Colch., Ham.
bed covering causes pain: Lach., Sul.
touch causes pain in abdomen and hypogastrium: Phos.
touch or pressure, sensitive to, on stomach or abdomen: Ars., **Lach.,** Phos.
bluish-red spots on parts upon which patient lies: Phos. ac.
blood stagnates, causing cyanotic blueness: Carbo v., Nux m.
blood stagnates, causing large purple spots, especially on feet: Sec.
blood stagnates, epidermic extravasation: Ars.
blood stagnates, ecchymosis on trunk: Arn., Ars., **Sul. ac.,** *Carbo v., Phos.,* Phos. ac., Pyr.
blood stagnates, red spots like blood stains, or petechiæ, on face, neck, chest, abdomen: Bell.
blood stagnates eruption, like flea bites: Puls.
petechiæ: Ars., Bap., Bry., Phos., Pyr., Rhus, Sec., Stram., Sul. ac., Ter.
petechiæ, small, shining, star-shaped on face, throat, chest: Stram.
petechiæ, with extreme weakness, complete loss of strength: Rhus.

Skin, petechiæ, small red, itching spots on body, here and there: Op.
sudamina, small transparent vesicles in the morning on various parts of the body: Mer.
sudamina, white rash: Apis, Lach., Mur. ac.
white miliary rash: Ars.
white miliary rash in beginning, with anxiety in region of heart: Bry.
miliary rash: Rhus.
miliary rash on the trunk: Phos.
miliary rash about the neck, chest, back, gradually extends over limbs to feet: Phos. ac.
miliary purulenta with anasarca: Sul.
red rash on the: Phos., Pyr.
red rash scattered, insufficient: Lyc., Phos. ac.
red miliary spots on chest and back: Cinch.
red rash appears on the back with sweating: Stram.
red rash breaking out repeatedly, short breathing: Ars.
cuticular red spots, with small vesicles in the centre: Rhus.
numerous roseola spots: Ars., Hyos., Phos., Pyr., Rhus, Stram., Sul., Sul. ac.
exanthem delayed, on the fourteenth day fever rising with new symptoms of brain irritation, delirium, twitchings, frightful visions, or great anguish (with or without diarrhea): Cal.

Decubitus: *Arn.,* Ars., **Bap.,** Carbo v., **Carb. ac.,** Cinch., **Fluor. ac.,** Ham., **Mur. ac.,** Nux, **Nux m.,** Phos. ac., **Pyr.,** Sec., **Sul. ac., Zinc.**
on sacrum and trochantur: Zinc.
bed sores on sweating parts: Fluor. ac.
gangrenous, rapidly: Carbo v., Carb. ac., **Pyr.**
ulcerations: **Bap.,** Carb. ac.
with abscess or boils: Hep., Mer., Psor., Sil.

Sweat of typhoid and typhus.
cold: Ars., **Camph., Carbo v.,** Carb. ac., **Colch.,** *Sec.,* **Ver.**
cold, over the whole body: **Camph.,** Carbo v., Ver.

Sweat, cold, on the forehead: Coc., *Colch.*, Ver.
cold, on the forehead and face: Sec.
cold, on face: **Bell.**, *Ver. v.*
cold, face and extremities: Carbo v.
cold, face and extremities with heat of trunk: Phos.
cold, only on head and trunk: Ver.
cold, with trembling of whole body: Puls.
cold, and clammy: Ars., Pyr.
cold, and partial or dry burning skin: Apis.
cold, and viscid, constant: Ars., Phos. ac., Sec.
from head to the epigastrium: Sec.
critical on forehead and face: Bap.
covers the face: Colch.
profuse, debilitating: Mer.
profuse, retarding convalescence: Psor.
profuse, great debility, with desire to be magnetized: Sil.
sour, or sour smell of body: Bry.
sour, at noon, sour diarrhea in daytime: Rhus.
sour, mostly in P. M., on upper part of body: Fluor. ac.
sour, makes patient thirsty: Iod.
offensive: Ars., *Bap.*, **Psor.**, **Pyr.**
offensive and sour: Ars.
offensive, and breath offensive: Arn., Psor.
cadaverous odor, scents the whole atmosphere: *Ars.*, Bap., Carbo v., **Psor.**, *Pyr.*
without any >: *Lach.*, **Mer.**, Phos., *Pyr.*
gentle, wishes to be covered: Hep., Nux, **Rhus.**
anxious, preventing sleep, with sighing, short cough, pressure in chest: Bry.
with great weakness and stupidity: Hyos.
with great dryness, followed by hot sweat, without >, not Mer., but Stram.

Tissues, complaints which go from above downward: Sel.
complaints spreading upwards: Fluor. ac.
neuralgic pains leave suddenly: Phos.

Tissues, great irritability of all the organs: Bell.
sensation of lead in the blood vessels, < when sitting: Mer.
stiffness of muscles, first stage: Bry.
rheumatic pains: Bry., Camph., Pyr., Rhus.
rheumatic pains, dull, stitching, tearing, < from motion and opening the eyes: Bry.
rheumatic pains, shooting in some part of the body, < when the part is at rest: Rhus.
rheumatic pains, intense, of bones and muscles, compelling patient to move: Bap., Eup., Lac c., Phyt., Puls., Pyr.
rheumatic pains, throbbing, beating: Bry.
rheumatic pains, the more in first stage, the more certain abdominal localization. The patient will call pains rheumatic, but they are nervous (spinal) and decrease when thinking about them: Camph.—JAHR.
throbbing in vessels, veins enlarge in places: Iod.
hemorrhages: **Alumen,** Arn., Ars., Bry., **Crot.,** *Carbo v., Carb. ac.,* Cinch., **Nit. ac., Phos.,** Rhus, Sul., **Ter.**
hemorrhages from beginning: *Crot.,* **Nit. ac.**
hemorrhages, exhaustion from loss of vital fluids: Carbo v., **Cinch.,** Chin. s., Phos. ac., Phos.
hemorrhages, with decomposition of fluids: Ars., *Bap., Crot.,* **Lach.,** Pyr., Rhus, *Sec.*
hemorrhages, with decomposition of, and great prostration: Bap., Mur. ac., Pyr.
little or no affection of mucous membranes of intestines, no dissolution: Hell., Mur. ac.

Constitutional and general; at the very onset all further progress may be cut off, in persons inclined to grow fat by: Cal. —HERING.
with a history of eczema, quinsy, asthma, hay fever or suppressed eruptions further progress may be cut off, the attack aborted, by: Psor.
weak, debilitated persons, in childhood or old age, when vitality is low: Ars., Bar., Op.

Constitutional and General; during epidemic cholera or when cholera ends in typhus: Ars., Cup., Psor., Sul., Ver.
in chronic alcoholism: Agar.
when the best selected remedy fails to arrest the progress of typhoid: Psor., Pyr., Sul., Tub.
with rapid course, tending to malignancy: Camph., Carbo v., Carb. ac., Psor.
after abuse of Mercury: Nit. ac., Sul.
after abuse of Bryonia: Alum., Bap., Mur. ac.
after abuse of Opium: Hell.
after over-mental and physical exertion: Coc.
after mental anxiety and worry: Cal.
after shock from financial losses: Staph.
great thirst, but fluids caused pain and gurgled through the intestines, as through an empty cask: Hydro. ac.

INDEX.

INDEX TO REPERTORY.